NURSING RESEARCH USING CASE STUDIES

Mary de Chesnay, PhD, RN, PMHCNS-BC, FAAN, is a professor at Kennesaw State University, School of Nursing, Kennesaw, Georgia. She has received 13 research grants and has authored two books: *Sex Trafficking: A Clinical Guide for Nurses* (Springer Publishing) and the AJN Book of the Year Award winner, *Caring for the Vulnerable: Perspectives in Nursing Theory, Practice and Research,* now in its fourth edition. Dr. de Chesnay has published more than 21 journal articles in *Qualitative Health Research, Journal of Nursing Management, International Journal of Medicine & Law,* and others. A former dean and endowed chair, she reviews for a variety of professional journals. Dr. de Chesnay is a noted expert on qualitative research and a founding member and first vice president of the Southern Nursing Research Society.

NURSING RESEARCH USING CASE STUDIES

QUALITATIVE DESIGNS AND METHODS IN NURSING

Mary de Chesnay, PhD, RN, PMHCNS-BC, FAAN

EDITOR

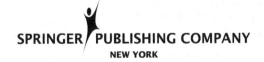

SPRINGER PUBLISHING COMPANY
NEW YORK

Springer Publishing Company, LLC
11 West 42nd Street
New York, NY 10036
www.springerpub.com

Acquisitions Editor: Joseph Morita
Senior Production Editor: Kris Parrish
Composition: Newgen KnowledgeWorks

ISBN: 978-0-8261-3192-8
e-book ISBN: 978-0-8261-3193-5

16 17 18 19 20/ 5 4 3 2 1

The author and the publisher of this Work have made every effort to use sources believed to be reliable to provide information that is accurate and compatible with the standards generally accepted at the time of publication. Because medical science is continually advancing, our knowledge base continues to expand. Therefore, as new information becomes available, changes in procedures become necessary. We recommend that the reader always consult current research and specific institutional policies before performing any clinical procedure. The author and publisher shall not be liable for any special, consequential, or exemplary damages resulting, in whole or in part, from the readers' use of, or reliance on, the information contained in this book. The publisher has no responsibility for the persistence or accuracy of URLs for external or third-party Internet websites referred to in this publication and does not guarantee that any content on such websites is, or will remain, accurate or appropriate.

Library of Congress Cataloging-in-Publication Data
Names: De Chesnay, Mary, editor.
Title: Nursing research using case studies / Mary de Chesnay, editor.
Other titles: Qualitative designs and methods in nursing.
Description: New York, NY: Springer Publishing Company, LLC, [2017] | Series: Qualitative designs and methods in nursing | Includes bibliographical references.
Identifiers: LCCN 2016013700| ISBN 9780826131928 | ISBN 9780826131935 (e-book)
Subjects: | MESH: Nursing Research--methods | Evidence-Based Nursing | Research Design | Case Reports
Classification: LCC RT81.5 | NLM WY 20.5 | DDC 610.73072--dc23
LC record available at http://lccn.loc.gov/2016013700

Special discounts on bulk quantities of our books are available to corporations, professional associations, pharmaceutical companies, health care organizations, and other qualifying groups. If you are interested in a custom book, including chapters from more than one of our titles, we can provide that service as well.

For details, please contact:
Special Sales Department, Springer Publishing Company, LLC
11 West 42nd Street, 15th Floor, New York, NY 10036–8002
Phone: 877-687-7476 or 212-431-4370; Fax: 212-941-7842
E-mail: sales@springerpub.com

Printed in the United States of America by Gasch Printing.

QUALITATIVE DESIGNS AND METHODS IN NURSING

Mary de Chesnay, PhD, RN, PMHCNS-BC, FAAN, Series Editor

Nursing Research Using Ethnography: Qualitative Designs and Methods in Nursing

Nursing Research Using Grounded Theory: Qualitative Designs and Methods in Nursing

Nursing Research Using Life History: Qualitative Designs and Methods in Nursing

Nursing Research Using Phenomenology: Qualitative Designs and Methods in Nursing

Nursing Research Using Historical Methods: Qualitative Designs and Methods in Nursing

Nursing Research Using Participatory Action Research: Qualitative Designs and Methods in Nursing

Nursing Research Using Data Analysis: Qualitative Designs and Methods in Nursing

Nursing Research Using Case Studies: Qualitative Designs and Methods in Nursing

For Judy Weismann, for all the help and friendship over the years.

—MdC

CONTENTS

Contributors   *ix*

Foreword   Barbara A. Anderson, DrPH, RN, CNM, FACNM, FAAN   *xv*

Series Foreword   *xvii*

Preface   *xxiii*

Acknowledgments   *xxv*

1 Overview of Case Study Research   *1*
   Patricia Hentz

2 State of the Art of Qualitative Case Study Methodology
   in Nursing Research   *11*
   Johnathan D. Steppe

3 Proposal for Case Study of Obstetric Fistula   *43*
   Mary de Chesnay, Jessica Ellis, and Tracey Couse

4 Case Study Research: A Methodology for Nursing   *55*
   Camille Cronin

5 Case Study of Creation of a New Social Service Organization:
   The Hope Box   *73*
   Mary de Chesnay, Sarah Koeppen, and Tiffany Turolla

6 Conducting Case Study Research: An Exemplar   *89*
   Esther Sangster-Gormley

7 Coming Home: Veterans With PTSD Adapting to Life at Home   *99*
   Patricia Hentz

8 Enabling Systems Raising Awareness of Breast Cancer
   Among Muslim Omani Women: A Case Study Exemplar   *115*
   Esra Al Khasawneh and Michael C. Leocadio

9 Case Study Methods for Graduate Students   139
   Mary de Chesnay and Genie E. Dorman

10 Canine Partners in Health Care   145
   Leslie Himot, Tanya Gordon, Rhonda L. Harrison, and Mary de Chesnay

11 From the Horse's Mouth: Case Study of a Handler's Perspective
   of Equine-Facilitated Therapy   155
   Christopher Hayes and Christopher R. Walker

12 "I'm the Guy With the Dog": Life History of a
   Combat Veteran Suffering From PTSD and TBI   169
   Stacey Tatroe and Laura D. Elledge

13 "Cheering Myself On": Bella's Story   185
   Melissa Anderson and Nancy Chambers

14 Loss of a Child to an African Family: A Phenomenological
   Case Study   199
   Jacqueline Kigundu and Titus Sairo

15 Tragedy to Triumph: Life History of an Older
   Woman Living With AIDS   221
   Tracey Couse and Kelly Heard

16 The Under-12 Rule: A Review on the Pediatric
   Lung Allocation Policy   239
   Amy P. Pope

17 The Health Consequences of Mothers Using Drugs and the
   Legal System's Call to Action   251
   Kathy Barnett

Appendix A   *List of Journals That Publish Qualitative Research*   261
   Mary de Chesnay

Appendix B   *Essential Elements for a Qualitative Proposal*   265
   Tommie Nelms

Appendix C   *Writing Qualitative Research Proposals*   267
   Joan L. Bottorff

Appendix D   *Outline for a Research Proposal*   275
   Mary de Chesnay

Appendix E   *Qualitative Software Comparison*   279
   Paul Mihas

Index   287

Contributors

Esra Al Khasawneh, DNsc, RN, is dean and associate professor at the College of Nursing at Sultan Qaboos University, Sultanate of Oman. Dr. Al Khasawneh has achieved many funded research projects from Jordanian, American, and Omani institutes. Her interests in teaching are women's health, problem-based learning, and simulation. She has taught nursing research and maternal–child health in various institutions. She is one of the few nursing scholars who received the His Majesty Strategic Trust Fund Grant in the Sultanate of Oman.

Barbara A. Anderson, DrPH, RN, CNM, FACNM, FAAN, owns a consultation business focusing on curricular development for public health programs, nurse-midwifery education, and DNP education. She has been a university professor and an administrator at all academic levels. She has worked in more than 100 countries in program development including curricular design based on the case study approach. She has edited and authored numerous works and serves on the board of directors of the American College of Nurse-Midwives.

Melissa Anderson, MSN, APRN, FNP-C, is a family nurse practitioner who has spent her career working with chronic care pediatric patients in both the intensive care setting and school health setting. Her research interests include adolescents and young adults managing chronic illness, specifically in school and work environments.

Kathy Barnett, RN, MSN, is a clinical instructor at Kennesaw State University. Her specialty is women's health and has focused her research on substance abuse and addiction, perinatal loss, and instruction of baccalaureate nursing students in the clinical setting. She has worked for the past 7 years providing community training in emergency preparedness and CPR, training more than 2,000 health care professionals and lay people.

Nancy Chambers, MSN, APRN, FNP-C, is a family nurse practitioner who specializes in pediatrics, both in hospital and outpatient settings. Her research interests include gastrointestinal chronic illnesses with a focus on Crohn's disease and colitis diagnosis and management in the pediatric population.

Tracey Couse, MSN, APRN, FNP-C, is a graduate of Kennesaw State University's family nurse practitioner program and a member of the American Association of Nurse Practitioners (AANP) and Sigma Theta Tau International (STTI). Before her nursing career, she spent 10 years in basic medical research, teaching quantitative research techniques. Since starting her nursing career, she has participated on a nursing research committee, informally presented and implemented numerous practice improvement projects, and was selected as a nursing research scholar resulting in a poster presentation at a local conference.

Camille Cronin, PhD, MEd, MSc, BSc(Hons), RN, SFHEA, is a lecturer and program lead for foundation degree in health sciences at the University of Essex, Southend-on-Sea campus. She has conducted case study research and qualitative studies in health service research in the United Kingdom and Ireland. She teaches research across programs and is the research lead for the oral health sciences group at the Southend campus.

Mary de Chesnay, PhD, RN, PMHCNS-BC, FAAN, is professor of nursing at Kennesaw State University and secretary of the Council on Nursing and Anthropology (CONAA) of the Society for Applied Anthropology (SFAA). She has conducted ethnographic fieldwork and participatory action research in Latin America and the Caribbean. She has taught qualitative research at all levels in the United States and abroad in the roles of faculty, head of a department of research, dean, and endowed chair.

Genie E. Dorman, PhD, APRN, FNP-BC, is a professor of nursing and the associate director of graduate-degree nursing programs at Kennesaw State University. She has codirected study-abroad programs in Mexico, Haiti, Puerto Rico, and the United Arab Emirates designed to enhance students' cultural competence through experiential learning. Her research interests include the provision of health care to the underserved and the development of cultural competence in both undergraduate and graduate students. She has made numerous presentations on these topics at both national and international conferences.

Laura D. Elledge, MSN, APRN, FNP-C, is a graduate nursing student at Kennesaw State University in the family nurse practitioner program. She is a member of Sigma Theta Tau, Society for Applied Anthropology (SFAA) and United Advanced Practice Registered Nurses of Georgia (UAPRN). She was an invited presenter at the National Lamaze Convention in 2013 and will be a presenter at the 2016 Society for Applied Anthropology-CONAA conference in Vancouver, British Columbia, Canada. She has been a labor and delivery nurse at Northside Hospital in Atlanta, Georgia, for more than 18 years and is a clinical educator for a department of more than 400 personnel.

Jessica Ellis, MSN, RN, CNM, is a clinical assistant professor of nursing at Kennesaw State University and an active member of the American College of Nurse-Midwives. Her research is focused on women's health, pregnancy, and health disparities. She has taught nursing at the undergraduate and graduate levels.

Tanya Gordon, MSN, APRN, FNP-C, is a certified rehabilitation registered nurse (CRRN) with 10 years of experience working with spinal cord injury and traumatic brain injury rehabilitation patients. She is a recent graduate of the Kennesaw State University family nurse practitioner program.

Rhonda L. Harrison, MSN, APRN, FNP-C, spent the first 13 years of her career in the operating room and 7 years in a private orthopedic office. She is a recent graduate of Kennesaw State University's family nurse practitioner track in the master's degree program.

Christopher Hayes, MSN, APRN, FNP-C, is a student at Kennesaw State University. He has worked in several areas within the health care field, including the intensive care unit (ICU), public health, and case management. He also holds a bachelor's degree in finance from Auburn University and worked in finance and accounting before changing his profession to nursing.

Kelly Heard, MSN, APRN, RN, FNP-CBSN, is a recent graduate of Kennesaw State University's family nurse practitioner program and a member of United Advanced Practice Registered Nurses (UAPRN) and Sigma Theta Tau International (STTI). She has been a nurse since 1987, working in both inpatient and outpatient pediatric settings, and as an allergy nurse for two ear-nose-throat (ENT) offices.

Patricia Hentz, EdD, PMHNP-BC, CRNP, is a clinical associate professor at Rutgers University School of Nursing. Her research areas include loss and psychological trauma. Dr. Hentz has taught for more than 30 years and has extensive experience in curriculum and program development at the graduate and undergraduate levels. Her expertise is in qualitative research; she has presented her research at national and international conferences in the areas of phenomenology, grounded theory, and case study research, along with publications in research journals and books.

Leslie Himot, MSN, RN, CNE, is a lecturer of nursing at Kennesaw State University and a certified nurse educator. She is the co-coordinator of the Dedicated Education Unit at WellStar Kennestone Hospital in Marietta, Georgia, and has written on the subject of animal-assisted therapy in vulnerable populations.

Jacqueline Kigundu, MSN, APRN, FNP-C, was born in Nairobi, Kenya, in the mid-1980s. She relocated to the United States with her family in the early 2000s, where she completed her early studies. She started her nursing career in 2005 when she graduated from J. F. Drake Technical College as a licensed practical nurse. In 2009, she graduated with her associate's degree in nursing from Calhoun Community College in Alabama. She earned her bachelor's degree in nursing from Kennesaw State University in 2013, and her master's degree in nursing from the same institution in 2015. She has a strong interest in the subject of cultural diversity.

Sarah Koeppen is a child, family, and marriage advocate and mentor. With profound spiritual insight, wisdom, and depth of knowledge on adoption matters, Sarah cofounded The Hope Box in 2014, which became a vital source of community impact offering safe options for abandoned children.

Michael C. Leocadio, DNM, RN, RM, CRN, is the assistant dean of training and community service at the College of Nursing at Sultan Qaboos University, Sultanate of Oman. His research interests include health promotion, nursing education, theory, and conceptual developments and leadership and management. He has taught nursing research at all levels in the Philippines and South Korea and is currently the faculty coordinator of the nursing administration course at Sultan Qaboos University. He is the recipient of several research awards.

Amy P. Pope, MSN, RN, PCCN, is a clinical assistant professor at Kennesaw State University. She has previously worked in a coronary intensive care unit where she acted as relief charge nurse and preceptor. She is currently working on her doctorate in nursing science at Kennesaw State University and is scheduled to graduate in 2017. Her research interests include transgender health, health disparities, and palliative and end-of-life care.

Esther Sangster-Gormley, PHD, RN, is an associate professor of nursing at the University of Victoria in Victoria, British Columbia, Canada. She has conducted case study research in Canada and is the author of case study research and mixed methods designs incorporating case study research.

Titus Sairo, MSN, APRN, FNP-C, graduated from the University of Nairobi in 1987 with a BSc in Zoology. Mr. Sairo relocated to the United States in 2001, graduated with a BSN from Kennesaw State University in 2006, and earned an MSN (primary care nurse practitioner) from the same institution in 2015. Mr. Sairo's research interests include family systems of immigrants from various cultures and how they cope with loss and grief.

Johnathan D. Steppe, MSN, RN, CCRN, is a clinical assistant professor of nursing at Kennesaw State University, where he is also pursuing a doctorate in nursing science. His clinical background is primarily in critical care. His current program of research focuses on health disparities in rural Nicaragua.

Stacey Tatroe, MSN, APRN, FNP-C, is a family nurse practitioner graduate student at Kennesaw State University and a member of Sigma Theta Tau and the Society for Applied Anthropology (SFAA). She spoke at the 2016 SFAA annual meeting in Vancouver, British Columbia, Canada. She left a career in law enforcement to begin a career in nursing as a licensed practical nurse. She worked as a staff nurse and resource nurse on a neuro/telemetry unit before transferring to the emergency department. She has been an emergency room nurse for the past 8 years.

Tiffany Turolla is executive director and cofounder of The Hope Box, Inc. She is also a Christian minister, musician, and songwriter. She has traveled internationally to minister and perform musically. In 2014 she began The Hope Box to help educate the community on the issue of newborn abandonment and create a solution for this problem.

Christopher R. Walker, MSN, APRN, FNP-C, is a staff nurse at WellStar Cobb Hospital in the emergency department. He is a recent graduate of the family nurse practitioner program at Kennesaw State University.

FOREWORD

TELL ME A STORY

Human history is embedded in stories—tapestries of culture, belief, and the commonality of human experience. The *story*, as prototype, explains, guides, and gives voice to experience. "Stories have to be told or they die, and when they die, we can't remember who we are or why we're here" (Kidd, 2002, p. 107).

The case study is an educational tool using the *story* in the context of causal links, interventions, outcomes, and ethics. It unveils dilemmas, social inequity, and cultural dimensions behind decisions and choices. It is a powerful tool to examine evidence-based practice around patient care, family dynamics, professional roles, and organizational systems. However, as a pedagogical method, it has not always been regarded highly in the health professions, which tend to rely on numbers and facts rather than listening and capturing the embodied story. It took the profession of anthropology, especially medical anthropologists and nurses with education in anthropology as well as Madeleine Leininger's work (1985), to show us how to use the themes in the *story* to explain health care–related phenomena.

Oliver Sacks, renowned author and neurologist, once said, "If we wish to know about a man, we ask 'what is his story—his real, inmost story?'—for each of us is a biography, a story" (Sacks, n.d.). The case study approach allows us to reach that story, beyond the numbers and facts. Its salience is the voice and perspective of the characters in interaction with other characters and the environment.

The case study methodology, sometimes referred to as the clinical case narrative, has been examined pedagogically and employed in the education of advanced practice nurses and doctor of nursing practice (DNP) students. Smolowitz, Honig, and Reinisch (2010) outlined an extensive framework for this approach in DNP education in the translation of research to practice.

Recently, Smolowitz and Honig operationalized this approach, using multiperspective analyses, in the translation of research to practice (Smolowitz & Honig, 2015). Analyzing the story, the case study as a research method for informing best practices has achieved a place in health science pedagogy. This book on case studies, the eighth in the series *Qualitative Designs and Methods in Nursing*, edited by Dr. Mary de Chesnay, makes a substantial contribution to this pedagogy.

Tell me a story—your story.

Barbara A. Anderson, DrPH, RN, CNM, FACNM, FAAN
Board Member
American College of Nurse Midwives
Retired Professor of Nursing and Public Health,
Riverside, California

REFERENCES

Kidd, S. (2002). *The secret life of bees.* New York, NY: Penguin Press.

Leininger, M. (Ed.). (1985). *Qualitative research methods in nursing,* New York, NY: Grune Stratton.

Sacks, O. (n.d.). Quote retrieved from http://www.azquotes.com/quote/449182

Smolowitz, J., & Honig, J. (2015) The clinical case narrative: Preparing the DNP nurse to deliver comprehensive care. In B. Anderson, J. Knestrick, & R. Barroso (Eds.), *DNP capstone projects: Exemplars of excellence in practice.* New York, NY: Springer Publishing Company.

Smolowitz, J., Honig J., & Reinisch, C. (Eds.). (2010). *Writing DNP clinical case narratives:Demonstrating and evaluating competency in comprehensive care.* New York, NY: Springer Publishing Company.

Series Foreword

In this section, which is published in all volumes of the series, we discuss some key aspects of any qualitative design. This is basic information that might be helpful to novice researchers or those new to the designs and methods described in each chapter. The material is not meant to be rigid and prescribed because qualitative research by its nature is fluid and flexible; the reader should use any ideas that are relevant and discard any ideas that are not relevant to the specific project in mind.

Before beginning a project, it is helpful to commit to publishing it. Of course, it will be publishable because you will use every resource at hand to make sure it is of high quality and contributes to knowledge. Theses and dissertations are meaningless exercises if only the student and committee know what was learned. It is rather heart-breaking to think of all the effort that senior faculty have exerted to complete a degree and yet not to have anyone else benefit by the work. Therefore, some additional resources are included here. Appendix A for each book is a list of journals that publish qualitative research. References to the current nursing qualitative research textbooks are included so that readers may find additional material from sources cited in those chapters.

FOCUS

In qualitative research the focus is emic—what we commonly think of as "from the participant's point of view." The researcher's point of view, called "the etic view," is secondary and does not take precedence over what the participant wants to convey, because in qualitative research, the focus is on the person and his or her story. In contrast, quantitative researchers take pains to learn as much as they can about a topic and focus the research data collection on what they want to know. Cases or subjects that do not provide information about the researcher's agenda are considered outliers and are discarded or treated as aberrant data. Qualitative researchers embrace outliers and actively seek diverse points of view from participants to enrich the data. They sample for diversity within groups and welcome different perceptions even if they seek fairly homogeneous samples. For example, in Leenerts and Magilvy's (2000) grounded theory study to examine self-care practices among women, they narrowed the study to low-income, White, HIV-positive women but included both lesbian and heterosexual women.

PROPOSALS

There are many excellent sources in the literature on how to write a research proposal. A couple are cited here (Annersten, 2006; Mareno, 2012; Martin, 2010; Schmelzer, 2006), and examples are found in Appendices B, C, and D. Proposals for any type of research should include basic elements about the purpose, significance, theoretical support, and methods. What is often lacking is a thorough discussion about the rationale. The rationale is needed for the overall design as well as each step in the process. Why qualitative research? Why ethnography and not phenomenology? Why go to a certain setting? Why select the participants through word of mouth? Why use one particular type of software over another to analyze data? Other common mistakes are not doing justice to significance and failure to provide sufficient theoretical support for the approach. In qualitative research, which tends to be theory generating instead of theory testing, the author still needs to explain why the study is conducted from a particular frame of reference. For example, in some ethnographical work, there are hypotheses that are tested based on the work of prior ethnographers who studied that culture, but there is still a need to generate new theory about current phenomena within that culture from the point of view of the specific informants for the subsequent study.

Significance is underappreciated as an important component of research. Without justifying the importance of the study or the potential impact of the study, there is no case for why the study should be conducted. If a study cannot be justified, why should sponsors fund it? Why should participants agree to participate? Why should the principal investigator bother to conduct it?

COMMONALITIES IN METHODS

Interviewing Basics

One of the best resources for learning how to interview for qualitative research is by Patton (2002), and readers are referred to his book for a detailed guide to interviewing. He describes the process, issues, and challenges in a way that readers can focus their interview in a wide variety of directions that are flexible, yet rigorous. For example, in ethnography, a mix of interview methods is appropriate, ranging from unstructured interviews or informal conversation to highly structured interviews. Unless nurses are conducting mixed-design studies, most of their interviews will be semi-structured. Semi-structured interviews include a few general questions, but the interviewer is free to allow the interviewee to digress along any lines he or she wishes. It is up to the interviewer to bring the interview back to the focus of the research. This requires skill and sensitivity. Some general guidelines apply to semi-structured interviews:

- Establish rapport
- Ask open-ended questions. For example, the second question is much more likely to generate a meaningful response than the first in a grounded theory study of coping with cervical cancer.

> Interviewer: Were you afraid when you first heard your diagnosis of cervical cancer?
>
> Participant: Yes.

Contrast the aforementioned with the following:

> Interviewer: What was your first thought when you heard your diagnosis of cervical cancer?
>
> Participant: I thought of my young children and how they were going to lose their mother and that they would grow up not knowing how much I loved them.

- Continuously "read" the person's reactions and adapt the approach based on response to questions. For example, in the interview about coping with the diagnosis, the participant began tearing so the interviewer appropriately gave her some time to collect herself. Maintaining silence is one of the most difficult things to learn for researchers who have been classically trained in quantitative methods. In structured interviewing, we are trained to continue despite distractions and to eliminate bias, which may involve eliminating emotion and emotional reactions to what we hear in the interview. Yet the quality of outcomes in qualitative designs may depend on the researcher–participant relationship. It is critical to be authentic and to allow the participant to be authentic.

Ethical Issues

The principles of the Belmont Commission apply to all types of research: respect, justice, and beneficence. Perhaps these are even more important when interviewing people about their culture or life experiences. These are highly personal and may be painful for the person to relate, though I have found that there is a cathartic effect to participating in naturalistic research with an empathic interviewer (de Chesnay, 1991, 1993).

Rigor

Readers are referred to the classic paper on rigor in qualitative research (Sandelowski, 1986). Rather than speak of validity and reliability, we use other terms, such as accuracy (Do the data represent truth as the participant sees it?) and replicability (Can the reader follow the decision trail to see why the researcher concluded as he or she did?).

DATA ANALYSIS

Analyzing data requires many decisions about how to collect data and whether to use high-tech measures such as qualitative software or old-school measures such as colored index cards. The contributors to this series provide examples of both.

Mixed designs require a balance between the assumptions of quantitative research while conducting that part and qualitative research during that phase. It can be difficult for novice researchers to keep things straight. Researchers are encouraged to learn each paradigm well and to be clear about why they use certain methods for their purposes. Each type of design can stand alone, and one should never think that qualitative research is *less than* quantitative; it is just different.

Mary de Chesnay

REFERENCES

Annersten, M. (2006). How to write a research proposal. *European Diabetes Nursing, 3*(2), 102–105.

de Chesnay, M. (1991). *Catharsis: Outcome of naturalistic research.* Presented to Society for Applied Anthropology, Charleston, SC.

de Chesnay, M. (1993). Workshop with Dr. Patricia Marshall of Symposium on Research Ethics in Fieldwork. Sponsored by Society for Applied Anthropology, Committee on Ethics. Memphis, March 25–29, 1992; San Antonio, Texas, March 11–14, 1993.

Leenerts, M. H., & Magilvy, J. K. (2000). Investing in self-care: A midrange theory of self-care grounded in the lived experience of low-income HIV-positive white women. *ANS. Advances in Nursing Science, 22*(3), 58–75.

Mareno, N. (2012). Sample qualitative research proposal: Childhood obesity in Latino families. In M. de Chesnay & B. Anderson (Eds.), *Caring for the vulnerable* (pp. 203–218). Sudbury, MA: Jones and Bartlett.

Martin, C. H. (2010). A 15-step model for writing a research proposal. *British Journal of Midwifery, 18*(12), 791–798.

Patton, M. Q. (2002). *Qualitative research and evaluation methods* (3rd ed.). Thousand Oaks, CA: Sage.

Sandelowski, M. (1986). The problem of rigor in qualitative research. *Advances in Nursing Science, 8*(3), 27–37.

Schmelzer, M. (2006). How to start a research proposal. *Gastroenterology Nursing: the Official Journal of the Society of Gastroenterology Nurses and Associates, 29*(2), 186–188.

PREFACE

Qualitative research has evolved from a slightly disreputable beginning to wide acceptance in nursing research. Long a tradition in anthropology, approaches that focus on the stories and perceptions of the people instead of what scientists think the world is about created a body of knowledge that cannot be replicated in the lab. The richness of human experience is what qualitative research is all about. Respect for this tradition was long in coming among the scientific community. Nurses seem to have been in the forefront, though, and though many of my generation (children of the 1950s and 1960s) were classically trained in quantitative techniques, we found something lacking. Perhaps, because I am a psychiatric nurse, I have been trained to listen to people tell me their stories, whether the stories are problems that nearly destroy the spirit, or uplifting accounts of how they live within their cultures or how they cope with terrible traumas and chronic diseases. It seems logical to me that a critical part of developing new knowledge that nurses can use to help patients is to find out first what the patients themselves have to say. Viewed this way, qualitative research is the first step in developing an evidence-based practice.

In this volume, we explore case study as a qualitative method of particular usefulness to nurses who wish to describe richness and depth of a person's experience, a disease process, an organization, or a group. Similar to life history, ethnography, or evaluation research, case study is an in-depth treatment that provides a picture of experience. Similar to ethnography and evaluation research, case study might use a variety of approaches, including both quantitative and qualitative methods, in order to meet the goals of the researcher. However, in this book, qualitative methods are emphasized.

Case study is a particularly useful design for nurse practitioners and doctor of nursing practice (DNP) students who typically do not conduct research in the same way that PhD students do. Two focused life histories by nurse practitioner students are included to show how case studies can be used to teach the research process in such a way that students see direct relevance to their clinical practice. The chapter on animal-assisted therapy is coauthored by two nurse practitioner students who completed their study as a requirement of graduation. We hope that the case studies included here inspire other students to make use of this method.

Mary de Chesnay

ACKNOWLEDGMENTS

In any publishing venture, there are many people who work together to produce the final draft. The contributors kindly shared their expertise to offer advice and counsel to novices and the reviewers ensured the quality of submissions. All of them have come up through the ranks as qualitative researchers and their participation is critical to helping novices learn the process.

No publication is successful without great people who not only know how to do their own jobs but also how to guide authors. At Springer Publishing Company, we are indebted to Margaret Zuccarini for the idea for the series, her ongoing support, and her excellent problem-solving skills. The person who guided the editorial process and was available for numerous questions, which he patiently answered as if he had not heard them a hundred times, was Joseph Morita. Also critical to the project were the people who proofed the work, marketed the series, and transformed it from the Web to hard copies, chief among these being Rachel Landes, Jenna Vaccaro, and Kris Parrish.

At Kennesaw State University, Dr. Tommie Nelms, director of the WellStar School of Nursing, was a constant source of emotional and practical support in addition to her chapter contribution to the *Phenomenology* volume. Her administrative assistant, Mrs. Cynthia Ellery, the "Indispensible One," helped in significant ways. For this last volume of the series, I would like to extend my gratitude to those who reviewed various drafts in all the books and gave the editor excellent advice for improving this series: Dr. Nancy Anderson, Dr. Karen Breda, Dr. Ellen Buckner, Dr. Nicole Mareno, Dr. Tommie Nelms, Dr. Patricia Hart, Dr. Joan Lockhart, and Dr. Susan Stevens.

CHAPTER ONE

OVERVIEW OF CASE STUDY RESEARCH

Patricia Hentz

Case study methods are well suited when the aim of a study is to retain the holistic and meaningful characteristics of real-life events (Yin, 2009). In addition, it may also be the method of choice when the researcher plans to investigate contemporary phenomena or contemporary problems in their natural or "real-world context" (Yin, 2014, p. 2). Key factors for choosing case study approaches include the following: (a) when the researcher has little or no control over the phenomenon of interest and/or the behavioral events and (b) when the contemporary phenomenon is inseparable from the social or contextual conditions related to the phenomenon. Case study research provides an in-depth and inside view of the phenomenon within its social context, sensitizing the reader to the issues, problems, and processes. In doing so, its aim is to foster a deeper understanding of the complexity of the phenomenon. An example of this depth and complexity can be seen in the case study by Hentz (2015), which focuses on the experiences of veterans returning from war. The cases uncovered processes that expand our understanding of veterans' experiences beyond the diagnosis of posttraumatic stress disorder (PTSD) or a list of PTSD-related symptoms. The reader is provided with an inside view of the veterans' lives after returning home. It is relevant to the study how the social contexts, both in war and then returning home, are critical to understanding the experiences of veterans. In this multiple case study, single cases are presented within their social context, highlighting the veterans' experiences after they have returned home. The cases examine in depth some of the challenges veterans faced, including a heightened fear process, compensatory survival behaviors, social disengagement, attachment difficulties with family and friends, and attachment bonds related to the military world. Data were obtained from the researcher's clinical work with veterans; interviews with veterans; discussions with a veteran who was a key informant; historical accounts, literature, films, and research; and theories in the areas of trauma, PTSD, and emotional processing.

CASE STUDY RESEARCH: WHAT IT IS AND WHAT IT IS NOT

When we are presented with the concept, *case study*, it is important to understand that a single definition does not exist. Within the social sciences, it has been very broadly defined and divided into four categories. Only the fourth category exclusively focuses on case study as a research approach. The first category is the *teaching case*. The teaching case study does not need to accurately depict a specific individual, event, or process because its primary aim is to enhance learning. The teaching case is illustrative, and although it often has been derived from case study observations, it does not necessarily comply with any specific research methodology. For example, case studies depicting specific psychiatric disorders are grounded in research. These case studies are often developed using a combination of diagnostic criteria and clinical observations. The second category, *case histories*, is used for the purposes of record keeping. Here again, the primary aim is not research; however, these cases may be useful as data in a research study. *Case work*, the third category, is used to describe the management of health care for a patient or a population. The fourth category, *case research* or *case study research*, is intended for the purpose of "investigating activities or complex processes that are not easily separated from the social context within which they occur" (Cutter, 2004, p. 367). Case study research maintains rigor in its research methodology and its attention to presenting findings that accurately and reliably represent the data.

OVERVIEW OF CASE STUDY RESEARCH

Philosophical Derivation

There is still no standardization or formula on how to conduct case study research (McKee, 2004; Yin, 2014). As stated by Rosenberg and Yates, "The methods used in case study research are pragmatically-rather and paradigmatically-driven" (2007, p. 448). In essence, the phenomenon of interest and the research question(s) determine the method and design. Thus, case study research may be developed at any level of research, including exploratory, descriptive, and explanatory designs. Furthermore, from a qualitative perspective, case study research might draw from phenomenological, ethnographical, and grounded theory research approaches depending on the aim of the study and the research question(s). It should be noted that even though case study research designs are quite flexible, they derive their rigor by creating the research designs in accordance with the research aims, hypotheses, or questions. A clearly developed phenomenon of interest along with the key questions to be explored form the basis for case study design. In case study research, as in any other research method, the researchers must justify their research approach and clearly identify the significance of the study whether the focus is on a single individual, a group of individuals, an organization, processes, neighborhoods, institutions, or events. The emphasis is on identifying the object of study within its social context and the importance of the bond between the object of study and the social context. To illustrate the object of study within its social context, the study by Hentz (2015) explored the experiences of veterans after returning home. The object of study involved exploring their processes of adapting back to "life at home." Foundational philosophical underpinnings for the case study research approach was adapted from ethnography and grounded theory research methods and an interviewing approach involved constant comparison of data as an ongoing process of data analysis.

The strength of case study research is its adaptability and flexibility. For example, the classic descriptive case studies, "Tally's Corner" (Liebow, 1967) and "Street Corner Society" Whyte (1955), provide in-depth, inside views of the life of these small groups. The concept used in case study research, *unit of analysis,* distinguishes the boundaries of the case. In these studies, the unit of analysis included the group of individuals who lived in the specifically defined neighborhood. This is certainly a contemporary phenomenon for its time. These studies illustrate the key aspects of case studies: investigation of a contemporary phenomenon in depth within its real-life context and the obvious interconnection between the phenomenon and the unit of analysis. Another example of a case study that clearly illustrated the interconnection or blurring of the social context and the phenomenon was the 2003 film, *Monster* (Theron, Damon, Peterson, Kushner, & Wyman, 2003). The film depicts the life story of the first female serial killer. The process of becoming a serial killer and how it is inseparable from her life experiences are strikingly apparent in this portrayal. A tragic and tortured history of dysfunctional and abusive relationships was portrayed. The rich contextual detail of her life story provided insights into how and why she became a serial killer. Here again, the strength of the case study method is apparent. The producers invite the viewer to understand the relevant details and "how" and "why" of her life path.

Because case study research focuses on a unit of study or phenomenon rather than any one specific research methodology, it can be used at any level of knowledge development, including exploratory, descriptive, or explanatory. The rigor of the design is reflected in the congruity and constancy of the research components within the research design. Therefore, the data collection approaches and data analysis strategies all need to be tailored to consistently reflect the research question and the research aims. Given the broad nature of case study method, researchers need to familiarize themselves with the data collection and analysis approaches appropriate for the level or type of case study. Thus, descriptive studies that focus on understanding an individual's experience regarding a specific phenomenon might consider incorporating a phenomenological approach. These case studies will be rich in description and focus on the lived experience. If the purpose of the study is to understand how individuals respond or adapt when faced with a challenging situations, the focus may be on the process within the social context. The researcher may choose a multiple-case approach, incorporating a constant-comparison approach as seen in grounded theory research. An ethnographic case study might be an approach of choice when the object of study is an organization or a group and may incorporate interviews and participant observation. Inherent in all case study research is the need for the researcher to clearly explain the logic behind the method being applied, show the research process, and clearly present how it is conforming to a rigorous methodological approach (Yin, 2014, p. 3). In essence, "The research design is the logic that links the data to be collected to the initial question of study" (p. 26).

ETHICAL ISSUES

A critical component in the planning process is the attention to the ethical issues and, most specifically, the protection of human subjects. If the research involves sensitive topics or vulnerable groups, the process for obtaining institutional review board (IRB) approval can be challenging. In addition, many members on the IRB may not be very familiar with case study research and may require that the researcher provide additional explanation of the research approach. The researcher needs to be clear on how the participants or cases will be informed fully about the research, informed of any potential risks in participating in the research, and the process of consent. For example, interviewing prisoners about their drug use history may place prisoners at risk legally. Such data need to be carefully collected, coded, and then presented to maintain anonymity. A strategy in this situation and similar cases for maintaining anonymity might be to present the multiple case studies as a cross-case analysis, and thus not depicting any identifiers from a single case (Yin, 2014, p. 196). Such an approach maintains the integrity of the data but it is presented as a case study that does not reflect any single individual's experience. Yin also discusses creating an exemplary case study when anonymity is a major concern. Given the importance of protection of human subjects, and to some extent the challenges presented in the IRB process, presenting the data as an exemplary case could offer a credible approach for reporting significant findings while maintaining the highest level of protection for those participating in the research. Exemplary case studies still adhere to the rigor of case study analysis and meet the general characteristics of case study research, including justifying the relevance and significance of the study, attending to the case and the social context, having awareness and exploring alternative perspectives that might challenge the findings, finding in-depth and sufficient evidence to support the findings, and presenting in an engaging manner so that the reader is able to "arrive at an independent conclusion about the validity" (Yin, 2014, p. 205). In addition, while adhering to the standards for protecting human subjects, the use of exemplary case study provides for an increased level of anonymity and offers an option for researchers who would like to pursue research on sensitive topics and with vulnerable populations.

CASE STUDY RESEARCH: A REVIEW

Although early studies may not have coined the term *case study research*, they certainly have served as models for case study research over the years. As discussed, case study research designs may be descriptive, exploratory, or explanatory. Case study research may also be used to describe processes, generate theory, and test theory.

Case study research may involve multiple data collection strategies. Yin (2009, 2014) presented six common types of research evidence: documents, archival records, interviews, direct observation, participant observation, and physical artifacts. The type of evidence depends on the research question and the methodological approach. For example, for a phenomenological case study, we may use open-ended interviews. Ethnographical case studies may draw on several different types of data, including observation, structured interviews, focus interviews, open-ended interviews, archival records, and documents. The use of multiple types of data, termed triangulation of data, provides different vantage points, which can help in providing depth as well as increased credibility to the case study (Figure 1.1)

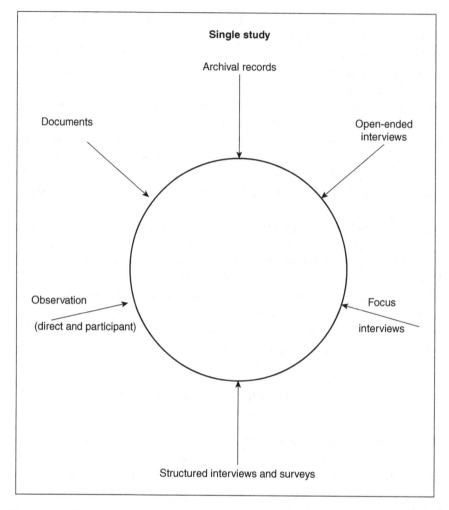

Figure 1.1 *Convergence of evidence (triangulation). Adapted from Yin (2003).*

The "Object of Study" Examples

The first step for case study research is to identify the *object of study* and to define its *boundaries*. This unit or object of study could be an individual, group, or process with its social context clearly defined. The following exemplars illustrate the object of study and the social context.

- Single-case example: In *The Jack-Roller*, Shaw (1930) presents comprehensive data on one individual, a juvenile delinquent who is the object of study. The case study is presented as a life history, written by him, with material about him from several other sources. The boundaries of this case study is clear; a single juvenile delinquent. The social context of his life is presented in depth.

- Multiple case study: In *Street Corner Society*, Whyte (1943/1955) focuses in detail on two gangs with the social context, a street corner. The object of the study is the "street corner gangs." The research is exploratory in nature using participant observation as the primary data collection approach. The boundaries of this case study is clear, two specific gangs with the location, a specific street corner.

- Multiple case study synthesis to identify themes and patterns: In *The Family Encounter of Depression*, Angell (1936/1965) focuses on the experiences of university students whose families had suffered a loss of income during the Depression. This case study presented a synthesis of the individual cases, which is an early example of how to offer greater anonymity and confidentiality.

- Case study with emphasis on social process: In *Boys in White*, Becker, Greer, Hughes, and Strauss (1961) focus on the effect of medical school on students. The object of study is medical students and the social context is medical school. Participant observation was the primary data collection strategy in this study. There was also longitudinal component. Researchers focused on different points of time in medical school rather than on the study of individuals in medical school (Platt, 1992).

- Case study with emphasis on culture: Goffman's (1961) classic study of mental institutions provided an in-depth description of the cultural "underlife" that exists in mental institutions and has been instrumental in understanding similar institutions.

- Explanatory case study: A group of educators in the late 1950s and 1960s wanted to understand why the changes they had made in educational approaches did not improve test results (Yin, 2003). Case by case, they explored the complexity of the teaching process in practice, widening the lens from the classroom activity to the organization, cultural, economic, and policy contexts in which learning and teaching occur. The object of study involved the educational approaches.

SUMMARY

This chapter offers an overview on the case study method. It is an approach that has evolved and continues to be developed. Its strengths include its holistic nature, depth of investigation, and its rich description. The case study method is a versatile and flexible approach well suited when studying phenomenon that is inseparable from its social context. Case studies can range from a single case to multiple cases. Single case studies are valued and can stand on their own, but they also require careful attention to reliability issues. Researchers who engage in single case study research need to remain vigilant regarding their biases and pre-understandings. Although unintended, novice researchers may experience difficulty separating what "they believe they know" from what is to be discovered. This might be described as the research bias, "believing is seeing" (Hentz, 2012). Thus, one needs to be aware that the inductive process inherent in qualitative approaches requires the researcher to be ever vigilant with the awareness that what is discovered is very often different from what was anticipated.

In addition to the single case study design, there are several case study research designs that involve more than one case. According to McDonnell, Jones, and Read (2000), case studies are chosen because they are viewed as an illustrative. When several cases are used in a multiple case study design, the cases need to represent a phenomenon. This requires that the cases be as homogeneous as possible. If the phenomenon is too broad, too loosely defined, and/or the social context is too varied, the study resembles an exploratory study but not a case study. The concept of *replication* is key in a multiple case study design. Each case needs to be carefully selected with the expectation that there will be similar findings. The rationale for multiple case study is to enhance the credibility of the findings and its validity and reliability.

With the range of research approaches from which to choose, case study research is well suited when the phenomenon of interest is best studied within its social context. Nurses are certainly witness to a variety of human conditions and social problems and case study may be a means of expanding our knowledge as well as contributing to research and practice.

REFERENCES

Angell, R. C. (1965). *The family encounters the Depression*. Gloucester, MA: Peter Smith. (Original work published 1936)

Becker, H. S., Greer, B., Hughes, W. C., & Strauss, A. L. (1961). *Boys in white: Student culture in medical school*. Chicago, IL: University of Chicago Press.

Cutter, A. (2004). Methodical failure: The use of case study method by public relations research. *Public Relations Review, 30*, 365–375.

Goffman, E. (1961). *Asylums: Essays on the social situation of mental patients and others inmates*. Garden City, NY: Anchor Books.

Hentz, P. (2012). Case study: Method. In P. L. Munhall (Ed.), *Nursing research: A qualitative perspective* (5th ed., pp. 359–369). Sudbury MA: Jones & Bartlett.

Hentz, P. (in press). *Nursing research using case study design*. New York, NY: Springer.

Liebow, E. (1967). *Tally's corner*. Boston, MA: Little, Brown.

McDonnell, A., Jones, M. L., & Read, S. (2000). Practical considerations in case study research: The relationship between methodology and process. *Journal of Advanced Nursing, 32*(2), 383–390.

McKee, A. (2004). Getting to know case study research: A brief introduction. *Work Bases Learning in Primary Care, 2*, 6–8.

Platt, J. (1992). Case of cases...of cases. In C. C. Ragin & H. S. Becker (Eds.), *What is a case?* New York, NY: Cambridge University Press.

Rosemberg, J. P., & Yates, P. M. (2007). Schematic representation of case study research designs. *Journal of Advanced Nursing, 24*, 447–452.

Shaw, C. (1930). *The Jack-Roller*. Chicago, IL: University of Chicago Press.

Theron, C., Damon, M., Peterson, C., Kushner, D., & Wyman, B. (Producers), & Jenkins, P. (Director). (2003). *Monster*. [Motion picture]. United States: Columbia Tristar Films.

Whyte, W. F. (1955). *Street corner society: The social structure of an Italian slum*. Chicago, IL: University of Chicago Press. (Original work published 1943)

Yin, R. K. (2003). *Case study research* (3rd ed.). Thousand Oaks, CA: Sage.

Yin, R. K. (2009). *Case study research: Design and methods* (4th ed.). Los Angeles, CA: Sage.

Yin, R. K. (2014). *Case study research: Design and methods* (5th ed.). Los Angeles, CA: Sage.

CHAPTER TWO

STATE OF THE ART OF QUALITATIVE CASE STUDY METHODOLOGY IN NURSING RESEARCH

Johnathan D. Steppe

Qualitative case study methodology (QCSM) is an approach to research that has become increasingly popular in nursing inquiry. Originating in the field of social sciences, QCSM offers a means to holistically explore complex phenomena within real-world contexts (Anthony & Jack, 2009). This holistic approach aligns well with the nursing perspective, which is often characterized by its holistic view of health and well-being. In an article meant for novice researchers, Baxter and Jack (2008) provided an excellent introduction to QCSM, which examined the philosophical roots that inform the approach. Although several theoretical views of QCSM exist, Baxter and Jack noted that the approaches of Yin (2014) and Stake (1995) predominate. Both of these approaches situate QCSM within a constructivist paradigm (Baxter & Jack, 2008) and both consider multiple sources of data as a defining characteristic of the case study approach (Anthony & Jack, 2009). Conversely, Yin (2014) defines case study methodology in terms of the empirical process, whereas Stake (1995) views the approach in terms of the unit of study (Anthony & Jack, 2009). Nevertheless, both approaches acknowledge the value of QCSM in conducting deep exploration of phenomena that cannot be manipulated or removed from their real-world context (Baxter & Jack, 2008; Stake, 1995; Yin, 2014).

Focusing specifically on nursing research, Anthony and Jack (2009) conducted an excellent integrative review of nursing studies published from 2005 to 2007 that employed a qualitative case study approach. The purpose of this review was to critically appraise the use of QCSM by nurse scholars. Anthony and Jack noted that QCSM has become increasingly prevalent in nursing inquiry, a fact that necessitated such a review. Using a defined set of criteria to produce a manageable yet representative sample of QCSM nursing studies, Anthony and Jack identified a total of 42 such studies to include in their review. The authors discovered that nurse scholars were employing QCSM in a broad range of nursing contexts, including acute care, long-term care, nursing education, community health, nursing research, family care, nursing management, adolescent health, and mental health. Furthermore, their review revealed that nurse scholars were paying increasing attention to issues of rigor within the context of QCSM. Still, confusion surrounding the nature of such inquiry persists, a fact that presents challenges to QCSM implementation (Anthony & Jack, 2009). Anthony and Jack recommended that further appraisal of the use of QCSM in nursing inquiry was warranted. Chan (2009) supported this recommendation, citing the increasing prevalence of QCSM in nursing research as the impetus to continue the work of Anthony and Jack and to further explore QCSM within a nursing context. As Chan (2009) noted:

> The case study approach has great potential in nursing research and yet there is still a great deal that we need to understand about what QCSM is, why it is being adopted, and how it is being conceptualized and implemented. (p. 1774)

Clearly, QCSM presents both challenges and opportunities for nurse scholars. When used appropriately, QCSM can be employed to conduct rigorous and empirically based studies that take into account the impact and implications of real-world contexts on the phenomena or concept in question. Furthermore, through the use of several data sources, QCSM allows scholars to investigate phenomena from multiple perspectives. Nevertheless, Yin (2014) cautions that QCSM poses unique challenges to novice researchers who may underestimate the complexity of conducting such research in an appropriately systematic and rigorous manner. Confusion over the nature of QCSM may further complicate the research process for neophyte scholars. To facilitate understanding of how QCSM can be employed by nurse researchers in the generation of new knowledge, the following section offers a review of the current body of nursing research that has used a qualitative case study approach. This section is then followed by a discussion of common trends in QCSM within nursing contexts. Through an exploration of contemporary QCSM nursing inquiry, it is our hope that readers considering QCSM for their own research will be better positioned to take advantage of the unique benefits the approach offers.

CURRENT STATE OF NURSING INQUIRY USING
CASE STUDY METHODS

In this section, we offer a review of current nursing studies that have been conducted using a QCSM approach. Initially, the search criteria used by Anthony and Jack (2009) guided a literature review of QCSM that spanned from 2009 to 2015. Databases included in the search were CINAHL, MEDLINE, and PsychInfo. Meaningful keywords and search phrases used to identify relevant articles included "qualitative case study," "case study," "qualitative," and "nursing." The initial search returned more than 140 articles that met the original criteria set, and so additional exclusionary criteria were established. To generate a manageable yet representative sample of studies, this review was further limited to research that was published in nursing journals during a 3-year period, from 2013 to 2015. Furthermore, only studies that listed a nurse as the primary author were included in the review. Incorporating these criteria, a modified search generated a total of 50 articles for inclusion in this review.

Results from the review are summarized as follows. Much like Anthony and Jack (2009), this review identified a broad range of nursing settings and issues in which QCSM has been employed as a research methodology. These settings included acute care, long-term care, mental health, community health, nursing education, peripartum/perinatal care, and professional/workplace issues. When a study overlapped two nursing areas, that study was categorized based on its primary focus. For example, a study conducted in the community health setting that explored implementation of an undergraduate learning strategy was categorized as nursing education.

Acute/Inpatient Care

QCSM studies conducted in acute care settings represented a large percentage of the studies identified for this review. First, Dionne-Odom, Willis, Bakitas, Crandall, and Grace (2015) chose a qualitative case study design to examine surrogate decision making (SDM) within the context of end-of-life issues in the intensive care unit (ICU). The case study approach allowed the researchers to make within- and cross-case comparisons to provide a deeper understanding of the complex psychological processes underlying SDM for terminally ill patients. The researchers recruited 19 informants who had served as SDMs for adult patients who had died in the ICU setting. Cognitive task analysis was used to conduct and analyze semi-structured interviews, which were digitally recorded and evaluated for common themes. Findings were then organized into a conceptual model that represented the SDM process. Results from this study have the potential to inform development of interventions designed to support SDM during end-of-life care.

Adams, Bailey, Anderson, and Thygeson (2013) also examined end-of-life issues in the ICU setting using a QCSM approach, this time from the perspective of both health care providers (HCPs) and family members. The study's stated purpose was to "describe the behavior of HCPs and responses of family members through the lens of Adaptive Leadership in a prospective case study of a patient transitioning from curative to palliative care" (Adams et al., 2013, p. 330). The researchers used a single case study design that focused on four family members, a nurse, and two physicians of one terminally ill patient. Data were collected using family group conferences and narrative interviews. During data analysis, the researchers employed Adaptive Leadership as a framework for understanding behaviors employed by health care providers to assist families during end-of-life care. The Adaptive Leadership model views organizations and individuals as complex adaptive systems that must confront technical and adaptive challenges through successful self-organization (Adams et al., 2013; Bailey et al., 2012; Thygeson, Morrissey, & Ulstad, 2010). The study findings supported the use of Adaptive Leadership behaviors to facilitate successful adaptation and coping in families facing the loss of a loved one.

Furthermore, within an ICU context, Nesbitt (2013) investigated nurses' experiences with journal clubs and how such participation influenced professional development. Using a two-site, multiple case study design, the researcher recruited 70 health care professionals (64 nurses) who participated in journal clubs in two Canadian ICUs for a 6-month period. Data-collection methods included six semi-structured interviews with each informant, two focus groups, field notes, anonymous surveys, and document review. Five major themes emerged from data analysis: community, incentive, confidence, impact on practice, and reflection. Findings demonstrated that participation in journal clubs increase nurses' confidence, competency, and motivation to read research articles, as well as foster an atmosphere of community. Gains in competency were thought to be modest. The researchers concluded that implementation of journal clubs in conjunction with other educational strategies would have a greater impact on competency than just journal clubs alone.

Similar to the study by Adams et al. (2013), Rudolfsson (2014) used a single case study design to elucidate one nurse's perception of the perioperative patient experience. Rudolfsson selected a QCSM approach for its advantages in providing an in-depth description of a particular phenomenon within specific real-world contexts (Rudolfsson, 2014; Stake, 1995; Yin, 2014). A unique characteristic of this particular study was that the researcher was both the narrator/informant of the case as well as the interpreter/researcher. Thus, the study not only focused on the perception of the perioperative nurse, but also on how that nurse interpreted the situation. The researcher adopted a hermeneutic approach to data analysis, which permitted new insights to arise from the experience. A key finding of this study was that patients experience shame related to body image even before arriving in the operating room.

Four studies used QCSM to explore complex experiences and challenges faced by nurses working in acute care settings. First, Hoyle and Grant (2015) conducted a study that aimed "to understand nurses' views and experiences of four treatment targets in the emergency department and how this impacts clinical decision making throughout acute secondary care hospitals" (p. 2211). The researchers interviewed 31 informants from three acute care specialties at a large hospital in Scotland. Employing a case study approach informed by Yin (2014) to provide a holistic perspective within a real-world context, the researchers used the hospital as the case unit for the study. Overall, informants perceived treatment time targets as unhelpful and potentially detrimental to patient care. Informants reported breaching treatment target guidelines in cases where acutely ill patients required more care. Emergency nurses bore the most responsibility in meeting treatment targets, a fact that created significant burden for these nurses. The researchers recommended that policy makers reevaluate implementation of treatment time targets to ensure appropriateness. In addition, health care providers breaching such targets to ensure patient safety should be immune from negative repercussions, and the burden arising from these target programs should be more evenly distributed.

A second study that examined experiences of acute care nurses was conducted by White, Pesut, and Rush (2014). In this study, the researchers explored the experiences of post-anesthesia care unit (PACU) nurses caring for ICU patients within the PACU setting. The researchers recruited six PACU nurses who participated in semi-structured interviews designed to elicit information about informant experience with ICU patients. Findings revealed that these nurses caring for ICU patients in a PACU setting often felt unable to provide the appropriate level of care given the limitations of the setting. This inability was related to nurses having the knowledge to provide appropriate care but lacking the resources to do so. The researchers noted that the study highlights the need for a planned change process that could provide PACU nurses access to resources and support needed to care for overflow ICU patients within the PACU setting.

A third study by Droskinis (2013) explored issues faced by diploma nurses working in acute care settings. Droskinis selected a QCSM approach because of its potential to provide authentic empirical data about complex issues within a real-life context. A single informant was recruited for the study, and phenomenological interviews were conducted via e-mail using semi-structured, open-ended questioning. Findings from the study revealed two major themes. The first theme, progressive transformation, related to changing educational requirements and increased responsibilities within the nursing profession. The second theme, technological innovation, represented informant experience with technological revolutions that have transformed nursing care. Overall, the researcher concluded that awareness of the needs of diploma-prepared nurses could contribute to better integration of these nurses within the current health care environment.

Finally, Powell (2013) investigated the experiences of night-shift nurses, with a particular focus on work satisfaction and professional relationships in an acute care setting. The researchers adopted a case study approach that was informed by the perspective of constructivist theory to provide night-shift nurses the opportunity to voice their own unique reality. Fourteen nurses participated in semi-structured interviews that were reinforced and collated with self-completed diaries. Four major themes emerged during data analysis: the importance of work relationships, the impact of the working environment, common work practices, and the personal impact of working nights. Informants reported feeling less supported by leadership than dayshift nurses, with fewer opportunities for engagement and professional development. In addition, working conditions for night-shift nurses appeared inferior to those experienced by day shift. Nevertheless, findings also demonstrated strong collegial relationships among night-shift nurses. The researchers concluded that facilities should capitalize on these strong relationships, while implementing strategies to improve support and working environments of night-shift nurses.

Turning to issues of nursing leadership, this literature review uncovered two studies that dealt with the relationship between nursing leadership and implementation of best-practice/evidence-based quality improvement programs. First, a study by Fleiszer, Semenic, Ritchie, Richer, and Denis (2015) aimed to describe the impact of nursing leader actions on the sustainability of best practice initiatives in the acute care setting. Thirty-nine informants participated in a multiple case study that used semi-structured interviews, document analysis, and field observations.

The study's purpose was to provide insight into the influence of nursing leader actions on the long-term success of best practice guideline programs across four acute care units. Data analysis revealed that successful strategies for sustaining such programs included those that maintained priorities and reinforced program expectations. In doing so, these strategies promoted learning and accountability in the workplace. A key implication of the study was the importance of nursing leadership actions in addressing issues of patient care through implementation and maintenance of best practice initiatives.

Stetler, Ritchie, Rycroft-Malone, and Charns (2014) also explored the impact of nursing leader actions on quality improvement programs, this time from the perspective of institutionalizing evidence-based practice (EBP) guidelines. The study used a multiple case study design that presented two contrasting acute care cases. The first case was a hospital widely known for its successful implementation and use of EBP guidelines, while the second case was a hospital characterized as a beginner in the use of formalized EBP. Data collection included multiple interviews with nurse leaders as well as focus groups with staff nurses. Findings demonstrated the complexity of leadership behaviors and actions that influence successful implementation of EBP. These actions cut across hierarchical levels, and included the efforts of both nurse administrators and staff nurses.

Another study related to quality improvement was conducted by Ireland, Kirkpatrick, Boblin, and Robertson (2013), who investigated the implementation of fall-prevention initiatives in three acute care hospitals located in Ontario, Canada. The researchers defined the case unit as implementation of best practice fall-prevention guidelines, while the three hospitals served as the contextual boundaries of the case. As with many of the previously discussed studies, Ireland et al. (2013) identified the appropriateness of a QCSM approach to investigate complex real-world situations within a specific context. Ninety-five nurses (both administrative and bedside) participated in interviews and focus groups, and also provided documentation and artifacts for data analysis. The researchers noted that triangulation via multiple data sources enhanced rigor of study findings, a claim supported by Stake (1995). Data analysis suggested four recommendations related to falls-prevention interventions:

- The need to listen to and recognize the expertise and clinical realities of the staff
- The importance of keeping the implementation process simple
- The need to recognize that what seems simple becomes complex when meeting individual patient needs

- The need to view the process as one of continuous quality improvement (Ireland et al., 2013, p. 95)

Related to the subject of nursing leadership, Maxwell, Baillie, Rickard, and McLaren (2013) studied the impact of social identity in achieving acceptance and workplace jurisdiction within two acute care hospitals. Using a multiple case study design, the researchers defined each hospital as a separate case, while two new specialty nursing roles constituted embedded units within the study. According to the researchers "the use of data from different sources is a classic strength of case study design" (Maxwell et al., 2013); accordingly, this study used a significant number of data collection methods, including semi-structured interviews, nonparticipant observation, partial-participant observation, organizational document review, and follow-up interviews. Two distinct role types were identified during data analysis: a "fixer" role and a "niche" role, each of which faced distinct challenges in establishing workplace jurisdiction. Furthermore, workplace jurisdiction was influenced by four different types of workplace identities. These included professional, specialty, organizational, and relational identities. These findings illustrate the need for facilities to support social processes that facilitate acceptance and legitimacy of new nursing roles within acute care settings.

Continuing with research conducted within acute care contexts, Velloso, Ceci, and Alves (2013) explored power configurations within a Brazilian emergency care system with the aim of understanding how such configurations impacted development of the new health care system. Semi-structured interviews and field observations comprised the data-collection strategies of this qualitative case study, which was informed by the work of Foucault (1979). The 31 informants participating in the study included nurses, nursing assistants, ambulance drivers, and physicians. Discourse analysis of the data highlighted the impact of hierarchical surveillance in shaping emergency care practices, which in turn influenced the nature of power relationships within the system. The researchers noted that study findings suggested that supporting flexibility in power relations within health care systems may be necessary in creating a system responsive to the dynamic health issues of contemporary society.

Tobiano, Chaboyer, and McMurray (2013) employed QCSM to understand family member perceptions of bedside shift reports in an Australian hospital. The researchers recruited eight informants who had a family member admitted to an inpatient rehabilitation ward. Data-collection methods included observations, field notes, and guided interviews using open-ended questioning. This combination of data collection methods was employed as a recognized strategy to enhance rigor of study findings (Yin, 2014). Data gathered from individual informants were regarded as separate cases, leading to a multiple case study design. Analysis of common threads among cases revealed three major themes: understanding the situation, interaction with nursing staff, and finding value. In turn, each of these major themes had several associated subthemes. The researchers concluded that families value inclusion and the chance to participate in their loved one's care, and that effective use of bedside shift reports can support a family-centered nursing approach.

Another study identified in the literature review addressed issues faced by older patients being discharged after hip fracture surgery. Popejoy, Marek, and Scott-Cawiezell (2013) conducted a longitudinal, multiple case study that investigated problems experienced by older adults transitioning through different levels of care following a hip fracture. A total of 21 informants were recruited for the study, and data were collected using participant interview and chart reviews. Interviews were conducted in person or by phone, and were scheduled during the immediate postoperative period, and that at post-discharge intervals of 2 weeks, 3 months, and 12 months. Three major transition patterns were identified: from home to hospital to inpatient rehabilitation, from home to hospital to nursing home, and from nursing home to hospital. Common problems experienced at all levels of transition included depression, delirium, pressure ulcers, weight loss, urinary incontinence, and falls. The researchers recommended that transitional care should enhance patient and family involvement during transitions.

Finally, parents experience significant stress when faced with the hospitalization of their child, and these challenges are exacerbated when one of the parents is a nurse. Lines, Mannix, and Giles (2015) considered the unique experiences of nurses who have had a child hospitalized for an acute illness. For this case study, the researchers recruited six nurses who participated in semi-structured interviews. The results of these interviews were thematically analyzed to identify commonalities among informant experiences. Informants characterized their situation as taking on a dual role, that of the parent–nurse; role conflict often emerged as the informants felt torn between these roles. The expertise of the informants compelled them to seek higher levels of care for their children, a fact that increased stress levels. The researchers concluded that health care professionals need to acknowledge and respond to the unique needs of the nurse–parents of pediatric patients.

Long-Term/Elder Care

Two studies investigated issues of long-term care placement using a QCSM approach. First, Mamier and Winslow (2014) used a single case study design to examine divergent perspectives of a family caregiver and a health care professional within the context of long-term care placement decision making. Informants in the study included a woman caring for her husband, who had been diagnosed with Alzheimer's disease, as well as a social worker who led a support group attended by the couple. The researchers constructed this revelatory case study from data collected during three interviews (two with the caregiver and one with the social worker). Data analysis was conducted from a grounded theory perspective and revealed 11 major categories in which divergent perspectives of decision making fell. Although some congruence between the perspectives of the social worker and the caregiver was identified, significant differences were also evident. A key finding of this study was that health care professionals may not be aware of the particular needs of caregivers facing long-term placement decisions, and that caregivers could benefit from anticipatory guidance before events necessitate long-term placement.

A second study by Koplow et al. (2015) explored caregiver experiences after long-term care placement of a loved one. Two caregivers were recruited as informants and constituted two separate, contrasting cases made up of a caregiver–care recipient dyad. Informants were purposefully selected to exemplify a smooth transition and a difficult transition within the context of long-term care placement. Data were collected through interviews conducted shortly after placement and again 3 months later. Similarities and differences between the two cases centered around four major issues: the relationship between caregiver and his or her loved one before long-term placement, factors contributing to the placement decision, continuing involvement in the loved one's care after placement, and available support systems for the caregiver. Implications of the study included the need for nurses and other health care professionals to understand caregiver perspective and the issues that can facilitate smooth transition for families facing long-term placement of a loved one.

Also, within the long-term care context, Tayab and Narushima (2015) used a QCSM approach to explore perceptions and practices of cultural competence among personal support workers (PSWs) working in a long-term care facility in Ontario, Canada. The long-term care facility constituted the case of the study, while six of the facility's employees served as key informants. The researchers employed multiple methods of data collection to increase study rigor; these methods included focus groups, document review, and semi-structured interviews of key informants. Findings from the study revealed a strong link between cultural competence and patient-centered care, multiple definitions of cultural competence that existed among PSWs, and organizational factors that impacted the development of cultural competence among employees. The researchers concluded that further education and research is needed to elucidate the meaning of cultural competence for PSWs and how their understanding of the concept impacts patient care.

Abrahamson, DeCrane, Mueller, Davila, and Arling (2015) investigated a long-term care quality improvement project designed to reduce pain in nursing home residents. The stated purpose of the study was to "closely examine processes for successful nursing home QI [quality improvement] with particular focus on pain management" (p. 262). This case study approach used implementation of the quality improvement project as the case unit. Informants included 24 nursing home employees from eight facilities that had implemented the quality improvement project. Data collection was accomplished via in-depth, semi-structured interviews. Findings identified five major facilitators of successful project implementation, including adequate training, participation by nursing assistants, leadership support, and interdisciplinary communication. Barriers to implementation included challenges with measuring outcomes, increased documentation, and resistance to change. The findings of this study suggest avenues for facilitating successful implementation of pain management projects within the long-term care setting.

Challenges to implementing long-term care research aimed at quality improvement was the focus of the next study to be discussed. Zapka et al. (2014) used QCSM in a study designed to explore factors that impacted willingness of caregivers and nursing home administration to participate in research seeking to determine the efficacy of feeding alternatives among patients with dementia. This multilevel case study employed multiple methods of data collection, including caregiver focus groups and in-person and electronic interviews with nursing home administrators. Data analysis revealed key challenges to caregiver participation in efficacy research including lack of clarity in research design, caregiver understanding of dementia prognosis, and caregiver perception of feeding needs of their loved one. Challenges to nursing home participation included legal issues, corporate approval, and previous relationships with researchers. The researchers noted that enhancing caregiver participation in such research should include comprehensive education about dementia as well as research purpose, design, and protocols. Such education should also take into consideration literacy levels of potential informants. Improving the likelihood of nursing home participation in research could be accomplished by preliminary work to develop a trusting relationship with nursing home administration, address potential legal issues, and navigate corporate policies and requirements for researchers.

Community/Outpatient Care

Six studies using QCSM were identified that explored issues in community/ outpatient care settings. In one of these studies, Sandy, Kgole, and Mavundla (2013) explored the needs of family caregivers of children with learning disabilities living in an impoverished province of South Africa. The researchers employed two phases of semi-structured interviews to elucidate issues faced by three case study families, all of whom had at least one child with a learning disability. Six major themes emerged from the study's findings, including caring as a stressful experience, working in partnership with health professionals, education and training needs, the need for support through professional supervision, the need for financial assistance, and experiences with discrimination arising from stigma associated with learning disabilities. The researchers concluded that support programs and policies are needed to assist families in the complex task of caring for children with learning disabilities within a resource-poor setting. Furthermore, such programs must be individualized to the needs of each family, and should include training and education as a major component of support.

Another study by Mizutani et al. (2015) also examined community health issues within a resource-poor area of rural Indonesia. The purpose of this study was to construct a model of healthy behaviors of rural Muslim Indonesians living with hypertension. Twelve married couples were recruited for the study, which used semi-structured interviews to provide the desired data. The researchers used Yin's (2014) method of data analysis to identify specific health promoting behaviors practiced by study informants. In doing so, the researchers also examined informant reasons for adopting these behaviors. Some of the healthy behaviors reported by informants included dietary choices, exercising, stress management, caring for others, and fulfilling one's duty to God. Reasons for practicing such behaviors related to personal beliefs and perceived competence. Conversely, challenges to health promoting behaviors included personal, environmental, and social barriers. The researchers recommended that health professionals working with the target population should reinforce reasons for adopting health promoting behaviors, while also finding ways to mitigate negative factors that formed barriers to healthy lifestyles.

Whiffin, Bailey, Ellis-Hill, Jarrett, and Hutchinson (2015) employed a longitudinal case study design to explore the narratives of noninjured family members of persons who suffered traumatic head injury. The researchers recruited nine family members from three families to participate in the 12-month study. Although recruitment took place in the acute care setting, whereas data collection was primarily conducted after patient discharge, which allowed the researchers to explore family reaction and adjustment in the post-injury period through a series of three unstructured narrative interviews. From these interviews, the researchers identified five interconnected narratives that included experiences related to trauma, recovery, autobiography, suffering, and family. An analysis of these narratives revealed that turbulence and disruption characterized family life during the first year following a traumatic head injury of a family member. The study illuminated the importance of addressing the needs of the family as a whole when caring for those with traumatic head injury. Supporting these families would include listening to their stories and validating their experiences.

Implementation of a patient-centered model of nursing care in outpatient radiation oncology was the subject of an instrumental case study conducted by Rose and Yates (2013). The stated purpose of this study was "to describe clinical staff perceptions of implementing a person-centered model of nursing in an outpatient radiotherapy treatment department, using a Primary Nursing/Collaborative Practice framework" (Rose & Yates, 2013, p. 554). The study sample included 13 clinical staff, including physicians, nurses and radiotherapists, who participated in semi-structured interviews over a 6-month period. Major themes that emerged from the study included changes in traditional practices, dominance of a profession-centric approach, operationalization of primary nursing, and ensuring an interdisciplinary approach. Findings from the study revealed that the person-centered model was generally well received, and resulted in increased nursing autonomy and satisfaction; nevertheless, challenges to providing holistic care within the interdisciplinary environment were also made evident. The researchers noted that the study highlighted the potential benefits of a person-centered model, as well as the integral role that communication and education play in the success of such a model.

Abbott, Fuji, and Galt (2015) used a qualitative case study approach to examine engagement among nurses working in a rural ambulatory setting that had implemented electronic health records (EHRs) and electronic prescribing system. Lewin's (1951) Change Theory provided a framework for the study, which employed an exemplar critical case design to allow for generalization to similar cases. Twelve informants, including eight nurses and four physicians, participated in semi-structured interviews that were constructed to identify common themes related to engagement with the EHR system. The researchers identified six major themes: nurses maintaining patient focus, lack of nursing involvement with the EHR, the influence of physician preference on nurses' use of EHR, nursing bypass of the EHR system, increased workload related to the EHR, and EHR impact on efficiency of nursing care. A notable conclusion of this study was that EHRs appeared to increase workloads while also contributing to new patient safety issues.

The final study conducted within a community setting sought "to explore, identify, and characterize the origins, processes and outcomes of effective chronic disease management models and the nursing contributions to such models" (Procter, Wilson, Brooks, & Kendall, 2013, p. 633). Six community case study sites that represented three different models of care for chronic conditions participated in the study. Models of care included case management, disease management, and supported self-care. Data were collected using semi-structured interviews with nurses working at each of the participating sites. Overall, the study found that nurses at all sites possessed high levels of clinical expertise. In addition, nurses working in community matron settings were also successfully accomplishing their goal of reducing hospital admissions. The researchers noted that structural factors and power relationships within integrated care models may constrain effective nursing care. Addressing this problem requires changes that reexamine and reconfigure traditional power structures.

Mental Health Nursing Care

Five of the identified studies focused on issues of mental health nursing using QCSM. First, the role of stigma in the formation of mental health nurses' professional identities was explored in a qualitative case study by Sercu, Ayala, and Bracke (2015). Using a multiple case study design that integrated ethnographic data collection from two psychiatric hospitals, the researchers sought to understand the role that stigma played in giving meaning to the mental health nursing role. Thirty-three nurses participated in the study, which used semi-structured interviews and intensive participant observation to explore the phenomenon of interest. Findings from the study suggested that overcoming stigma and resisting a reductionist approach that focused on diagnosis rather than patient was a major motivator to becoming a mental health nurse. Thus, stigma appeared to be enmeshed in the turbulent relationship between mental health nursing and the traditional psychiatric model of care. Many informants described a desire to resist what they felt to be stigmatizing practices found in general health care, which focus on illness rather than person. The researchers concluded that the concept of stigma should be integrated in future research focused on exploring the identity crisis currently experienced by mental health nurses.

Next, McKeown, et al. (2014) used a multiple, comparative case study design to explore relationships between professional mental health care providers and independent mental health advocates. Although nurses often serve as advocates for patients with mental health issues, the advocacy role of nursing is often unsupported and weakly delineated. Conversely, independent mental health advocacy groups represent and champion patient interests from a position unencumbered by co-allegiances to employers. An expansive case study that covered eight geographical regions and included 214 informants, the study also included a variety of inpatient, outpatient, and community settings. The researchers used informant interviews and a survey of available advocacy services to collect data. From their findings, the researchers concluded that the extent to which professionals understand and appreciate the advocacy role influences relationships between health care professionals and independent advocates.

Recovery, a familiar concept within the field of mental health, was the focus of a study by McKenna, Furness, Dhital, Park, and Connally (2014). The purpose of the study was to describe the impact of a recovery-oriented approach on service care delivery in an inpatient, Australian, mental health facility. An illustrative case study design was employed. Informants included 20 stakeholders, all of whom worked in a 26-bed mental health unit of a large urban hospital in Melbourne. Data collection methods included interviews and focus groups. Findings from the study demonstrated that stakeholders embraced the recovery-oriented approach, which they characterized as collaborative, holistic, engaged, strength based, and supportive of patient autonomy. Overall, the case illustrates the recovery-oriented approach of action, and could potentially guide other agencies wishing to adopt such an approach.

Seeking to identify strategies that could prevent involuntary admission for patients with mental illness, de Jong, Schout, and Abma (2014) designed a naturalistic case study approach informed by Stake (1995) that examined the impact of a Family Group Conferencing (FGC) approach on such compulsory admissions. This single case study used semi-structured interviews with 17 informants who had participated in one FGC that addressed the family concerns of a man living with schizophrenia. The 17 informants represented four stakeholder groups, including the man's neighbors, family, and other social acquaintances, the FGC coordinator, and mental health professionals involved with the case. Four themes emerged from the data analysis phase: a history of avoiding care and involuntary treatment, prevention of compulsory admission following the FGC, optional participation of the patient in FGC, and resolution of conflict between neighbors and the involved case managers. Overall, the case supported the use of FGC to avoid involuntary admissions due to mental illness, and to improve relationships of those involved.

Shifting focus to pediatric mental health, a final identified study by Morris (2014) used a case study approach to explore how parental perceptions of mental illness change after a child is diagnosed with such a disorder. For this study, the researcher recruited one informant, the father of a 7-year-old boy who had received several possible diagnoses, including attention deficit hyperactivity disorder, bipolar disorder, mood disorder, and low-grade autism. The informant participated in two semi-structured interviews that were recorded and thematically analyzed. Six themes emerged from this analysis: alienation from peers, ambivalence toward the diagnosis and outcome, an evolving orientation toward mental illness, stigmatization within the school system; conflict with mental health care, finding specialists, and finally acquiring new peers. Factors impacting parental perception included the educational and mental health systems and interactions with peers. The researcher concluded that further research is needed into parental experiences with the diagnosis and illness trajectory of pediatric mental illness. Such research could assist health care professionals in supporting family adaptation in such cases.

Peripartum/Perinatal Care

Peripartum/perinatal care was another nursing context in which QCSM was used to explore a variety of health care issues. First, De Rouck and Leys (2013) investigated how the illness trajectory of neonates admitted to an ICU impacted parents' use of online sources for health information. The study used a longitudinal, multiple case study design, in which the unit of analysis was the parental dyad of each infant. Data were collected over a 10-month period using in-depth, in-person interviews with 40 dyads. Initially, parents were interviewed every 2 weeks for the first 2 months following admission. Afterward, interviews were conducted on a monthly basis. Data analysis revealed multiple factors influencing parental use of the internet as a health information source along the illness trajectory, including the parent–health provider relationship. Information-gathering behaviors also changed as parents moved along the illness trajectory and became more proficient with comprehending complex medical information. An important theme emerging from this study was the use of online information gathering as a part of the coping process for the informants. In addition, illness labels associated with an infant's condition significantly influenced the success of online search strategies employed by parents; vague labels tended to confound searches, while precise terminology facilitated them.

Another study that examined perinatal issues within the neonatal intensive care unit (NICU) context was one by Johnston (2014), which explored a high-risk father's experiences following the hospitalization of his low-birth-weight infant. The study combined a single case study design with a hermeneutical, phenomenological approach. The defined case for the study was a young black man from a high-risk background characterized by violence and loss. Over a 10-week period, the informant participated in three semi-structured, in-depth interviews at specific points in time: shortly following his child's birth, a week before discharge, and 2 weeks post-discharge. Themes that emerged during data analysis can be characterized by feelings of loss and unmet needs and the need to appear strong in the face of adversity. Supportive themes were also identified, including support through communication, the benefits of finding a mentor, and adopting a new perspective as a father. Male nurses may be well suited as mentors for these fathers, who often lack positive male role models. Findings demonstrated the important role that health care workers using caring practices can play in meeting the needs of these fathers.

Chang, Rowe, and Goopy (2014) also used a longitudinal case study design to explore how nonfamily support influenced breastfeeding in Taiwanese career women. Low breastfeeding-maintenance rates in Taiwan justified the study. In addition, the researchers chose a case study design because of the highly contextualized nature of phenomenon in question. Fourteen women participated in a series of two to three in-depth interviews, which took place at three significant times: shortly after participation in a culturally important postpartum ritual, before returning to work, and shortly after resuming work responsibilities. The informants were interviewed alone, without inclusion of their partners. Data analysis identified several significant nonfamilial factors contributing to breastfeeding maintenance, including collegial support, onsite workplace services, and online resources. Overall, these findings provide insight into possible ways of sustaining breastfeeding within this population.

Professional Development/Workplace Issues

A remarkable number of recent QCSM studies have investigated the experiences of newly graduated nurses transitioning into professional practice. This literature review identified four such studies published in nursing journals within the past 3 years. The first such study, conducted by Al Awaisi, Cooke, and Pryjmachuck (2015), focused on new graduate nurses living and working in Oman during their first year of practice. The researchers defined the case of this study as "new graduate nurses' transition experiences while working at a tertiary hospital in Oman" (Al Awaisi et al., 2015), while the experiences of individual nurses were embedded units within the overlying case. A case study approach was adopted because of its ability to illuminate complex and contextual factors influencing transition experiences of new nurses. The researchers acknowledged the use of triangulation using multiple methods of data collection, including interviews, focus groups, participant observation, and document review. Findings revealed that Omani nurses often have negative views of nursing, particularly basic patient care. Furthermore, informants reported experiencing a reality shock as they transitioned from school to professional practice. The study highlighted the impact of the cultural view of the status of nursing in Oman, and elucidated the need for strategies to bridge the theory–practice gap experienced by newly graduated nurses.

Another study that examined the experiences of newly graduated nurses was undertaken by Stacey, Pollock, and Crawford (2015). The stated purpose of this study was to explore how entry-level nurses respond to new structures (Stacey et al., 2015). The researchers noted that, in the United Kingdom, a critical movement has argued that nursing has become too academic to the detriment of clinical competency. This movement has led to the adoption of competency-based education models in nursing education, which some feel compromises the progression of the nursing profession. Furthermore, newly graduated nurses often must navigate encounters with anti-intellectualist stereotypes of nursing among established practitioners. For this study, the researchers employed a longitudinal case study design that spanned a 2-year period and included eight newly graduated nurses. As in other previously discussed studies, the researchers noted their use of triangulation strategies using multiple methods of data collection, including interviews, diaries, focus groups, and document review. A key finding of this study was that informants developed methods to achieve acceptance among established practitioners, including the use of fundamental care as a currency, while also demonstrating skills competence in a manner that would not be perceived as arrogant or threatening. Furthermore, informants displayed significant resilience to hostility they encountered from established practitioners by not taking personally such hostile encounters. The study findings suggest the need for a supportive environment that fosters and encourages student and new graduate learning. In addition, the researchers noted that the study further advances the current debate over the use of competency-based models in nursing education.

Lea and Cruickshank (2015) also conducted a study that focused on the newly graduated nursing experience. The purpose of this exploratory case study was to investigate ways of supporting newly graduated nurses transitioning to rural nursing practice in Australia. The researchers collected data via in-depth interviews with 16 experienced rural health nurses, all of whom had previous experience working with new graduates. Thematic analysis of the data revealed that support for new graduate nurses transitioning to rural practice is significantly impacted by staffing allocation and the skill mix of RNs working within a specific rural health service. Furthermore, many of the informants felt that experienced rural nurses were unaware of how to best support newly graduated nurses. Findings of this study could be used to inform interventions aimed at providing timely support for new graduates entering rural nursing practice.

The impact of preceptorship on newly graduated nurses transitioning to acute care practice was the focus of a study conducted by Whitehead, Owen, Henshaw, Beddingham, and Simmons (2015). Fifty-two informants, all of whom were involved with one hospital's preceptorship program, were recruited for the study. Informants included preceptors, preceptees, administrators, hospital nurse educators, and nurse managers. Data were triangulated using focus groups, semi-structured interviews, and documentation review. The researchers identified multiple factors that influenced the outcomes of the preceptor program, including recognition of the preceptor role, preceptor selection and preparation, managerial support of preceptors, and time out from patient care for preceptors to fill the additional responsibilities of preceptorship. These findings suggest points at which interventions could be implemented to facilitate the success of a preceptorship program.

Turning to issues of professional collaboration and interpersonal relationships, Moore, Prentice, and McQuestion (2015) investigated the impact of social factors on collaboration between nurses in inpatient and outpatient oncology settings. Specifically, the study examined how social interactions among nurses facilitated professional collaboration. The study employed a single case study design with embedded units. The researchers chose a case study approach because "it supports an interpretive approach to gaining an understanding of the phenomenon of interest" (Moore et al., 2015, p. 52). Data were collected from 14 nurses working at an inpatient/outpatient oncology clinic using telephone interviews and online document review. Documents reviewed included job descriptions from the clinic, regulatory provisions, and frameworks from professional oncology nursing organizations, and guidelines and competencies issued by Canadian licensing agencies. Findings showed that knowing someone personally as well as professionally facilitated collaboration. Furthermore, getting to know colleagues on a personal level occurred within the professional setting as well as at planned events occurring outside the workplace. The researchers concluded that nurse leaders should encourage and promote the development of positive social interactions, as well as develop educational opportunities to enhance interpersonal skills.

Hoyle (2014) explored how nurses providing direct care for the National Health Service of Scotland perceived senior managers who were not nurses. An initiative promoting hands-on management within the organization was the impetus for the study. A single case study design that employed an interpretive approach grounded in adaptive theory was used. Through the use of semi-structured interviews with 31 direct care nurses, the researchers discovered that nurses were often uncertain of the roles and responsibilities of non-nurse managers, and that many of the informants felt the number of managers employed by the agency was unnecessary. Furthermore, informants voiced concerns related to the competency of managers who had no previous clinical experience and who may not understand pressures associated with direct care nursing. These findings underscore the need to understand nurses' perceptions of nonclinical managers in order to identify and resolve conflicts between the two groups, conflicts which could negatively impact patient care.

A final study that addressed professional/workplace issues from a QCSM was conducted by Salami, Nelson, Hawthorne, Muntaner, and McGillis Hall (2014). This study considered the motivations of Filipino nurses who chose to migrate to Canada to work as domestic caregivers. Using a single case study methodology that defined the case as nurses migrating from the Philippines to Canada to participate in the Live-in Caregiver program, the study included a total of 15 informants for their study. Although the researchers noted the importance of multiple data collection methods to address the numerous contextual factors in case study research, it appears that informant interviews were the sole method of data collection. Findings revealed that many informants initially migrated to Middle Eastern countries before reaching their final destination in Canada. Surprisingly, none of the informants cited financial gain as a motivator for moving to Canada, as salaries in the Middle East tended to be higher than those in Canada. The most significant motivators included increased social status associated with living in North America, increased personal freedoms, access to long-term benefits, and the opportunity to permanently relocate family members to Canada. Recommendations reached from the study included policy changes that create adequate premigration education for nurses going abroad, as well as creation of policies that can prevent the deskilling of international nurses by supporting successful integration of these nurses within the health systems of their destinations.

Nursing Education

Issues of nursing education are well represented in studies using QCSM; a total of eight were identified in the literature review and are described here. First, Krumwiede, Van Gelderen, and Krumwiede (2015) employed QCSM to assess the effectiveness of using a Community-Based Collaborative Action Research (CBCAR) framework to enhance learning for students implementing a community health needs assessment as part of a service–learning project. Fifteen nursing students participated in this study, which used student observational field notes, faculty observations, minutes from collaborative meetings, and reflective narratives as the sources of data collection. Results were qualitatively analyzed to evaluate student knowledge and their fidelity to the CBCAR framework. The researchers concluded that students effectively implemented the community needs assessment within the CBCAR framework. Furthermore, students achieved significant learning and skills acquisition in six of eight public health competency domains. These findings support the use of a CBCAR framework to promote student learning in undergraduate community health courses.

QCSM has also been used to explore ethical issues within the context of nursing education. This review identified two such studies. First, Ramos et al. (2013) sought to understand ethical education and content within Brazilian nursing programs through the experiences of nurse educators. The researchers chose a multiple case study approach "because case studies allow exploration, description, and explanation of unique phenomenon or of a set of situations and/or experiences that present a relative empirical unity among themselves, giving value to the real and complex context in which the phenomenon is located an occurs" (Ramos et al., 2013, p. 1125). For this study, six schools from five geographical regions constituted six separate cases. Data were collected using focus groups that included a total of 50 nurse educators. Three categories of factors influencing ethics in nursing education emerged from data analysis. The first category described educator motivation to teach ethical content. The second category centered on local and global changes that demand changes in approaches to ethical discourse. The final category

represented barriers to teaching values and ethics within the nursing education context. The researchers concluded that, rather than focusing strictly on
content and pedagogical approaches, educational ethics in nursing should
facilitate development of a professional identity with a commitment to core
nursing values.

In a second study that focused on ethical issues in nursing education,
Ramos et al. (2015) used QCSM to examine the experiences of Brazilian nursing students facing ethical conflicts during clinical rotations at a primary
care setting. The researchers sought to identify situations in which students
perceived a moral conflict as well as to describe ethical decision-making
processes used by these students. Fifty students participated in the study,
which employed focus groups and a questionnaire to gather information
about the students' experiences. Data analysis revealed that students perceived ethical conflicts in the primary care setting as being primarily related
to workplace processes, confidentiality, and failure to protect patients' rights
to adequate health care. The researchers also found that the decision-making
process that informed a student's choice to intervene in observed ethical conflicts consisted of three phases: realization, reflection, and intervention. The
researchers concluded that clinical education should incorporate aspects of
ethical decision making in the learning environment in order to encourage
the development of a higher level of critical moral reflection within nursing
students.

Another study conducted in Brazil sought to explore the gaps in education and practice of nurses prescribing medications in a primary care setting (Martiniano et al., 2015). As of 2013, advanced practice nurses in Brazil
were granted the ability to prescribe medications, however it is uncertain
how well current curriculum guidelines ensure adequate training in pharmacology for these nurses. To investigate this concern, Martiniano et al.
(2015) employed an exploratory case study design that investigated the phenomenon of medication prescribing by nurses in Brazil using the primary
care setting as the bounding context. In total, 37 nurses participated in the
study, which used focus groups as the data collection method. All informants felt that they had received inadequate education in pharmacology to
allow them to safely prescribe medications. Furthermore, a number of informants voiced the need for postgraduate education, as well as the vital role
of clinical experience. Findings supported the need for curriculum changes
to provide nurses with the education necessary to safely and confidently
prescribe medications.

Pront, Kelton, Munt, and Hutton (2013) used QCSM to identify significant factors influencing student learning in a rural nursing environment in

Australia. The researchers selected a case study approach to provide a holistic view of the myriad determinants of student learning within a specific context. During the study, the researchers recruited two clinical preceptors and five nursing students, all of whom lived within the same rural environment in which they studied or worked. Data were collected via semi-structured interviews with the seven informants. Much like the study by Lea and Cruickshank (2015), which investigated new nurses' transition to rural practice in Australia, the findings from this study revealed that preceptor workload, clinical site staffing, and preceptor skill mix significantly influenced student learning. In particular, inadequate staffing often left students unsupervised during the clinical experience. In addition, the unique situation of living and studying within a small rural community impacts the formation of relationships and can impact learning and the capacity to link theory to practice. The researchers concluded that support for nursing students studying in rural environments is urgently needed.

Exploring the congruency between nurse educators' teaching philosophies and the use of EHRs as a learning strategy was the topic of a qualitative case study by Bani-issa and Rempusheski (2014). Citing the benefits of QCSM to explore phenomena in real-world contexts, the researchers used a collective case study approach that employed open-ended interviews and observational field notes to explore the experiences of seven nurse educators. Two collective case studies emerged that were characterized by contrasting teaching beliefs. The first case study embodied a constructivist belief that was student centered and focused on experiential learning. This case study was associated with enthusiasm toward incorporating EHR learning strategies within the classroom. The second case study was characterized by an objectivist philosophy in which the need to control the learning environment predominated. An objectivist view was associated with resistance to integration of EHR learning strategies within the curriculum. The researchers recommended that strategies be adopted to encourage nurse educators to adopt a constructivist approach to teaching, which would better support innovation in nursing education.

Another study that used a case study approach to examine the impact of teaching philosophy on student learning was conducted by Waterkemper, do Prado, Medina, and Reibnitz (2014). The purpose of the study was to identify how a critical pedagogical approach to teaching fundamentals of professional care course impacted the development of critical attitudes in graduate nursing students. Fourteen students participated in interviews, the results of which were triangulated with nonparticipant observation and document analysis of student portfolios. Thematic analysis revealed three common threads: feeling free, admiring by curiosity, and reflecting about the admired object. The researchers noted that students require learning contexts that provide the freedom to be responsible for their own learning. Such a freedom affords students the opportunity to view themselves as incomplete individuals, a view that supports the development of criticality. Furthermore, educators should provide students the chance to cultivate and exercise their curiosity, which in turn provides impetus for self-directed learning. Finally, by considering concepts from a standpoint of freedom and curiosity, students begin to critically reflect on those concepts. The researchers concluded that critical pedagogy can foster the development of critical attitudes in students, but only if institutions actively construct learning contexts that support such development.

Hegenbarth, Rawe, Murray, Arnaert, and Chambers-Evans (2015) used a multiple case study design to explore the perceptions and beliefs of hospital nurse managers and unit preceptors about nursing student clinical experiences. In doing so, the study aimed to describe unit-level processes and beliefs that impacted clinical learning. Four hospital units were included in the research, with each unit forming a separate case. Two of the units chosen demonstrated consistent acceptance of nursing students, while the other two units were actively trying to improve the student clinical experience. Through semi-structured interviews and focus groups with nurse managers, staff nurses, and advanced nurse practitioners, two major themes emerged. The first theme, influencing factors, related to the unit's conception of what constituted a positive learning environment, as well as to the unit's ability to provide such a context for students. The second theme was characterized as willingness of a unit to invest in the student experience. The researchers recommended that hospitals would benefit from developing a common institutional vision and approach to ensure a positive student learning environment. Such an approach would allow units to successfully manage contextual factors that facilitate student learning.

DISCUSSION

Methodological Considerations

The number of studies identified in the preceding review corroborates assertions that QCSM has become an increasingly popular methodology in nursing inquiry. In considering the above studies, several trends in the literature are evident. First, many of the studies offered similar reasons for choosing QCSM for their research. When an explicit rationale for using QCSM was given, these rationales most commonly included the desire to explore complex phenomena within real-world contexts. Furthermore, many of the researchers also cited the need to gain deep and/or holistic understanding of phenomena as the justification for choosing a case study approach. These rationales align with expert opinions on QCSM application, which view the methodology as a means of studying complex phenomena that cannot be easily removed or separated from the contexts in which they occur (Anthony & Jack, 2009; Baxter & Jack, 2008; Stake, 1995; Yin, 2014).

In addition, the majority of researchers used either Yin's or Stake's theoretical approaches to QCSM to inform their studies, a fact that corroborates Baxter and Jack's (2008) assertion that these two theoretical views predominate in case study research. Of the 50 studies reviewed, 19 cited Yin, nine cited Stake, and seven credited both. The remaining 15 studies offered no explicit discussion of the guiding theoretical framework employed. Considering that different approaches to case study research may exacerbate confusion about the use of case study design, it may be beneficial for researchers new to QCSM to compare and contrast the works of Yin and Stake before delving into case study research. Baxter and Jack (2008) provide such a comparison, which may offer greater clarity with respect to the methods and applications of QCSM.

Turning to issues of data collection, both Yin (2014) and Stake (1995) identify the use of multiple data sources as a defining characteristic of QCSM. As Yin asserts, case study inquiry "relies on multiple sources of evidence, with data needing to converge in a triangulating fashion" (Yin, 2014, p. 17). Thus, the use of multiple data sources is a feature of case study research that contributes to rigor. Indeed, in a study examining methods of enhancing rigor in QCSM in nursing research, Houghton, Casey, Shaw, and Murphy (2013) identified the use of multiple data sources as one of the major ways to ensure rigor in such research. Of the studies previously reviewed in this chapter, only 22 used multiple sources of evidence in their study design. The most common sources of data included interviews, nonparticipant observation, focus groups, and document review. Of the studies that employed a single data collection method, 26 used interviews and two used focus groups. Arguably, those studies that relied on one source of data could have benefited from inclusion of other forms of evidence. Nevertheless, the majority of studies included in this review explicitly or implicitly addressed issues of rigor, a finding that is consistent with Anthony and Jack's (2009) assertion that nurse scholars generally employ rigorous methods when implementing case study research.

Common and Emerging Themes

The studies included in this review represented the breadth of nursing contexts, and included research from a diverse range of international settings, such as Australia, Belgium, Brazil, Canada, Indonesia, the Netherlands, Oman, South Africa, Sweden, Taiwan, the United Kingdom, and the United States. Yet, in spite of this diverse range of international settings, common themes between the studies emerged. First, many of the studies used informant experiences within specific contexts as the case unit for the study. The majority of these studies focused on the experiences of nurses in specific settings or situations, For example, Powell (2013) explored the experiences of night-shift nurses, while Awaisi et al. (2015) focused on the experiences of new graduate nurses practicing in Oman. Studies that explored family member experiences were also well represented, including families' experiences with bedside shift report (Tobiano et al., 2013) and parental experiences with the hospitalization of infants with critical illnesses (De Rouck & Leys, 2014; Johnston, 2014).

Studies that evaluated the implementation of quality and/or workplace improvement initiatives also represented an emerging trend in nursing research using QCSM. For example, Ireland et al. (2013) investigated implementation of a fall-prevention program at three hospitals, while Abrahamson et al. (2015) evaluated a program for pain control in nursing home residents. Within the realm of nursing education, Krumwiede et al. (2015) examined the effectiveness of an educational intervention aimed at enhancing learning within the context of community health nursing. Using QCSM as evaluative research is a creative use of the methodology that may offer a more holistic appraisal of quality improvement initiatives.

A third emerging trend in QCSM identified by this review was the exploration of interprofessional dynamics and issues of collegiality and collaboration. Several studies investigated how nurses construct and maintain professional and social relationships in the workplace, as well as examined factors that facilitated these relationships. For example, Moore et al. (2015) explored collaboration among oncology nurses, while Maxwell et al. (2013) investigated the construction of social identity among new specialty nurses. Powell (2013) also examined professional relationships, this time within the context of nurses working night shift.

A final trend that emerged from this review was the use of QCSM to investigate new nurses transitioning to professional practice. Four studies were identified that explored transition to practice issues in several settings, including rural nursing, acute care nursing, and nursing within the Sultanate of Oman (Awaisi et al. 2015; Lea & Cruickshank, 2015; Stacey et al. 2015; Whitehead et al. 2015). Given the complexity of factors that influence new nurses' adjustment to professional nursing, QCSM appears to be a logical choice for studies investigating this multifaceted phenomenon.

SUMMARY

Clearly, QCSM has gained significant popularity within the realm of nursing inquiry, a fact that is not surprising given the increasingly complex nature of contemporary nursing situations. Through QCSM, nurse scholars can conduct in-depth, comprehensive, and holistic studies that explore nursing issues across the breadth of care settings and nursing contexts. Given the advantages the QCSM for specific types of inquiry, it is important that nurse scholars gain an understanding of the uses and benefits of this scholarly approach. Furthermore, because of the increased presence of QCSM in nursing literature, scholars must be able to critically appraise evidence generated by case study research.

REFERENCES

Abbott, A. A., Fuji, K. T., & Galt, K. A. (2015). A qualitative case study exploring nurse engagement with electronic health records and E-Prescribing. *Western Journal of Nursing Research, 37*(7), 935–951.

Abrahamson, K., DeCrane, S., Mueller, C., Davila, H. W., & Arling, G. (2015). Implementation of a nursing home quality improvement project to reduce resident pain: a qualitative case study. *Journal of Nursing Care Quality, 30*(3), 261–268.

Adams, J. A., Bailey, D. E., Anderson, R. A., & Thygeson, M. (2013). Finding your way through EOL challenges in the ICU using Adaptive Leadership behaviours: A qualitative descriptive case study. *Intensive & Critical Care Nursing: The Official Journal of the British Association of Critical Care Nurses, 29*(6), 329–336.

Al Awaisi, H., Cooke, H., & Pryjmachuk, S. (2015). The experiences of newly graduated nurses during their first year of practice in the Sultanate of Oman—A case study. *International Journal of Nursing Studies, 52*(11), 1723–1734.

Anthony, S., & Jack, S. (2009). Qualitative case study methodology in nursing research: An integrative review. *Journal of Advanced Nursing, 65*(6), 1171–1181.

Bailey, D. E., Docherty, S. L., Adams, J. A., Carthron, D. L., Corazzini, K., Day, J. R.,...Anderson, R. A. (2012). Studying the clinical encounter with the Adaptive Leadership framework. *Journal of Healthcare Leadership, 2012*(4), 83–91.

Bani-issa, W., & Rempusheski, V. F. (2014). Congruency between educators' teaching beliefs and an electronic health record teaching strategy. *Nurse Education Today, 34*(6), 906–911.

Baxter, P., & Jack, S. (2008). Qualitative case study methodology: Study design and implementation for novice researchers. *The Qualitative Report, 13*(4), 544–559.

Chan, Z. C. (2009). In response to: Anthony, S. & Jack, S. (2009). Qualitative case study methodology in nursing research: An integrative review. *Journal of Advanced Nursing, 65*(8), 1774.

Chang, S. M., Rowe, J., & Goopy, S. (2014). Non-family support for breastfeeding maintenance among career women in Taiwan: A qualitative study. *International Journal of Nursing Practice, 20*(3), 293–301.

de Jong, G., Schout, G., & Abma, T. (2014). Prevention of involuntary admission through Family Group Conferencing: A qualitative case study in community mental health nursing. *Journal of Advanced Nursing, 70*(11), 2651–2662.

De Rouck, S., & Leys, M. (2013). Illness trajectory and Internet as a health information and communication channel used by parents of infants admitted to a neonatal intensive care unit. *Journal of Advanced Nursing, 69*(7), 1489–1499.

Dionne-Odom, J. N., Willis, D. G., Bakitas, M., Crandall, B., & Grace, P. J. (2015). Conceptualizing surrogate decision making at end of life in the intensive care unit using cognitive task analysis. *Nursing Outlook, 63*(3), 331–340.

Droskinis, A. (2013). A case study exploring the current issues faced by diploma-prepared nurses. *Journal for Nurses in Professional Development, 29*(1), 30–34.

Fleiszer, A. R., Semenic, S. E., Ritchie, J. A., Richer, M., & Denis, J. (2015). Nursing unit leaders' influence on the long-term sustainability of evidence-based practice improvements. *Journal of Nursing Management, 15*(1), 535. doi:10.1111/jonm.12320

Foucault, M. (1979). *Discipline and punish: The birth of the prison.* New York, NY: Vintage.

Hegenbarth, M., Rawe, S., Murray, L., Arnaert, A., & Chambers-Evans, J. (2015). Establishing and maintaining the clinical learning environment for nursing students: A qualitative study. *Nurse Education Today, 35*(2), 304–309.

Houghton, C., Casey, D., Shaw, D., & Murphy, K. (2013). Rigour in qualitative case-study research. *Nurse Researcher, 20*(4), 12–17.

Hoyle, L. (2014). Nurses' perception of senior managers at the front line: People working with clipboards. *Journal of Advanced Nursing, 70*(11), 2528–2538.

Hoyle, L., & Grant, A. (2015). Treatment targets in emergency departments: Nurses' views of how they affect clinical practice. *Journal of Clinical Nursing, 24*(15–16), 2211–2218.

Ireland, S., Kirkpatrick, H., Boblin, S., & Robertson, K. (2013). The real world journey of implementing fall prevention best practices in three acute care hospitals: A case study. *Worldviews on Evidence-Based Nursing/Sigma Theta Tau International, Honor Society of Nursing, 10*(2), 95–103.

Johnston, D. A. (2014). Releasing the flood: A qualitative case study of one high-risk father's journey through the labor unit and neonatal intensive care unit. *The Journal of Perinatal & Neonatal Nursing, 28*(4), 319–331.

Koplow, S. M., Gallo, A. M., Knafl, K. A., Vincent, C., Paun, O., & Gruss, V. (2015). A case study approach to nursing home placement: Smooth and difficult cases and implications for nursing. *Journal of Gerontological Nursing, 41*(7), 58–64.

Krumwiede, K. A., Van Gelderen, S. A., & Krumwiede, N. K. (2015). Academic-hospital partnership: Conducting a community health needs assessment as a service learning project. *Public Health Nursing (Boston, Mass.), 32*(4), 359–367.

Lea, J., & Cruickshank, M. (2015). The support needs of new graduate nurses making the transition to rural nursing practice in Australia. *Journal of Clinical Nursing, 24*(7–8), 948–960.

Lewin, K. (1951). *Fields theory in social science: Selected theoretical papers.* New York, NY: Harper & Row.

Lines, L. E., Mannix, T., & Giles, T. M. (2015). Nurses' experiences of the hospitalisation of their own children for acute illnesses. *Contemporary Nurse, 50*(2–3), 274–285.

Mamier, I., & Winslow, B. W. (2014). Divergent views of placement decision-making: A qualitative case study. *Issues in Mental Health Nursing, 35*(1), 13–20.

Martiniano, S. C., de Castro Marcolino, E., Barros de Souza, M., Alves Coelho, A., Arcêncio, R. A., Fronteira, I., & da Costa Uchôa, S. A. (2015). The gap between training and practice of prescribing of drugs by nurses in the primary health care: A case study in Brazil. *Nurse Education Today, 36*, 304–309. doi:10.1016/j.nedt.2015.07.017

Maxwell, E., Baillie, L., Rickard, W., & McLaren, S. M. (2013). Exploring the relationship between social identity and workplace jurisdiction for new nursing roles: a case study approach. *International Journal of Nursing Studies, 50*(5), 622–631.

McKenna, B., Furness, T., Dhital, D., Park, M., & Connally, F. (2014). Recovery-oriented care in a secure mental health setting: "Striving for a good life". *Journal of Forensic Nursing, 10*(2), 63–69.

McKeown, M., Ridley, J., Newbigging, K., Machin, K., Poursanidou, K., & Cruse, K. (2014). Conflict of roles: A conflict of ideas? The unsettled relations between care team staff and independent mental health advocates. *International Journal of Mental Health Nursing, 23*(5), 398–408.

Mizutani, M., Tashiro, J., Maftuhah,, Sugiarto, H., Yulaikhah, L., & Carbun, R. (2015). Model development of healthy-lifestyle behaviors for rural Muslim Indonesians with hypertension: A qualitative study. *Nursing & Health Sciences, 18*(1), 15–22. doi:10.1111/nhs.12212

Moore, J., Prentice, D., & McQuestion, M. (2015). Social interaction and collaboration among oncology nurses. *Nursing Research & Practice, 201*, 51–57.

Morris, M. (2014). Diagnosis in young children: How a father's perceptions of mental health change. *Journal of Child and Adolescent Psychiatric Nursing: Official Publication of the Association of Child and Adolescent Psychiatric Nurses, Inc, 27*(2), 52–60.

Nesbitt, J. (2013). Journal clubs: A two-site case study of nurses' continuing professional development. *Nurse Education Today, 33*(8), 896–900.

Popejoy, L. L., Dorman Marek, K., & Scott-Cawiezell, J. (2013). Patterns and problems associated with transitions after hip fracture in older adults. *Journal of Gerontological Nursing, 39*(9), 43–52.

Powell, I. (2013). Can you see me? Experiences of nurses working night shift in Australian regional hospitals: A qualitative case study. *Journal of Advanced Nursing, 69*(10), 2172–2184.

Procter, S., Wilson, P. M., Brooks, F., & Kendall, S. (2013). Success and failure in integrated models of nursing for long term conditions: Multiple case studies of whole systems. *International Journal of Nursing Studies, 50*(5), 632–643.

Pront, L., Kelton, M., Munt, R., & Hutton, A. (2013). Living and learning in a rural environment: A nursing student perspective. *Nurse Education Today, 33*(3), 281–285.

Ramos, F. S., Brehmer, L. F., Vargas, M. A., Trombetta, A. P., Silveira, L. R., & Drago, L. (2015). Ethical conflicts and the process of reflection in undergraduate nursing students in Brazil. *Nursing Ethics, 22*(4), 428–439.

Ramos, F. S., de Pires, D. P., Brehmer, L. F., Gelbcke, F. L., Schmoeller, S. D., & Lorenzetti, J. (2013). The discourse of ethics in nursing education: Experience and reflections of Brazilian teachers—Case study. *Nurse Education Today, 33*(10), 1124–1129.

Rose, P., & Yates, P. (2013). Person centered nursing care in radiation oncology: A case study. *European Journal of Oncology Nursing: The Official Journal of European Oncology Nursing Society, 17*(5), 554–562.

Rudolfsson, G. (2014). Being altered by the unexpected: understanding the perioperative patient's experience: A case study. *International Journal of Nursing Practice, 20*(4), 433–437.

Salami, B., Nelson, S., Hawthorne, L., Muntaner, C., & McGillis Hall, L. (2014). Motivations of nurses who migrate to Canada as domestic workers. *International Nursing Review, 61*(4), 479–486.

Sandy, P. T., Kgole, J. C., & Mavundla, T. R. (2013). Support needs of caregivers: Case studies in South Africa. *International Nursing Review, 60*(3), 344–350.

Sercu, C., Ayala, R. A., & Bracke, P. (2015). How does stigma influence mental health nursing identities? An ethnographic study of the meaning of stigma for nursing role identities in two Belgian psychiatric hospitals. *International Journal of Nursing Studies, 52*(1), 307–316.

Stacey, G., Pollock, K., & Crawford, P. (2015). A case study exploring the experience of graduate entry nursing students when learning in practice. *Journal of Advanced Nursing, 71*(9), 2084–2095.

Stake, R. E. (1995). *The art of case study research.* Thousand Oaks, CA: SAGE Publications.

Stetler, C. B., Ritchie, J. A., Rycroft-Malone, J., & Charns, M. P. (2014). Leadership for evidence-based practice: Strategic and functional behaviors for institutionalizing EBP. *Worldviews on Evidence-Based Nursing / Sigma Theta Tau International, Honor Society of Nursing, 11*(4), 219–226.

Tayab, A., & Narushima, M. (2015). "Here for the residents": A case study of cultural competence of personal support workers in a long-term care home. *Journal of Transcultural Nursing: Official Journal of the Transcultural Nursing Society / Transcultural Nursing Society, 26*(2), 146–156.

Thygeson, M., Morrissey, L., & Ulstad, V. (2010). Adaptive leadership and the practice of medicine: A complexity-based approach to reframing the doctor–patient relationship. *Journal of Evaluation in Clinical Practice, 16*(5), 1009–1015.

Tobiano, G., Chaboyer, W., & McMurray, A. (2013). Family members' perceptions of the nursing bedside handover. *Journal of Clinical Nursing, 22*(1–2), 192–200.

Velloso, I., Ceci, C., & Alves, M. (2013). Configurations of power relations in the Brazilian emergency care system: Analyzing a context of visible practices. *Nursing Inquiry, 20*(3), 256–264.

Waterkemper, R., do Prado, M. L., Medina, J. L., & Reibnitz, K. S. (2014). Development of critical attitude in fundamentals of professional care discipline: A case study. *Nurse Education Today, 34*(4), 581–585.

Whiffin, C. J., Bailey, C., Ellis-Hill, C., Jarrett, N., & Hutchinson, P. J. (2015). Narratives of family transition during the first year post-head injury: Perspectives of the non-injured members. *Journal of Advanced Nursing, 71*(4), 849–859.

White, C., Pesut, B., & Rush, K. L. (2014). Intensive care unit patients in the postanesthesia care unit: A case study exploring nurses' experiences. *Journal of Perianesthesia Nursing: Official Journal of the American Society of Perianesthesia Nurses / American Society of Perianesthesia Nurses, 29*(2), 129–137.

Whitehead, B., Owen, P., Henshaw, L., Beddingham, E., & Simmons, M. (2015). Supporting newly qualified nurse transition: A case study in a UK hospital. *Nurse Education Today, 36*, 58–63.

Yin, R. K. (2014). *Case study research: Designs and methods.* (5th ed.). Thousand Oaks, CA: SAGE.

Zapka, J., Amella, E., Magwood, G., Madisetti, M., Garrow, D., & Batchelor-Aselage, M. (2014). Challenges in efficacy research: The case of feeding alternatives in patients with dementia. *Journal of Advanced Nursing, 70*(9), 2072–2085.

CHAPTER THREE

PROPOSAL FOR CASE STUDY OF OBSTETRIC FISTULA

Mary de Chesnay, Jessica Ellis, and Tracey Couse

*I*n a sense, case studies are the most elemental form of qualitative research in that they provide an in-depth analysis of one or more cases—individuals who represent a phenomenon of interest. Case studies have a long tradition in medicine and nursing having developed from practitioners sharing information about the presentation of illness in a patient, the progression of the disease, and successful and unsuccessful treatment outcomes. Case studies might involve one or more cases and researchers use a variety of methods to address the research question. Methods include interviews, physiological measurements, psychological tests, and analysis of the patients' diaries or journals.

The following proposal is an example of how one might design a study and how one presents such a study to an institutional review board (IRB). For this example, a fictional woman is described because we do not have access to a real patient, but wanted to bring the problem of obstetric fistula to the attention of the nursing community.

PURPOSE

The purpose of the proposed case study is to document the progression of obstetric fistula in a pregnant early adolescent who was married at the age of 8 years to a 30-year-old man from South Sudan. An obstetric fistula is a tearing of the vaginal or rectal wall that adjoins the urethra, resulting in leakage of urine and/or feces. The hole is always in the vaginal wall and may join either the rectum or the bladder leaking either urine or feces. Fistulas are of high risk in early adolescents in whom the pelvis is not developed enough to carry a child to birth a full-term infant. Prolonged labor results in excessive stress in the pelvis and perineum and can result in fistula. The prevalence of child brides in many cultures results in early childbirth soon after menarche and fistula related to pelvic underdevelopment with long, unsuccessful labor. The result is often a stillborn infant with subsequent tearing of the mother's urethra. Included in this case study are the sociocultural and medical history of a child bride, how she became pregnant, progression of the pregnancy, how she was delivered, how the fistula was treated, and social and psychological impact on the child and family.

REVIEW OF LITERATURE

Qualitative research focusing on patient perspectives of obstetric fistulas appears to have increased over the past few years. Much of the research has been performed in Africa where there is a high incidence of obstetric fistulae. One retrospective observational study describes the factors leading up to fistula development and fistula treatment based on survey data obtained at a hospital in Goma of the Democratic Republic of Congo (Benfield, Young-Lin, Kimona, Kalisya, & Kisindja, 2015).

Researchers have used structured interviews of hospitalized women in Tanguieta, Benin, to explore the nature of obstetric fistulae, specifically cause, care obstacles, prevention, and reintegration (Nathan, Rochat, Grigorescu, & Banks, 2009). A different qualitative study performed in five fistula repair hospitals in Niger and Mali used obstetric fistula patient real-life experiences of hospital care to assess how the women's views impacted care uptake and coping (Maulet, Berthe, Traore, & Macq, 2015).

Lived-experience qualitative research has been used to explore obstetric fistula experiences of African women in Ghana and Malawi (Mwini-Nyaledzigbor, Agana, & Pilkington, 2013; Yeakey, Chipeta, Taulo, & Tsui, 2009). One study concluded on a number of obstetric fistula-contributing themes and the other study explored how the obstetric fistula experience affected the victims and their families (Mwini-Nyaledzigbor et al., 2013; Yeakey et al., 2009). Qualitative studies have used surveys to explore both positive and negative religious coping strategies of women who have suffered obstetric fistulae (Watt et al., 2014).

Community awareness regarding risk factors, presentation, and prevention of obstetric fistulae has been studied through the use of focus groups of both males and females (Kasamba, Kaye, & Mbalinda, 2013). A couple of recent qualitative studies have looked at quality of life of women before and after obstetric fistula repair (Imoto, Matsuyama, Ambauen-Berger, & Honda,

2015; Singh, Jhanwar, Mehrotra, Paul, & Sinha, 2015). Mixed-method studies have been used to explore the birthing experiences of women with obstetric fistulae and the barriers faced to access quality care during labor and delivery (Mselle, Kohi, Mvungi, Evjen-Olsen, & Moland, 2011).

Finally, insight into the challenges faced by women who underwent surgical repair of their obstetric fistula, the long-term effects of women from multiple dimensions of postsurgical repair, and documentation of women's health needs was accomplished through interviews and small focus groups in West Pokot, Kenya (Khisa & Nyamongo, 2012).

Although on the rise, qualitative studies focusing on obstetric fistula patient values, perspectives, and experiences as well as patient perspectives on reintegration needs remain scarce (Lombard, St. Jorre, Geddes, El Ayadi, & Grant, 2015). Also, there are few, if any, studies specifically looking at child brides and their unique perspectives. Much of the published quantitative demographic data describes age of patients, but qualitative studies of personal perspectives for this age group remain absent. The proposed case study adds to these research gaps by providing in-depth information from a person who has suffered fistula due to early adolescent pregnancy. Additionally, the proposed study offers a sense of relief and consolation for the numerous others who have suffered this isolating and devastating condition.

METHODOLOGY

Design

The design is case study research. Semi-structured interviews will be conducted with the participant, any of her family who agree to be interviewed, the surgeon who performed the fistula repair, and the health care workers who attended to her after the surgery. As the husband abandoned her, we will not attempt to interview him. With her permission, we will examine her medical records and the journal she kept during her treatment at the Fistula Clinic. If any family members accompany her, we will invite them to participate as well.

Sample

Onnab (pseudonym) is a 19-year-old Sudanese woman who was married as a child at 8 years, subjected to sexual intercourse by her husband before puberty, became pregnant at the age of 14 years, delivered a stillborn, and then suffered a vaginal fistula that resulted in abandonment by her husband after a surgery attempt to repair it failed. Raised in a village in South Sudan, she made her way home to her family of origin after her husband left and after a second surgical procedure failed to correct the fistula. However, the leakage of urine was constant and foul smelling, and her family required her to live apart from them in a small hut they built for her on the edge of the village. She was highly embarrassed and ashamed and soon became depressed. She returned to the fistula clinic and is currently recovering from a third surgery, which was successful. She was referred to the study by the American surgeon who attempted the first repair.

Setting

The interviews will take place in the fistula clinic where Onnab resides temporarily and where the staff are accessible. If any family members are nearby, they will be interviewed as well with Onnab's permission. The area in which Onnab lives is located in South Sudan.

There are reportedly 2.8 doctors for every 10,000 people in South Sudan (Fistula Foundation, 2015). For the 35 million Sudanese, there are 33 hospitals with only 16% of all health care facilities powered by electricity (Alder, Fox, Campbell, & Kuper, 2013). South Sudan has one of the world's highest maternal mortality rates and has an estimated 60,000 women who suffer from obstetric fistulae (Jacques, 2014; Modi Igga, 2015). It is unfortunate that there are limited fistula repair services in South Sudan to support the needs of these women (Alder et al., 2013). This is in part due a poor health care infrastructure, including political instability, lack of resources, and a scarcity of trained surgeons and support staff (Jacques, 2014).

The existing fistula clinics are sparse. The Dr. Abbo Khartoum Teaching Hospital Fistula Center in Khartoum is one of the longest running fistula programs in Africa, but the number of treated women is limited due to the poor health care infrastructure (Fistula Foundation, 2015; WAHA, 2011). A small fistula care team at Kassala Hospital provides limited routine services to obstetric fistula patients (Fistula Foundation, 2015). Nyala Hospital has a small ward, but it provides limited services due to a lack of resources (Fistula Foundation, 2015). Many of the described clinics are supported by grants from various organizations (Alder et al., 2013; Fistula Foundation, 2015). These agencies also fund fistula reparative clinics periodically in attempts to service these patients (Fistula Foundation, 2015; Jacques, 2014; Modi Igga, 2015). Between 2006 and 2011, eight campaigns were held, which resulted in fistula repairs for an estimated 150 women (Alder et al., 2013). Awareness and support are slowly improving. In 2012, more than 200 surgeries were performed at two of the fistula-supporting hospitals in South Sudan (Fistula Foundation, 2014).

Instruments

As in any ethnographic type of research, the primary instrument is the researcher and her or his skill at eliciting the story. Due to the sensitive nature of the data and need to protect the participant's privacy, tape recorders will not be used, but extensive field notes will be taken by the American interviewers, a nurse-anthropologist experienced in cross-cultural fieldwork and a nurse-midwife. Interviews will be conducted in English with the English-speaking staff, and a bilingual Sudanese woman referred by the staff will be hired as an interpreter for interviews with the participant and her family. The interviewer will be trained in techniques of research interviewing as well as confidentiality. Criteria for selection of the interpreter include the following: older than 18 years, not a family member of Onnab, experience interpreting for medical situations, and fluency in English and Onnab's dialect. The interpreter will sign a confidentiality agreement. Participant observation at the clinic will complete the data collection methods.

The semi-structured interview guides for the patient, health care staff, and family members are found in Tables 3.1, 3.2, and 3.3; however, it should be noted that this kind of research often digresses from the planned

Table 3.1 *Semi-Structured Interview Guide for Patients*

Tell me how you got this terrible condition.
How did/does it make you feel?
Where did you go to seek help?
How did your family learn of your condition?
What was their response?
How have you coped with everything?
Is your life better after surgery?
What are your plans for the future?

Table 3.2 *Semi-Structured Interview Guide for Staff*

How/why did you get involved in this specialty?

How did you come to know the patient?

What condition was she in when you met her?

Were you able to medically help her?

What was her biggest need next to medical treatment?

What do you see as your biggest role in helping this patient? Other similar patients?

What resources do the patients need?

What resources does the clinic need to improve outcomes for the patient and baby?

Table 3.3 *Semi-Structured Interview Guide for Family Members*

How did you learn about your daughter's condition?

Had you ever heard of this condition before your daughter?

How did her condition make you feel?

What do you think caused this for your daughter?

interviews as the participants have their own way of telling their stories and it is critical to respect their ownership of the interview.

Procedures

Once IRB approval is received, the plan for the study is to enter the field by introducing ourselves to the hospital directors and staff, recruit Onnab as the person whose story will be told, hire the interpreter, collect and analyze data, and terminate from the field. On arriving home in the United States, the study will be closed with the IRB, and manuscripts will be prepared.

Data Analysis

Content analysis with elaboration of themes is the method of data analysis. Raw data will be analyzed for key concepts and subconcepts, a typology will be constructed, and a narrative analysis of the woman's story will be the outcome (Table 3.4). The timeline provides an estimate of completion of expected activities for the study.

Table 3.4 *Timeline*

Task/Person Responsible	Month											
	1	2	3	4	5	6	7	8	9	10	11	12
Submit IRB protocol/MdC	X											
Make travel arrangements/MdC		X										
Prepare materials for interviews	X	X										
IRB approval (assume 2 months)			X									
Travel to Sudan and settle in city of fistula clinic				X								
Introductory visit to fistula clinic				X								
Recruit and train interpreter				X	X							
Conduct first interview with participant					X							
Conduct staff interviews					X	X	X	X				
Conduct more interviews with participant							X					
Travel to village for interviews with family							X	X				
Analyze interview and participant observation data						X	X	X	X	X	X	
Conduct follow-up interviews via e-mail to clinic staff											X	
Return to the United States										X		
Write final report										X	X	
Submit for publication/presentation												X

IRB, institutional review board.

49

SUMMARY

This chapter was presented as a sample IRB protocol to demonstrate some of the issues in case study research with a child bride who experienced fistula. Although many readers of the book will never encounter obstetric fistula, it is important for nurses to understand that this is an extensive problem among many women in developing countries and one of the best ways to educate ourselves is to the hear the stories of women who have endured. Case study research is a viable method for accomplishing this objective.

REFERENCES

Alder, A., Fox, S., Campbell, O., & Kuper, H. (2013). Obstetric fistula in Southern Sudan: Situational analysis and key informant method to estimate prevalence. *BMC Pregnancy and Childbirth, 13,* 64.

Benfield, N., Young-Lin, N., Kimona, C., Kalisya, L. M., & Kisindja, R. M. (2015). Clinical article: Fistula after attended delivery and the challenge of obstetric care capacity in the eastern Democratic Republic of Congo. *International Journal of Gynecology and Obstetrics, 130*(2),157–160.

Fistula Foundation. (2015). *Sudan.* Retrieved from https://www.fistulafoundation.org/countries-we-help/sudan

Imoto, A., Matsuyama, A., Ambauen-Berger, B., & Honda, S. (2015). Clinical article: Health-related quality of life among women in rural Bangladesh after surgical repair of obstetric fistula. *International Journal of Gynecology and Obstetrics, 130*(1),79–83.

Jacques, J. (2014). *Fistula campaign in South Sudan seeks lasting solutions.* Retrieved from http://www.unfpa.org/news/fistula-campaign-south-sudan-seeks-lasting-solutions

Kasamba, N., Kaye, D., & Mbalinda, S. (2013). Community awareness about risk factors, presentation and prevention and obstetric fistula in Nabitovu village, Iganga district, Uganda. *BMC Pregnancy & Childbirth, 13*(1), 1–19.

Khisa, A., & Nyamongo, I. (2012). Still living with fistula: An exploratory study of the experience of women with obstetric fistula following corrective surgery in West Pokot, Kenya. *Reproductive Health Matters, 20*(40), 59–66.

Lombard, L., St. Jorre, J., Geddes, R., El Ayadi, A., & Grant, L. (2015). Rehabilitation experiences after obstetric fistula repair: Systematic review of qualitative studies. *Tropical Medicine & International Health, 20*(5), 554–568.

Maulet, N., Berthe, A., Traore, S., & Macq, J. (2015). Obstetric fistula "disease" and ensuing care: Patients' views in West-Africa. *African Journal of Reproductive Health, 19*(1), 112–123.

Mselle, L. T., Kohi, T. W., Mvungi, A., Evjen-Olsen, B., & Moland, K. M. (2011). Waiting for attention and care: Birthing accounts of women in rural Tanzania who developed obstetric fistula as an outcome of labour. *BMC Pregnancy and Child-birth, 11*(75). Retrieved from http://dx.doi.org/10.1186%2F1471-2393-11-75. doi:10.1186/1471-2393-11-75

Modi Igga, L. (2015, March 19). *Fistula in South Sudan, the ghastly women tale.* Retrieved from http://www.atlascorps.org/blog/?p=7483

Mwini-Nyaledzigbor, P., Agana, A., & Pilkington, F. (2013). Lived experiences of Ghanaian women with obstetric fistula. *Health Care for Women International, 34*(6), 440–460.

Nathan, L., Rochat, C., Grigorescu, B., & Banks, E. (2009). Obstetric fistulae in West Africa: Patient perspectives. *American Journal of Obstetrics & Gynecology, 200*(5), e40–2.

Singh, V., Jhanwar, A., Mehrotra, S., Paul, S., & Sinha, R. J. (2015). A comparison of quality of life before and after successful repair of genitourinary fistula: Is there improvement across all the domains of WHOQOL-BREF questionnaire? *African Journal of Urology.* doi:10.1016/j.afju.2015.06.003

WAHA. (2011). *Sudan: 86 women with obstetric fistula treated in Dr. Abbo's National Fistula & Urogynaecology Centre.* Retrieved from http://www.waha-international.org/?what-we-do=1364&sudan-86-women-with-obstetric-fistula-treated-in-dr.-abbos-national-fistula-urogynaecology-centre

Watt, M., Wilson, S., Joseph, M., Masenga, G., MacFarlane, J., Oneko, O., & Sikkema, K. (2014). Religious coping among women with obstetric fistula in Tanzania. *Global Public Health, 9*(5), 516–527.

Yeakey, M. P., Chipeta, E., Taulo, F., & Tsui, A. O. (2009). The lived experience of Malawian women with obstetric fistula. *Culture, Health & Sexuality, 11*(5), 499–513.

APPENDIX 3.1 CONSENT FORM

It should be noted that sometimes people from developing countries may be reluctant to sign their names on any document not approved by their tribal elders, even if they are literate. The customary way to accomplish informed consent then is to read the consent, allow time for explanations and responses to concerns, and then to audiotape verbal consent even if the interview will not be taped. Alternatively, a witness can sign that the consent was given. The following serves as a typical format from an American IRB and is only an example.

[University letterhead]

Title: Obstetric Fistula: A Case Study of a Child Bride
Principal Investigator: [name and contact information]

Introduction:

Obstetric fistula (tearing of the internal organs after childbirth) is a common occurrence among new mothers who give birth in their early teenage years because their bodies are not developed fully and labor tends to be long and hard. We are nurses who work with these women and we need to know more about their experiences in order to give them the best care. We ask your help by agreeing to be interviewed for our study about what it is like to have a fistula.

Procedures:

If you agree to participate, we would ask you to share your story and give us permission to talk with the doctors and nurses at the fistula clinic where you had your surgery. Although we will not tape record the meetings, we will take extensive notes in order to accurately present what you tell us. If you are not comfortable speaking in English, we will hire a local interpreter, whom we will train.

Time Required:

There might be several interviews with you and they would last about an hour each. Then we will talk to others for about ½ hour each and the total number will be however many you give us permission to talk with.

Risks/Discomforts:

Some people we have interviewed about similar topics are somewhat embarrassed at telling their stories but as nurses we do not judge, we simply listen.

If at any time you feel too uncomfortable to continue or wish to stop the interview for any reason, we will respect your decision and withdraw you from the study without penalty.

Benefits:

Even though there are no direct benefits to you, many people we have interviewed for similar problems find it useful to confide in listeners who understand their situation and they express relief at knowing that sharing the story of their suffering will help others.

Compensation:

We will provide a small food basket for you.

Confidentiality:

We respect your privacy and will only identify you by a name other than your own that you can choose. We will keep all the materials for the study in a locked file cabinet at the office and disguise any information that could identify you when we publish the study.

Inclusion Criteria:

- Age 18 or older
- Child bride with resulting early childbirth and obstetric fistula
- Single participant from South Sudan

Withdrawal:
You may withdraw from the study at any time without penalty. You will receive the food basket even if you withdraw.

_____   _____

Signature of participant   Date

_____   _____

Signature of PI   Date

PLEASE SIGN BOTH COPIES OF THIS FORM, KEEP ONE AND RETURN THE OTHER TO THE INVESTIGATOR
Research at [xxxxxx] University that involves human participants is carried out under the oversight of an Institutional Review Board. Questions or problems regarding these activities should be addressed to the Institutional Review Board, [name, address, phone]

CHAPTER FOUR

CASE STUDY RESEARCH: A METHODOLOGY FOR NURSING

Camille Cronin

This chapter presents a personal perspective on using case study research for both novice and prospective nurse researchers. My doctoral thesis, *Workplace Learning—An Examination of Learning Landscapes* (Cronin, 2012) provides a reference point and an example of case study research (CSR). This chapter, after describing the study briefly, focuses on the underlying philosophy, definitions, and justifications for using CSR and why I chose this method. The opportunity to reflect on my work, postdoctoral, is a pleasure and will provide others with insight into a valuable methodology for researching complex health care issues.

A CASE STUDY

For my doctoral research I chose to examine five students' experiences of 15 health care placements as part of a health care program. As learning environments, these workplaces were explored through observations, interviews, and documents. This study reports on real-life context, which were examined over a 2-year period. This presented rich empirical data offering a pragmatic framework for investigating learning in the workplace.

From carrying out this research, I presented a number of findings, which offered a useful framework to review the complexities that exist within the health care learning environment, how they interact with each other, and the possible impact they may have on learning in the workplace. This piece of work also highlighted the relationship the learner has with the learning environment and learning over time. The work examined the type of individual; their self-awareness; and their level of willingness to learn, which is seen as equally important in the learning environment. I concluded some very suggestive but realistic findings from this study proposing that the learning environment is unpredictable and that learning experiences are random.

Through CSR, qualitative research methods were embraced in a rigorous and systematic manner. Each step of the research protocol was addressed. CSR can be both qualitative and rigorous. This study provided an example of a rigorous qualitative design in which CSR has been used to its full potential. The implications for nursing practice and for research in nursing are that real-life settings can be studied in a systematic and rigorous way and is certainly transferrable to other settings.

A PHILOSOPHY OF PRACTICE

I consider myself to be a learner at all times. There is always something more to discover, which is why life is so exciting and where my source of motivation lies. My interest in teaching has taken me through various paths and has always been a part of my role with colleagues, students, and patients. As a nurse, researcher, or manager, teaching and learning are essential prerequisites for these roles. My doctoral research is the culmination of various walks of my working life in nursing: practice, research, management, and education. With a number of experiences, this augmented the genesis of my work. A number of workplace visits and observations started to seam together. Although on a placement visit, I was observing a student and asked myself: Does this workplace affect practice? If so, how does this affect the students' learning? How does each work environment affect the student? What about the other students and the other placements? How do these placements help students in their pathway toward becoming a nursing professional? How many students actually make it? Does this then have an impact on nursing recruitment? What about the other health care professions? Do these learners feel adequately prepared? So, this led to my decision to examine learning in the workplace focusing on health care settings.

WHY CSR?

Once it became clear what I was going to research, choosing CSR became straightforward (but getting to this point can take some time). It suited the practical nature of this study (and me which is actually very important to find a design that fits one's own values and methods) and fitted very well with the variety of health care settings under investigation. CSR provides a practical and systematic way of collecting data in the naturalistic setting. This was very much a key issue as I wanted to be in each place of work collecting data. CSR assumes predetermined experience and knowledge and thus the literature review became a significant chapter in my thesis. Here, I could unload all my preconceptions and assimilate all I know from previous studies, practice, and pedagogy.

The focus of this research study was to conduct an exploration of learning in health care workplaces. The research question was: How do students engage in learning in real-life settings? I ensured a number of objectives were set for data to be collected comprehensively, but in different ways:

- To observe and report the learning context where every day face-to-face interactions of students take place in health care settings (hospitals, nursing homes, nurseries)
- To examine critical learning incidents
- To understand the different experiences and learning in the workplace

Choosing the right research methodology is obviously very important for a dedicated piece of work over a number of years. Although attention is paid to what the research question is asking, one must ensure that both question and method will keep your interest sustained. This was very important to me, so I devoted a great amount of time deciding which philosophical and ethical approach to take. Fundamentally, the research question needed to be answered in the best possible way in order to understand and develop knowledge in this area.

Personal philosophical beliefs were examined and how this world is constructed (a huge undertaking at the beginning of my thesis and I really did not know what it meant). But fundamentally I kept asking myself how students learn and engage in the workplace. However, the health care arena is complex; everyone is different and our expectations of each place differ. Are there patterns to learning or is it that we are individual and different? How does learning come together in this busy environment? Is it packaged differently to classroom learning? The workplace can be very different and yet in practice there is heavy reliance on this environment for learning. In practice-based disciplines, such as nursing, the importance of learning in the workplace provides up to half of the educational experience for students undertaking preregistration nurse education programs (Warne et al., 2010).

Although objective knowledge can be gained from direct experience, what are we to learn in a health care environment–only facts? The purpose of science is to help people understand the world and their surroundings satisfying the natural curiosity of human beings through empirical data. Although this is possible, this study looks at people's reality as represented through the eyes of the participants. Here, the importance of viewing the meaning of experience and behavior in *context* in its full complexity was the point of this study. CSR embraces this and the context becomes the focal point.

With this in mind and as an educator, much of the ideas and theory on social constructivism have influenced my own epistemological and ontological stance often influencing ongoing personal and professional development. Social constructivism emphasizes the importance of culture and context in understanding what occurs in society and constructing knowledge based on this understanding (Kukla, 2000). This perspective is closely associated with many contemporary theories, most notably the developmental theories of Vygotsky (1978) and Bruner (1999), and Bandura's (1989) social cognitive theory. Social constructivism is based on specific assumptions about reality, knowledge, and learning (Kukla, 2000). Here again, CSR embraces the reality where I wanted to collect my data.

Constructivism is a theory of knowledge that argues that humans generate knowledge and meaning from an interaction between their experiences and their ideas (Piaget, 1950). Piaget suggests that through the processes of *accommodation* and *assimilation*, individuals construct new knowledge from their experiences. According to the theory, accommodation is the process of reframing one's mental representation of the external world to fit new experiences. Accommodation can be understood as the mechanism by which failure leads to learning: When we act on the expectation that the world operates in one way and it violates our expectations, we often fail, but by accommodating this new experience and reframing our model of the way the world works, we learn from the experience of failure, or others' failure (Rogoff, 1999). Piaget's theory of constructivist learning has had wide-ranging impact on learning theory and teaching methods across disciplines.

Constructivism is not a particular pedagogy; it is a theory that describes one way of how learning happens; regardless of whether learners are, for example, using their experiences to understand a lecture or follow the instructions to build a model house. In both cases, the theory of constructivism suggests that learners construct knowledge out of their experiences. However, constructivism is often associated with pedagogic approaches that promote learning by doing. In this research, constructivism provides a philosophical framework that has informed the thought process and research strategy for exploring learning environments in health care settings.

How Did CSR Fit With My Exploration of Learning?

However, in developing this philosophy further, social constructivism views each learner as a unique individual with unique needs and backgrounds, and is seen as complex and multidimensional (Wertsch, 1997). Moreover, social constructivism encourages the learner to arrive at their own version of the truth, which is influenced by their cultural background. This also stresses the importance of the nature of the learner's social interaction with knowledgeable others. Without the social interaction with other more knowledgeable people (i.e., going to a work placement), it is impossible to acquire social meaning of important symbol systems and learn how to utilize them. From the social constructivist viewpoint, it is thus important to take into account the background and culture of the learner throughout the learning process, as this helps to shape the learner (Wertsch, 1997).

Interestingly, Glasersfeld (1989) argues that the responsibility of learning should reside with the learner. This is where the philosophy of social constructivism overlaps into the workplace, emphasizing the importance of the learner being actively involved in the learning process with an element of responsibility. With learning, therefore, being an active social process, Vygotsky's (1978) work strongly influences social constructivism, suggesting that knowledge is first constructed in a social context and is then appropriated by individuals viewing learning as an active process (Glasersfeld, 1989; Kukla, 2000). Furthermore, Vygotsky (1978) adds that the most significant moment in the social and practical elements of learning in intellectual development is when speech and practical activity, two previously independent lines of development, converge.

Most social constructivist models stress the need for collaboration among learners, which is a contradiction to traditional approaches. One Vygotskian notion that has significant implications for peer collaboration is that of the zone of proximal development in which guidance or collaboration is given with more capable peers, and this contrasts with the fixed biological nature of Piaget's stages of development. Through a process of "scaffolding" a learner can be extended beyond the limitations of physical maturation to the extent that the development process lags behind the learning process (Vygotsky, 1978).

Finally, the social constructivist paradigm views the context in which the learning occurs as central to the learning itself (Kukla, 2000). Knowledge should not be divided into different subjects or compartments, but should be discovered as an integrated whole (Kukla, 2000). This also again underlines the importance of the context in which learning is presented.

The world, in which the learner needs to operate, does not approach one in the form of different subjects, but as a complex myriad of facts, problems, dimensions, and perceptions (Wertsch, 1997). This is where Lave's and Wenger's (1991) notion of situated learning is directly relevant to learning, specifically those learners who have part of their curriculum taught in the workplace. This constructivist model of learning attempts to "invite learners to a community of practice" so that through authentic activity and social interaction a successful apprenticeship is formed with the learner. Meaningful learning occurs when individuals are engaged in social activities (Kukla, 2000).

Instructional models based on the social constructivist perspective stress the need for collaboration among learners and with practitioners in the society (Lave & Wenger, 1991; Kukla, 2000). Lave and Wenger (1991) assert that a society's practical knowledge is situated in relations among practitioners, their practice, and the social organization and political economy of communities of practice. For this reason, learning should involve such knowledge and practice (Gredler, 1997; Lave & Wenger, 1991).

Therefore, this study investigated workplaces where students go to learn. The health care workplace is one example of a complex and unpredictable environment and there is an assumption that learning is "situated" and that there is an application of "appropriated" learning. This is where the methodology of choice, CSR, *captured* the reality of learning in real-life complex health care settings, the context in which learners (who are also complex beings) go to learn. In this way, CSR can examine complex situations that unfold multifaceted realities.

Reality cannot be defined objectively, but subjectively; it is this interpretation of social reality that is important here. With this in mind the ontological stance takes precedence over the epistemological. Within the health care environment, the principles of the natural sciences are difficult to maintain; people cannot be treated as objects and measured objectively. Individual people are involved in the study sharing their views and experiences. Nonetheless, rigor and high-quality research must be applied in order to produce meaningful and pertinent research applicable to contemporary health care.

In terms of epistemological influence over this piece of research, the researcher found strong overlaps with some of the methodologies available, namely, phenomenology, ethnography, and grounded theory. Although they do not directly relate to the ontological stance, there are strong influences and similarities among these philosophical methods of inquiry, which were scrutinized at length and were consequently discarded.

A Brief Historical Perspective of CSR

A case study approach is one of the most frequent research designs applied in social sciences (Burton, 2000). Despite its widespread use, it has changed over time and varies between disciplines and individual researchers (Creswell, 2009; Denzin & Lincoln, 2000; Yin, 2003b). Historically, there have been marked periods of intense use and periods of disuse. During the 1930s, particularly in America with high levels of immigration, poverty, and unemployment, it was associated with The University of Chicago Department of Sociology and, as an approach, it was strongly associated with the field of sociology, but during this time frame, other disciplines raised many questions about its scientific worth. Consequently, this led to a decline in the use of case study as a research methodology.

The use of CSR in nursing has been similar to other disciplines, though its peak interest was in the 1960s followed by a rapid decline in its use (Burns & Groves, 1997). We are now seeing its revival, for example, with Newton, Billett, and Ockerby's (2009) Australian-based case study of six students from a nursing cohort, and my study. Another example is Houghton, Murphy, Shaw, and Casey's (2015) multiple case study exploring the role of the clinical skills laboratory in preparing students for the real world of practice. There has been some CSR in the further education (FE) sector, which shares some similarities with this area of exploration, namely, Colley et al. (2003) and Hodkinson and James (2003). Both these pieces of research resulted from a project "Transforming Learning Cultures in Further Education," which aimed to deepen the understanding of the complexities of learning across the FE sector (Hodkinson & James 2003). It was a collaborative partnership among four universities and four FE colleges in England following level 3 programs in child care, health care, electronics, and telecommunications. All the sites had a substantial amount of work-based learning included throughout and data were generated from a cohort and followed for 2 years (Colley et al., 2003).

Traditionally, quantitative researchers have argued that the CSR is anecdotal and nonscientific, dismissing the results and findings obtained by this method on the grounds that they lack validity and reliability. The controversy that surrounds its scientific nature is nothing new. Like others, Al Rubaie (2002) argues that the CSR is a completely legitimate method suited in both qualitative and quantitative dichotomies. In fact, Al Rubaie (2002) suggests that it is better suited to a holistic, democratic discipline dealing with the understanding and change of interwoven complexities associated with interpersonal processes that emerge and unfold within a wider social context. Hence, this is why this particular approach suits the complexities of the learning in the workplace.

It is somewhat of a paradox because much of what we know about the empirical world is drawn from case studies, and many disciplines still continue to generate a large number of case studies. Yet, according to Gerring (2004) and Burton (2000), the case study is held in low regard or is just simply ignored. A case study might mean that its method is qualitative, with small numbers of participants; that the research may be ethnographic, clinical, participant–observation, or otherwise "in the field" (Yin 2009); the research that is carried out is characterized by process tracing (George and Bennett 2004), in which, as in an audit trail, the steps in the research can readily be followed; and the research can investigate a single case or single phenomenon. Interpretation of CSR has led to arguments resulting in no particular agreement. Although this may be the case, any researcher using CSR must ensure that each step of the research process is transparent.

CASE STUDY RESEARCH

Definition

Defining case study remains problematic because it can constitute a design and a research method. The terms case study, case study method, and case method appear to be used interchangeably in the literature (Hamel, 1993; Yin, 2009). However, it is clear that CSR focuses on specific situations, providing a description of individual or multiple cases. In using this design, the researcher can investigate "everything" in that situation be it individuals, groups, activities, or a specific phenomenon. A distinguishing feature of case study is that although the number of cases may be small (or even one); the number of variables involved is large (Burns & Groves, 1997; Yin, 2009).

To start with, I used a definition from Walsh et al. (2000): in-depth data analysis from systematic investigation over time. It describes basically what I summarized and particularly stressed that the "systematic" approach is to be taken. On further reading, Yin's (2009) work on CSR became prominent in my reading. Yin's (2003a) definition of a case study "is an empirical inquiry that investigates contemporary phenomena within its real-life context, especially when the boundaries between phenomena and context are not clearly evident" (p. 13). Yin (2009) argues that one of the most powerful uses of the method is to explain real-life, casual links.

What this means is that the researcher can appreciate the subjective richness of individuals recounting their experiences in a particular context and the meanings embedded help guide practice. Yin developed his work further producing two research companion books (Yin, 2003a; 2003b), which provide rich and varied material. This has now been updated with a new fourth edition (Yin, 2009), which promotes CSR as a valid research tool. Many researchers quote Yin's work and arguably it remains at the forefront of case study research.

Advantages

Gomm et al. (2007) identify three advantages to conducting CSR. First, case studies can take us to places where most of us would not have access or the opportunity to go. They provide enriched experiences of unique situations. Second, case studies allow us to look through the eyes of the researcher. Glesne and Peshkin (1992) recommended that researchers should be as unobtrusive as the wallpaper. In this instance, a poignant piece of reflection comes to mind (see Box 4.1).

Although we do not in reality see through the researcher's eyes, we in fact share the researcher's perspective of the theoretical position in the study. Furthermore, by definition, theory simplifies our understanding of reality. Finally, the third reason why case studies may be preferable is that it is less likely to produce defensiveness and resistance to learning. It is more acceptable because the research reflects real life. All these issues raised bring together what case study is, and Hakim (1987) sums up how focused this CSR is like a spotlight on a unit of analysis. Thus the spotlight (or unit of analysis) is on a group of five learners participating in a 2-year study program in which the completion of work placements is compulsory.

BOX 4.1 Fieldwork

In conducting the fieldwork, during the observations, I recall the feeling of being "pinned to the corridor wall" in a central position, just observing the "goings on" or just sitting on a stool positioned with other corridor furniture. The feeling of disappearing or sinking back in to the wall was the ultimate experience in being an observer.

Unit of Analysis

CSR is a "systematic inquiry into an event or set of related events which aims to describe and explain the phenomenon of interest" (Bromley 1990, p. 302). The unit of analysis can vary from an individual to a group, in this case the individual student or the group of students. Although it has been applied as a method retrospectively, it is most commonly used prospectively as in this study. The goal of the case study is to describe as accurately as possible, the most complete description of the case. In this study, the unit of analysis was students studying on a health studies program. The phenomena under investigation are embedded in everyday real-life health care practice. In using CSR, how students engage in learning within the workplace is explored. The phenomena of learning and the nature of the workplace can be difficult to understand. When using CSR, it "copes with the technically distinctive situation in which there will be many more variables than data points" (Yin 2009, p. 13). The unpredictable nature of health care in itself presents numerous consequential variables. Every day is different; the learning environment can be so volatile that even the next working shift can be different. It typically becomes a system of "actions" rather than an individual or a group of individuals. Case studies can have multiple perspectives and tend to focus on one or two issues that are fundamental to understanding the system being examined (Jones & Lyons, 2004). This means that the researcher considers not just the voice and perspective of the actors, or the relevant groups of actors and the interaction between them, but also the context in which this happens. This one aspect is a salient point in the characteristic that case studies possess. They give a voice to the powerless and voiceless. And this is the crux of this piece of research, the context in which learning occurs. This is what I tried to illuminate in my work, not only the perspective of the students, and the interaction among them, but also the context in which this happens. In this CSR observation, interviews and documentation were used transcending through 2 years of study in which participation in workplaces formed a compulsory element of the program.

Methodology—How and Why

The focus of this in-depth study is to explore how students learn in real-life settings. The chosen settings were work-based health care settings (e.g., nurseries, nursing homes, and hospitals). The students were recruited from a program of study called National Diploma in Health Studies based at a local college. Through a case study approach, the data collected focused on the learning that took place in everyday face-to-face interactions of students in work-based health care settings. Learning was examined through observations, critical incident interviews, and documentation. The study was conducted over a 2-year period in set stages:

1. After initial contact and consent obtained; students were allocated placements and observations commenced thereafter.
2. Interviews took place at the end of each placement. In this time student journals were accessed (with student permission).
3. The first two stages took place throughout the duration of the students' study program until data saturation.
4. Documentation was collected during the 2-year period.

Reflexivity in the Research

The use of memos as a reflective tool to record the researcher's abstract thinking (or any thoughts that matter to the study) about the data is recommended (Alvesson & Sköldberg, 2009). There are a variety of memo styles advocated, and a need to separate the data and descriptions of the data out of the memos (Charmaz, 2006). Memos serve to place data within time or place. At times, the researcher needs to make personal entries either in a diary or in a notebook, to reflect on an experience whether good, bad, or indifferent. These entries are useful when retracing events and how they felt, or how a situation went (e.g. a difficult interview or confrontation in the field). Sometimes these notes are helpful in decision making. A written catharsis may help the researcher to externalize ideas, development one's thinking and the entry is then recorded and kept for a future date. I found this particularly useful at specific research events, for example, postethics committee meeting, after presenting at a research conference or after a supervision session. All these activities add to reinforcing the rigor in the research undertaken. Therefore, reflexivity forms an important part of the whole research process providing links among the methods used and reinforces the approach taken in qualitative research.

A striking feature of the research that builds theory from case studies is the frequent overlap of data analysis with data collection and the interaction of the researcher. As described by Van Maanen (1988) field notes are an ongoing commentary about both observation and analysis in the research. This forms an important running commentary and is an essential way in which to accomplish this overlap. A useful way to make notes is to write down impressions as they occur, just simply react as it happens. Sometimes you also need to ask yourself questions, for example, "Is this really happening?" or "Does this still happen?" Other important question to ask is "why" it is happening and look around. These notes and ideas can become useful in cross-case comparisons, or when patterns start to emerge. (My memos and my notes became immensely useful during my writing up, to replay events in my head or recall event.)

Other sessions that have been useful are regular supervisor sessions, student group sessions, and research conferences. Although neither has been involved with the data directly, they have served as an arena to externalize different thoughts rather than making abstract notes. For example, as the study progressed, in each supervisory session areas of research were discussed, it may have been about the way data was collected or discussion about the current stage of the analysis. This transferring of information from data analysis into meaningful discourse with other intellectual colleagues can often lead to triumph and excitement because it does actually mean something. The externalizing of ideas and rapid note making over repeated sessions during the duration of the study is essential. Other sessions with student groups have always proved useful because on many occasions you can see that you are not alone in your thinking (see Box 4.2).

Building the Case Study

Each stage of this CSR follows in sequence and leads directly to the next, unfolding and revealing a way of understanding how these students learn in the workplace. Eisenhardt (1989) describes this process of inducting theory in case study designs and argues that although some features of the process, such as problem definition and construct validation, are similar to hypothesis-testing research, others, such as within-case analysis as in this study, are unique to the inductive, case-orientated process, which Eisenhardt

---

BOX 4.2 Catharsis

I remember after receiving the first rejection of my ethics decision, I attended a student seminar. Well, the whole session turned into a cathartic session for all, I remember feeling engulfed by the session and hoped the topic would change. But on reflection it was important stage to go through (despite its relatively short period of pain).

(1989) describes as "highly iterative and tightly linked to the data" (p. 532). Consequently, this process is a useful route for investigating new areas, which Yin (2009) describes as a process of explanation building. The overlapping of data collection and analysis not only facilitates the process, but also allows the researcher some flexibility to make adjustments in data collection, or in the tools or take up opportune moments if the situation presents itself. Such alterations are legitimate in theory-building research because researchers are trying to understand each case in depth. The gradual building of an explanation is similar to the process of refining a set of ideas. Thus, if a new line of thinking emerges, it makes sense to take advantage of it (e.g., in the case of the deep observations). Nevertheless, this flexibility is by no means a license to become unsystematic; the researcher must remain transparent in the research process thus maintaining rigor. As such Yin (2009) suggests a number of safeguards including storing the entire array of data, and logging where and when it was collected, and having it available for inspection. I developed a data set grid for my study, which started as a list of names and placements evolving into a chain of evidence that becomes inherent in the explanation-building process.

The practice of theory building in CSR is begun as close as possible to the ideal of no theory. However, an attempt is made to approach this "ideal" because preconceived ideas of theories and propositions may bias and limit the findings. Thus, it is important when identifying the research problem to specify important variables and making this clear from the beginning. Thereafter, researchers should avoid thinking about this, putting it to one side so that the research process can begin.

Analyzing within-case data is the heart to theory building from case studies, but can be the most difficult part too. It is hard to impress the reader how a pile of data can be compressed into a conclusion. Within-case analysis typically involves immersing yourself in the data, detailing each case, and becoming intimately familiar with each case, each incident, and each observation made—becoming one with the data. This allows the unique patterns of each case to appear in front of the investigator before patterns are merged across cases. By immersing oneself with the data in this way, it facilitates the process of cross-case comparison. Here the data is looked at in many divergent ways. One way to do this is to look at categories or repeated themes and then look for similarities or differences among the cases. The tactic I used was the movement across cases and down methods like in a matrix pattern. My grid became very, very important here as a data set presented in a grid or matrix pattern allowed me to move across and down. Another tactic Eisenhardt (1989) suggests is to select pairs of cases and list subtle similarities and differences. Alternatively data can be divided among researchers, where one deals with interviews and another deals with observations. In this research, each method was dealt within sequence using the data set grid. This exploits the data further opening it up. When a pattern does emerge and is corroborated by evidence from another method, the findings become more valid and better grounded.

Overall the main idea behind cross-case analysis is to go beyond the initial findings, forcing the researcher deeper into the data to find new theory that is reliable and fits closely with the data. After this deep-repetitive process, one must systematically compare theory and data. This is to sharpen constructs and refine definitions. In using multiple sources of evidence to define and distinguish other constructs, the aim of the researcher is to ultimately achieve construct validity.

Before reaching closure of the research or theoretical saturation, a feature of theory building is to make comparisons of the emerging themes, patterns, and concepts with existing literature looking for similarities and contradictions. In this process, it is important to delve within a broad range of material and through a critical examination of the literature, one gains deeper insight in to the resultant theory and/or conflicting theory. This can result in a theory with stronger internal validity, sharper generalizability, and a higher conceptual level. Linking with a variety of literature in other contexts also raises confidence with the observed phenomena.

Although many researchers from other disciplines have undertaken their own variations and additions to earlier methodological works, acknowledging previous work and as a result developing their own research apply different techniques for building theory. Eisenhardt (1989) applied cross-case analysis on strategic decision-making data and developed a more complete roadmap of the process of building theory from case study identifying an eight-step framework. Pandit (1996) outlined an alternative approach to building theory in a project on corporate turnaround outlining three novel aspects: first, the systematic and rigorous application of the grounded theory method; second, the use of online computerized databases as a primary source of data; and, third, the use of a qualitative data analysis software package to aid the process of grounded theory building. Pandit (1996) identified five analytic (and not strictly sequential) phases of theory building: research design, data collection, data ordering, data analysis, and literature comparison. The work of Eisenhardt and Pandit shared many similarities and processes with this CSR.

By using CSR inductively as an all-encompassing theoretical method and philosophy, it captures the very essence of the researcher's work from the very beginning in developing a research question, in the field and data analysis, right the way through to the very end in completing the concluding paragraphs of the report (or thesis in this case).

SUMMARY

This chapter offers the novice and researcher an introduction to case study research. With an example of a case study, CSR philosophy, and personal reflective accounts, it is hoped that this chapter provides some insight is to a "really" useful methodology for nursing practice. It provides a methodology for investigating and exploring the realities and complexities of nursing.

REFERENCES

Al Rubaie, T. (2002). The Rehabilitation of the case study method. *European Journal of Psychotherapy & Counselling, 5*(1), 31–47.

Alvesson, M., & Sköldberg, K. (2009). *Reflexive Methodology* (2nd ed.). London, UK: Sage.

Bandura, A. (1989). Human agency in social cognitive theory. *The American Psychologist, 44*(9), 1175–1184.

Bromley, D. B. (1990). Academic contributions to psychological counselling. *Counselling Psychology Quarterly, 3*(3), 299–307.

Bruner, J. (1999). Culture, mind and education. In B. Moon & P. Murphy (Eds.), *Curriculum in context.* Open University Text Reader 1. London, UK: Paul Chapman.

Burns, N., & Groves, S, (1997). *The practice of nursing research: Conduct, critique and utilization* (3rd ed.). Philadelphia, PA: W. B. Saunders.

Burton, D. (2000). *Research training for social scientists.* London: Sage.

Charmaz, K. (2006). *Constructing grounded theory: A practical guide through qualitative analysis.* London, UK: Sage.

Colley, H., James, D., Tedder, M., & Dimen, K. (2003). Learning as becoming in vocational education and training: Class, gender and the role of vocational habitus. *Journal of Vocational Education and Training, 55*(4), 471–498.

Creswell, J. W. (2009). *Research design qualitative, quantitative, and mixed methods approaches* (3rd ed.). London, UK: Sage.

Cronin, C. (2012). *Workplace learning—An examination of learning landscapes.* Unpublished Thesis, Albert Sloman Library, University of Essex.

Denzin, N. K., & Lincoln, Y. S. (2000). *The handbook of qualitative research* (2nd ed.). London, UK: Sage.

Eisenhardt, K. M. (1989). Building theories from case study research. *Academy of Management Review, 14*(4), 532–550.

George, A. L, & Bennett, A. (2004). *Case studies and theory development in the social sciences.* Boston, MA: Massachusetts Institute of Technology Press.

Gerring, J. (2004). *Case study research: Principles and practices.* Cambridge, UK: Cambridge University Press.

Glasersfeld, E. (1989). Cognition, construction of knowledge, and teaching. *Synthese, 80*(1), 121–140.

Glesne, C., & Peshkin, A. (1992). *Becoming qualitative researchers.* New York, NY: Longman.

Gomm, R., Hammersley, M., & Foster, P. (2007). *Case study method.* London: Sage.

Gredler, M. E. (1997). *Learning and instruction: Theory into practice* (3rd ed.). Upper Saddle River, NJ: Prentice-Hall.

Hakim, C. (1987). *Research design: Strategies and choices in the design of social research.* London, UK: Unwin Hyman.

Hamel, J. (1993). *Case study methods* (2nd ed.). London: Sage.

Hodkinson, P., & James, D. (2003) Transforming learning cultures in further education. *Journal of Vocational Education and Training, 55*(4), 389–406.

Houghton, C., Murphy, K., Shaw, D., & Casey, D. (2015). Qualitative case study data analysis: An example from practice. *Nurse Researcher, 22*(5), 8–12.

Jones, C., & Lyons, C. (2004). Case study: Design? Method? Or comprehensive strategy? *Nurse Researcher, 11*(3), 70–76.

Kukla, A. (2000). *Social constructivism and the philosophy of science.* New York, NY: Routledge.

Lave, J., & Wenger, E. (1991). *Situated Learning: Legitimate peripheral participation.* Cambridge, UK: Cambridge University Press.

Newton, J. M., Billett, S., & Ockerby, C. M. (2009). Journeying through clinical placements—An examination of six student cases. *Nurse Education Today, 29*(6), 630–634.

Pandit, N. R. (1996). The creation of theory: A recent application of the grounded theory method. *The Qualitative Report, 2*(4) (December). Retrieved from http://www.nova.edu/ssss/QR/QR2–4/pandit.html

Piaget, J. (1950). *The psychology of intelligence.* London: Routledge and Kegan Paul.

Rogoff, B. (1999). Cognitive development through social interaction: Vygotsky and Piaget. In P. Murphy (Ed.), *Learners, learning and assessment.* London: Paul Chapman.

Van Maanen, J. (1988). *Tales of the field: On writing ethnography.* Chicago, IL: University of Chicago Press.

Vygotsky, L. S. (1978). *Mind in society: The development of higher psychological processes.* Cambridge, MA: Harvard University Press.

Walsh, M., de Souza, J., Scourfield, P., Stephens, P., & Price, G. (2000). *Research perspectives in health and social care.* Health and Social Care. London, UK: Harper Collins.

Warne, T., Johansson, U. B., Papastavrou, E., Tichelaar, E., Tomietto, M., Van den Bossche, K.,...Saarikoski, M. (2010). An exploration of the clinical learning experience of nursing students in nine European countries. *Nurse Education Today, 30*(8), 809–815.

Wertsch, J. V. (1997). *Vygotsky and the formation of the mind.* Cambridge, UK: Cambridge University Press.

Yin, R. K. (2003a). *Case study research: Design and methods.* London, UK: Sage.

Yin, R. K. (2003b). *Applications of case study research* (2nd ed.). London, UK: Sage.

Yin, R. K. (2009). *Case study research: Design and methods* (4th ed.). London, UK: Sage.

CHAPTER FIVE

CASE STUDY OF CREATION OF A NEW SOCIAL SERVICE ORGANIZATION: THE HOPE BOX

Mary de Chesnay, Sarah Koeppen, and Tiffany Turolla

One of the crucial factors in obtaining grant funding for a social service organization is sustainability after funding ends. The best way to document sustainability is in the evaluation plan in which the leaders show the effectiveness of the work done by the organization; that is, were the expected outcomes achieved? Evaluation begins when the organization is created and is performed at regular intervals throughout the life of the organization. In this chapter, the authors present a case study of the beginning phases of a faith-based social service organization and show how the founders made the decisions they did in order to create the organization, how they obtained support, and what factors they considered in structuring the organization. At the time of publication, The Hope Box office renovation has not yet been completed but is scheduled to open shortly thereafter. Meanwhile, an incredible amount of foundation work has been done: getting legal advice, making connections with social service, medical and legislative people, and recruiting an evergrowing number of volunteers who are also passionate about caring for the vulnerable.

In 2006, the state of Georgia Department of Human Services (DHS) publicized an initiative to support community and faith-based projects to address child abuse. Relieving the stress on the overburdened child welfare system, these organizations provide a variety of options to families (DHS, 2006). The Hope Box is an innovative approach to unwanted pregnancy that bypasses both abortion and the cumbersome traditional adoption process. The organization does this by providing a drop box in a public place in which mothers can literally place their infants without being seen and therefore having to explain themselves. The Hope Box replaces the need for mothers to place their infants on the steps of a church or in an alley behind a fire station, abandoning them without knowing they will be safe. Medical staff receive the infant anonymously and provide immediate assessment, rehydration, and medical intervention.

Functioning under the abandonment laws of the state of Georgia, The Hope Box stabilizes the child, and a partner organization that is chartered as an adoption agency assumes custody of the child to find "forever" homes for the infants in their care. One problem with the traditional legal channel for adoption is that the mother carries the baby to term and then changes her mind, leaving prospective adoptive parents in the distressful position of having to start over. The Hope Box works with a legal agency that has a waiting list of prospective parents, shortening the time and simplifying the adoption process.

ORGANIZATIONAL MISSION AND STRUCTURE

The Hope Box is a faith-based organization founded by two women, mothers themselves, who share a passion for the plight of sex trafficking victims and other young mothers who find themselves unable to care for their infants. The mission of The Hope Box is to provide a safe and anonymous place for a mother to give up her newborn without fear of reprisal. The structure is evolving to meet the needs of the 501c3 application (an application for nonprofit status) but currently consists of an all-volunteer staff comprised of the two founders (second and third authors) and a volunteer medical coordinator who is a baccalaureate-prepared nurse. As no staff are paid, all donations are directly applied to setting up the agency to provide direct service. Funding to date has been solely through donations of time, space, and small amounts raised to cover costs. The charitable organization status is expected to generate tax-deductible donations.

METHODOLOGY

Design

Case study as a qualitative design is used for the study. The usefulness of case study as the design for studying a new organization is that it provides beginning data the organization can use for its growth, evaluation, and funding since grant agencies like to see documentation of decision making, an evaluation plan, and a plan for sustainability. For this case study, the founders (Koeppen and Turolla) of the organization document their work and decision making. The other author (de Chesnay) is a researcher who recorded their story.

Sample

Participants

The primary participants are the two founders of the organization and key staff. Several physicians and nurses have been recruited and they will undergo intensive training for volunteer staffing. Other volunteers are students who assist with office functions, fundraising, and marketing. An attorney serves as legal counsel pro bono. The board of directors is in the process of being formed but includes a variety of professionals and community leaders.

Who Are the Founders?

The women who founded The Hope Box have dedicated their lives not only to their own families but also to facilitate happy adoptions by other families. They have extensive experience in international mission work and are educating themselves with the help of their advisory board to the intricacies of the abandonment laws and the adoption process. Partnering with an adoption agency, they match the infants with preapproved adoptive parents.

Impact on the Community

By providing a safe haven for mothers to give up their infants without reprisals, the women also are addressing the growing problem of domestic minor sex trafficking in their community. Sex trafficking is sometimes thought to be a problem "over there and far away" from the United States, but it is a major problem in the United States (de Chesnay, 2013). Worldwide, about 35.8 million people are trapped in slavery (Global Slavery Index, 2014), representing more than the trans-Atlantic slave trade of earlier centuries (UNESCO, 2016). Atlanta is one of several American cities with the highest rates of sex trafficking (Dank et al., 2014).

IRB Statement

For this case study, institutional review board (IRB) approval was given by the principal investigator's university and the co-investigators are the two founders of the organization.

Setting

The Hope Box is a newly renovated space in a strip mall next to an urgent care center, donated by a local business. It is being subdivided into an exam room, an office, and a waiting room. The total area is about the size of a small restaurant or insurance office. Visitors enter from the front of the building into a waiting area adjacent to a partially enclosed office and separated from the back of the space, which is dedicated to an exam room, nursery, and medical equipment storage for addressing the needs of the infants. The box itself is cut into the fire door, which opens to a small alley behind the strip mall. This enables mothers to drop off the infants privately and also allows for ambulance access if needed. The box will be cushioned and furnished with cameras and an alarm to alert the staff to open the box.

RESULTS

The founders are coauthors of the chapter and their stories comprise the data source. Following are their stories in their own words.

Tiffany Turolla

My name is Tiffany Turolla, I have co-founded The Hope Box, Inc. with my business partner Sarah Koeppen. To begin my story, I will share about my life prior to The Hope Box. I grew up as a pastor's daughter. Both my mother and father have been in ministry and pastoring for over 40 years. They raised our family to care for those in need, help those who are helpless, and honor the Lord in all that you put your hand to. They instilled in us to not only love God but to *go* and *do* greater things than Jesus. I was raised feeding the homeless, providing for the needy, praying for the sick, honoring the widows, and caring for the orphans. Many times throughout my life we hosted families, young adults, teenagers, and extended family members into our home. Although we were not a foster family, we surely took those in who needed a home and a family, together we became Christ's hands and feet extended. I have traveled to many countries on ministry trips, sharing the gospel, praying for healing, and being the extended arms of the Kingdom of Heaven to the lives of thousands of people. My parents have a non-profit called Hope Makes A Difference in which they support and care for orphanages, tribes, and communities around the world. They have extended the legacy of their parents into their generation while training their children to do the same. My mother's parents and grandparents were both foster families and ministers. They were one of the top-requested foster families in the State of Washington. They would take in the worst of the worst cases, whether it would be the handicapped, mentally challenged, babies born on drugs and alcohol; the ones others rejected quickly became family. They loved and cared for each child who came through their doors pouring into them the love of Jesus and praying them into their future adoptive homes. My father's parents and grandparents were ministers and travelling evangelists changing and shaping their generations for the Kingdom of God. As you can see, there is a history ingrained into my very core that reaches far beyond the depths of legacy I will ever truly understand.

The Lord really began my path through music. As a child I oozed worship. I would go to bed changing the lyrics to songs on the radio to reflect the love and worship to Jesus so much so my dad took it upon himself to listen at my door at night to then turn around to learn the songs I have re-written and play them for (my unintentionally embarrassment) the congregation at church on Sunday. Worship was and is my passion. I started officially leading on the worship team in my church at the age of 14, going on to becoming the worship leader by the age of 18. I took the summer after high school graduation to tour with a record label I was signed with and really get my feet wet into what I thought would be my music career. After touring, I quickly realized that performing music wasn't enough, I wanted more out of my time spent on stage and with people afterwards. It lacked the ministry and intimacy that happens in truly abandoning yourself before the Lord in worship. That true connection you get when you let your guard down and just love him through the music. As King David danced undignified before the Lord I too seek that experience with the Father each time I lead a song.

After that tour, I returned to do missionary trips to Brazil where the Lord opened several opportunities for me to lead worship for major influential international ministries to help release the Kingdom of Heaven into the streets and hearts of the people in Brazil. The Lord changed me, where I feel he actually began to truly shape me for my calling and destiny to begin to be fulfilled. Since those trips I attended different ministry schools to educate myself into this field I feel called to. Also, I was married to my husband, Lucas, of 8 years, and we have three beautiful children, Isabella, Liam, and Guinevere. I continued as the worship leader for my parent's church and started to self-publish my music.

Then 2½ years ago, the Lord called my husband and me to Atlanta, Georgia. Within 2 months of agreeing to move we were here living away from everyone, family, friends with only a few connections in this area. A year and a half ago I met Sarah. Through the development of our friendship we began to discover each other's dreams, passions, and desires. Sarah's testimony of her son Elijah is amazing. Sarah's son Elijah was abandoned at her doorstep when he was 3 years old, left by his mother with a car seat, bike, and back pack. Sarah had no prior contact with his mother. Sarah also comes from a family of ministers. Her father has been ministering and pastoring for over 40 years as well. She is the fourth of 12 children. Sarah and her husband Joel were leaders in their church and community really focusing on building strong families and counseling many in their community when Elijah's grandmother approached her. She explained to Sarah that her daughter wanted to ask Sarah and Joel to adopt her baby when she was pregnant 3 years prior but changed her mind after delivery. Her daughter was caught up in a tough lifestyle and decided that she wanted to pursue the Koeppens again to take her son Elijah. The Lord had already prepared Sarah and Joel 2 weeks earlier by speaking to them of a child who was not a newborn but a little older that was to be a part of their family although they did not know how this would happen. Sarah and Joel agreed to the grandmother's request from the daughter to take Elijah into their family. From this point, Sarah began to pursue social services requesting advocates for herself and Elijah and was told, "There's nothing illegal about her leaving him in a safe place, good luck." Stunned by the response, Sarah began researching the laws of Colorado and counseling with lawyers to become one in five in the state of Colorado to gain sole custody of a nonblood relative. The judge said to Sarah, "People like you do not exist." Again, stunned by this response, Sarah began to question why not? Why isn't the body of Christ stepping up and being what the body was intended for? That began a fire in her spirit to actively find a solution in the communities to help these children and babies being abandoned.

As she shared this testimony, she asked if I had heard of [the Drop Box in Seoul, Korea] and I quickly stopped her by replying that I had a year or two prior from a YouTube video. [Pastor Lee Jong-Rak of South Korea created a box in which mothers could leave their unwanted children. The story was told in a documentary film directed by Brian Ivie and released in March of 2015 (Ivie, 2015).] It was something that always stuck with me. I had not experienced firsthand abandonment, but I had just had my first baby pregnant with my second and my heart was captured. Longing to be an answer to abandoned babies in my area. Little did I know the Lord had divinely set up our friendship.

Then we meet. She explains her testimony and my heart was excited; my thoughts began to process as she kept talking until I looked at her and said, "We can do this." She responded, "Really?" I replied. "Yes!" and at that moment we both felt the spirit of the Lord increase in our midst and a divine shifting happened in our spirits. We both looked at each other realizing what had happened and that the Lord orchestrated our paths to do this.

Over the next few months Sarah and I began to figure out what it would look like. Finally, coming to an outline of a vision one inspired by personal experience and in part by Pastor Lee. We began researching baby boxes finding them in all parts of the world but not in the United States. We began consoling with many people, lawyers, social workers, pastors, and family members, to see if the vision the Lord had developed in us could work. Is this legal? Are we reading this correctly? Does this look right? Through our research, findings, and development, we decided to partner and work under Hope Makes a Difference and launch our vision of The Hope Box. We began our vision cast in November 2014 followed by an internet launch in December 2014 as a developing project under Hope Makes a Difference.

We quickly began to receive a response from the community. By January, we found ourselves with our first two volunteers, a nursing student and a lawyer. As we began to speak out into our community another lawyer who happens to be highly involved with rescuing girls and women out of sex trafficking approached us. As he began to share his personal experiences we quickly saw an additional need for what we were doing. He followed by saying that we were a solution to an unfortunate byproduct of this problem. This was such a devastating statement. One account of a situation really hit home to me as a young 4-year-old girl was sold into trafficking by her father. She was trafficked through 21 different states before being rescued at 6 years old. As a result of her trafficking she now is in rehabilitation for schizophrenia. As he shared her story my heart sank into my stomach and my emotions were filled with rage, disgust, sorrow, and heartbreak, as I have a young 5-year-old daughter sitting at home waiting for me to arrive from work. How could this happen to a child? From my new awareness of the realities of trafficking not only what is portrayed in movies I knew that we needed to help protect these babies even more. It ignited a fire in me that brought fierce determination to protect and save those who have no voice. He proceeded by sharing a firsthand account of assisting in the rescuing of a pregnant teenager from the Mexican cartel traffickers who kidnapped the girl after her pimp "boyfriend" learned she was pregnant and shipped her into Mexico. Along with his counsel and advice, we began more research into the area of sex trafficking. We began to speak with Georgia Bureau of Investigation (GBI) investigators, superior court judges, hospital employees, and other organizations that all fight against trafficking and were told time after time, "we don't know what happens to the babies."

Through further research, we learned there are several things that can happen to the babies of mothers in trafficking through unwanted pregnancies, here are a few examples;

- The mother will ask a friend to help deliver the baby somewhere so that there is no record of her or the baby from the hospital.
- The pimp claims the baby as his own and leverages her interaction with the baby for prostitution.
- The pimp will sell the baby back into trafficking.
- The mother or pimp will abandon the baby.

We have attended local trafficking awareness panels speaking to the communities consisting of top officials, investigators, and organization educating the awareness of trafficking in our communities that it is no longer a lower class or urban issue but one that extends into high class and suburbs. We have learned how traffickers groom their targets and that not only girls and women are lured into trafficking, but there is a rise in boys and men being taken. A state panel gave a national statistic of 50% girls to 50% boys are sold into trafficking now. With only one organization in North Carolina hosting three beds for rescued boys out of trafficking, there are no other places helping to get the boys and men out at this time.

We have also taken the opportunity to work alongside of organizations that are reaching out to and rescuing women and girls in trafficking and prostitution of Atlanta to hear firsthand the women's fear and hopelessness not only for themselves but their unborn babies. It was shocking to see that there would be anywhere from one to five pimps guarding a single girl/woman at a time.

· Within our research on abandonment we only saw the rise in numbers across the board in all minors. As our research continued we wanted to find specifics to the age group of 0 to 12 months. We learned that the statistics have been compiled of all ages 0 to 17 years as of 1980 and are categorized under abuse, neglect, and abandonment. We expanded our statistical research to include Georgia and national averages. The numbers are shocking. The Court-Appointed Special Advocates for Children (CASA) maintains statistics on child abuse and neglect. Here are a few of those statistics for Georgia. It is estimated 33 children daily are confirmed victims of abuse or neglect with 200 incidences filed daily of child abuse and neglect. There were 39 children who died in the fiscal year due to abuse and neglect. Nationally, 27% of victims are under the age of 3 and the highest rate of victimization is under 1 year of age (CASA, 2016).

With these findings, we began to research more into social services along with participating with social workers in seeing the issues of the abandoned, abused, and neglected in our communities. We even began to find articles regarding social services so desperate for foster families they have begun housing children in hotels in Atlanta. This story was covered by Channel 2 Action News (www.wsbtv .com/news/news/local/dfcs-using-local-hotels-house-foster-children/ nkzWT). Where do you think a trafficker operates their business? They lure children in with gifts and promises of a better life. We have spoken with hospital social workers that the children are being shipped to other counties in efforts to find foster homes. We have attended the local children's cabinet meetings to learn of the issues of homelessness, abandonment, abuse, and neglect of minors in our own cities and how the community efforts were just not enough for the need. We learned that the demand of heroin in our middle and high schools is on the rise surpassing cocaine and contributing to the rise in homelessness of students.

We also became educated in the issue of "boarder babies" within our own hospitals. Boarder babies are infants up to 12 months who remain in the hospitals after being medically discharged. These babies have been abandoned into the hospitals either after delivery or through the Safe Haven law. The hospitals then take on the responsibility of these babies for up to 11 months before turning them over to social services. We have spoken with local hospital employees that are aware their facilities are rejecting women trying to use the safe haven law because their hospitals are full. A few links regarding our findings on this issue are found in Table 5.1.

Table 5.1 *Helpful Websites*

News stories about The Hope Box:
    http://www.11alive.com/story/news/2015/11/17/hope-box-drop-
    abandoned-sex-trafficking-kennesaw-adoption/75872782
    http://mdjonline.com/view/full_story/26970835/article-Nonprofit-Hope-Box-
    aims-to-deliver-abandoned-newborns-to-new-families?instance=secondary_
    story_left_column

Safe Haven Law:
    http://aia.berkeley.edu/media/pdf/abandoned_infant_fact_sheet_2005.pdf
    https://books.google.com/books?id=RATyep8nF7EC&pg=PA5203&lpg=
    PA5203&dq=boarder+babies+georgia&source=bl&ots=u1XCes4RXS&sig=
    awr2HMp_fbsKxHQxtTIdPUqtS5Y&hl=en&sa=X&ved=0ahUKEwj6isLtuar
    JAhUJR4gKHRPSDnsQ6AEIWDAJ#v=onepage&q=boarder%20babies%
    20georgia&f=false

The Hope Box and supporting agencies:
    http://www.thehopebox.org/contact.html
    http://hopemakesadifference.com/
    http://outofdarkness.org
    http://www.albanyhouseofprayer.com

The Safe Haven Law for the State of Georgia is as follows:

O.C.G.A. § 19–10A-4 provides that a mother shall not be prosecuted for leaving her newborn child (defined as a no more than 1 week old) in the physical custody of an employee, agent, or member of the staff of a medical facility who is on duty in either a paid or volunteer position. The mother must show proof of her identity, if available, and provide her name and address to avoid prosecution. A medical facility is defined in O.C.G.A. §19–10A-2 as "any licensed general or specialized hospital, institutional infirmary, health center operated by a county board of health, or facility where human births occur on a regular and ongoing basis which is classified by the Department of Community Health as a birthing center, but shall not mean physicians' or dentists' private offices" (Safe Haven Law, n.d.)

Georgia's Safe Haven protections are aimed at providing legal protection to the mothers of the children as well as a liability shield to certain medical facilities in order prevent injury and death to newborns by providing a safe way for a mother to abandon a child.

As you can see we have a very limited Safe Haven law in Georgia. Through our efforts of bringing awareness of the issue of abandonment and educating the community that all of these issues are occurring in our own cities, we have begun to see the community want to get involved and help make a change. We have reached out to every legislator in our state to bring awareness of our efforts and to ask if any of them would be interested in getting involved. Through our most recent efforts in our television exclusive interview with 11Alive News on November 17, 2015, and news article in the *Marietta Daily Journal* on November 22, 2015, we were able to bring our organization to the attention of Georgia State Representative Judy Manning who has recently contacted our organization to learn more about us and to see how she can offer help. State Representative Manning fought for the "Safe Haven for Newborns Act 2002" to come to pass for Georgia. She is highly interested in our organization and how we are developing.

By May 2015, we found ourselves growing in our efforts and responses. In order to bring our vision to life, through legal counsel and discussion with the founders of Hope Makes a Difference, we decided to branch off into our own nonprofit entity. Over the next several months we developed our vision into what we feel will be the most successful and efficient solution to the issue of newborn abandonment at this time.

So, what exactly is The Hope Box doing? The Hope Box provides a safe and anonymous option for a mother who is unable or unwilling to care for her newborn, by acting as a receiving point for the child. After receiving a newborn, The Hope Box immediately contacts an adoption agency so that agency may place the child with an approved and waiting family who is ready to adopt. We also provide an emergency hotline number that a mother who is unable to make her way to our facility can call to set up a safe meeting location for our rescue team to then receive the newborn.

Our hearts are to provide these newborns the best chance at life. We have established our organization through forging partnerships in our community in order to establish that each baby that comes through our organization is placed through an adoption agency to become adopted, never to enter foster care. The Hope Box is not an orphanage, we are not an adoption agency, and we are not a foster system. We are a first responder and rescue.

Through our forged partnerships in the community, I would like to highlight four of them outside of our partnership with Kaylor Ministries/Hope Makes a Difference.

The first partnership we would like to highlight is Embracing Life Adoption Agency located in Lawrenceville, Georgia. Through development, visions, and goals, together we have established The Hope Box Adoption Program. It is through their expertise in adoption and similar culture to our own that we were able to develop a program for any newborn received through The Hope Box to be placed through Embracing Life Adoption Agency into an awaiting adoptive home.

The second partnership is with Out of Darkness located in Atlanta, Georgia. In their expertise in the field of rescuing girls and women in sexual exploitation by helping them into rehabilitation, we are partnering in many areas of outreach and awareness along with the development of The Hope Box rescue response.

The third partnership is Deakon Home Services located in Kennesaw, Georgia. Deakon Home Services is sponsoring The Hope Box office and first receiving location. With their similar culture and passion to create community unity and support we are proud to have Deakon Homes as a partner in helping bring the vision of The Hope Box into a physical reality.

The fourth partnership is with Albany House of Prayer located in Albany, Georgia. Through their passion for community outreach and restoration along with their similar culture and establishment within the community of Albany, Georgia, we have partnered together to bring our secondary hope box location to southwest Georgia.

With both locations under construction we do not officially have a receiving hope box. We could not be more pleased with the development of that has taken place within 1 year of start-up. We are beyond grateful and blessed with how the community support and encouragement to help bring this new option of life into a reality.

We feel strongly that the Lord is seeking those who will answer a call for help and that the Lord's heart is claiming back those in the world that have been left for dead to be rescued. It is this next generation who will become our future leaders and influencers and we get to the chance to give back to them a future and a hope to fulfill their lives by simply saying, Yes! Yes, to a call and helping save a generation that is being left unwanted.

Sarah Koeppen

The interview with Sarah started with the story of how she and her husband came to adopt a 3-year-old boy named Elijah, now 10 years old. As Tiffany recounted, Sarah described meeting a woman who asked her to take care of her grandchild because her daughter could not cope well and was willing to give him up as the best option for the child:

> She loved her son—she really loved him but she just couldn't take care of him. I watched her face [when she brought him to me] and it was the hardest thing she'd ever done. So then I called social services and explained I wanted an advocate for her, for me and for Elijah, and they said well there's nothing illegal so we aren't going to get involved. So Joel [Sarah's husband] and I had talked and prayed about it together and so I studied the law and found that if a child is in your home for 6 months, I could file for custody to full custody to sole custody. I was one in five in the state of Colorado to do what I did—to take a nonrelative child.

So I started hearing more stories from people who didn't know what to do—even the adoption lawyers said, "Sarah you know more than I do—this is a gray area in the law." In Georgia, many grandparents are fighting to get custody but hard to adopt a non-relative-but it would save the system a lot of money. So meanwhile I had seen the Drop Box film (Ivie, 2015) and realized this is an old idea. And this is something that's needed here—it is very much a European custom—all over the world and we need it here.

So I moved to Georgia from Colorado for my husband so he could go to school and I put [the idea for The Hope Box] on back burner. So, after a couple years I met Tiffany—mutual friends said you just have to meet. She asked me, "What are your dreams?" So I shared my dream about abandonment of children. For example, border babies are babies born with drug abuse or for any reason are abandoned; a girl in sex trafficking gets a friend to deliver her baby; anyone who lives in a place of fear or uncertainty might abandon their child. So abandonment might mean the best thing for the child—a girl who is in sex trafficking deals with incredible abuse every day. We don't know why they are in that situation of abandoning their baby.

We were not trained to do this [neither Tiffany nor Sarah]. I had one of my friends [a lawyer] sit in the back of the courtroom to make sure I am doing this right [court appearance to adopt Elijah]. I'm not a lawyer—I'm a mom! So much I found out about adoption and the process just by doing my research. If you want to do something you can do it. When I met Tiffany it was like an explosion—we found immediately we had the same dream. She said, "Sarah we can do this—with your knowledge and my background [worked in law office] we can do this."

Three times we tried to stop it or slow down—too busy, just too much, but something happened to make us continue. One time a lawyer contacted us and as a result he is our pro bono attorney, so literally we couldn't stop—it is bigger than us—so that continues to happen. There is power in realizing you can do something.

It's not that social services don't want to help—just no protocol for this. Border babies sit in hospital up to 11 months—then in social services system for 2 to 3 years—so not actually adopted out till 2 to 3 years old. They say, let's wait and see if someone from the family shows up. But would we really want to return the child to that family? So many families on adoption lists, but social workers cannot cross counties and families do, for whatever reason. Families get evicted and bounce from county to county, kids get lost in system.

Status of Hope Box today: Renovations are still going on but that is okay. We are trying to go about things correctly—working with government, medical people, social services. Goals for this year: Getting ready to meet with Judy Manning—she wrote the safe haven law. Having her on our side is huge—she wanted it more like Hope Box [but could not get support at the time]. Georgia has one of the worst safe haven laws: Right now, only a mother can abandon only at a hospital; the father can be prosecuted; they only accept the baby younger than 7 days old; the mother has to leave her information, but a girl in sex trafficking may not know her real name or address. Hospitals can refuse to accept the baby so even if a girl gets there she gets rejected, so the black market is thriving. People don't want to hear this but there is a big market for sex with infants. That is why black market is thriving—there is nowhere to go. Not to mention hospitals are scary—you cannot abandon anywhere else.

Now we want to connect with social services—they want to work with us—how to make it all work—a game plan. We are looking to partner with medical facilities so if someone could take us under their wing so we can work with them [we can ensure the babies are seen immediately]. We have a lot of doctors and nurses contact us. We are doing training—since we partnered with Out of Darkness and they do a great orientation, we ask all of our volunteers to go through that training to start.

Albany, Georgia, is blowing up—they have their mayor involved, emergency room people are completely trained. They are not affiliated with us, but when we came up with the idea, they asked to be part of it. She [the person spearheading the Albany efforts] is the director of a local house of prayer. We felt comfortable with her. She's amazing—she said we have a template for a small city and a large city [as programs develop].

People we've talked to have said they hope we do a national conference because no one has done this—we're dealing with abandonment in general but safe haven is specific to a mother who abandons, not others like black market babies. No one is uniting the safe haven laws—we want to identify what's working, what's not working.

The way we work together, Tiffany and I have a good division of labor and are true partners. She is very good at the details behind the scenes—writing things up. I carry the passion (both of us are passionate but I might be more verbal about it) and tend to be more of the face of the partnership— people attach to my passion—we carry two different gifts which balance very well: me speaking, her writing. We talk about everything—if we disagree we talk it out.

When asked about their main message to people, Sarah had this to say:

If you see a need, you can fulfill it—it is all about creating strong communities and inviting people into your story. Begin a healing within the communities—a lot of people see things but they don't know what to do so talk to people. We all change things together. People live in fear. I don't know what to do so they don't do anything. The whole process is scary. Do I know enough to get me in trouble? [When I went to court for Elijah] the judge covered the mic and said, "Sarah, people like you do not exist in society and I am so thankful for you and what you are doing for this boy." I was grateful for the compliment, but why am I unique? We can all do it.

SUMMARY

This case study documents what two individuals can do given their passion for the vulnerable and their commitment to their values. As a faith-based organization, The Hope Box is a social service agency that is founded on spirituality and a commitment to using the strengths and resources of the most favored to help the most vulnerable members of their community. The Hope Box represents what a small group of committed people can do in a short time. The idea was generated only a year ago with no funding. Unique in the United States, The Hope Box can be a model for other communities in.

which vulnerable young women, whether or not they are victims of human trafficking, and who see no other option than to abandon their infants.

Regardless of one's personal beliefs or religious practices, all have much to learn from the faith-based community on caring for the vulnerable. The basic idea in the mission of this organization is to find a way to bridge the gap between existing social services and highly vulnerable and somewhat invisible young women who, for whatever reason, cannot access services through regular channels. By inviting us into their story, the founders of The Hope Box inspire others to think about the most vulnerable members of their communities and find ways to bring the right people to the table to find solutions.

REFERENCES

CASA. (2016). *Statistics.* Retrieved from http://www.gacasa.org/statistics.php

Dank, M., Khan, B., Downey, P. M., Kotonias, C., Mayer, D., Owens, C.,...Yu, L. (2014). *Estimating the size and structure of the underground commercial sex economy in eight major US cities.* Research report from Urban Institute for the U.S. Justice Department. Retrieved from http://www.urban.org/research/publication/estimating-size-and-structure-underground-commercial-sex-economy-eight-major-us-cities/view/full_report

de Chesnay, M. (2013). *Sex trafficking: A clinical guide for nurses.* New York, NY: Springer Publishing Company.

DHS. (2006). DFCS promotes community and faith-based projects to prevent abuse and neglect. Retrieved from https://dhs.georgia.gov/dfcs-promotes-community-and-faith-based-projects-prevent-abuse-and-neglect

Global Slavery Index. (2014). Retrieved from http://www.globalslaveryindex.org

Ivie, B. *The Drop Box* (2015). Produced by Arbella Studios, Pine Creek Entertainment.

Safe Haven Law. (n.d.). GA Code Ann 19-10A-1,k2,3,4,5,6,7. Retrieved from http://safehaven.tv/states/georgia

UNESCO. (2016). *Trans-Atlantic slave trade.* Retrieved from http://www.unesco.org/new/en/culture/themes/dialogue/the-slave-route/transatlantic-slave-trade

CHAPTER SIX

CONDUCTING CASE STUDY RESEARCH: AN EXEMPLAR

Esther Sangster-Gormley

Nursing scholars use research to validate, refine, and extend nursing knowledge and test theories. Knowledge developed through research contributes to nurses' understand of the discipline and practice. This knowledge informs the development and implementation of nursing interventions that promote high-quality outcomes for patients, families, providers, and health care systems (Burns & Grove, 2001; Twinn, 2003). Today nurse researchers use quantitative and qualitative approaches, as well as mixed methods, in knowledge development (Twinn, 2003).

Qualitative research is relatively new to nursing; indeed early nurse researchers exclusively used quantitative research methods (Hutchinson, 2001; Morse & Richards, 2002). Over the years, nurse researchers have debated how best to pursue nursing knowledge development, and which approach (qualitative vs. quantitative) was more appropriate to generate knowledge of nursing's unique contributions to health care (Hutchinson, 2001). No doubt these debates continue today as some researchers continue to maintain a dualist position of privileging one approach over others (Johnson & Onwuegbuzie, 2004).

Quantitative and qualitative research each has distinct, classical methods associated with how research is conducted. For example, quantitative researchers employ standardized instruments and/or conduct randomized-controlled trials to measure the effects of variables or interventions on outcomes. Research findings are determined using odds ratios, inferential statistics, and other methods (Burns & Grove, 2001). Qualitative research is associated with methods such as grounded theory, phenomenology, and ethnography (Hutchinson, 2001). Qualitative researchers have sustained interactions with participants, use interviews, observations, and other unstructured approaches. Findings incorporate participants' language and perspectives (Guba & Lincoln, 1989).

Increasingly, nurse researchers are finding case study research (CSR) a useful method that allows the flexibility to mix qualitative and quantitative data, for example, surveys and interviews, to explain a phenomena (Stake, 1995; Yin, 2009). Nonetheless, what seems to be missing in nursing research is a clear definition of CSR and how it is conducted. In this chapter, I use my research to illustrate how I used CSR to explain nurse practitioner (NP) role implementation in one provincial health authority in Canada. At the time of this study, NP role implementation was in its early stages, having been introduced 4 years earlier. Thus, this was a unique opportunity to study the process of implementing a new role into the health care system in its early stages. The study was completed in partial fulfillment of my doctoral studies and was my first experience using CSR.

DEFINING CASE STUDY RESEARCH

Early sociologists described CSR as a collection and presentation of detailed, unstructured data obtained from multiple sources to analyze social phenomena in its natural setting, and at a specific time and place (Hammersley, 1989; Ragin, 1992). Today researchers continue to select CSR to study complex phenomenon in the environment in which participants exist, be that work place, home, or community. It allows researchers to obtain multiple perspectives, explore the meanings people attach to the phenomenon of interest, as well as contextual complexity (Creswell & Miller, 2000; Stake, 1995).

Defining the Case

Stake and Yin, two proponents of CSR, have been cited by nurse researchers as offering direction for conducting CSR (Gangeness & Yurkovich 2006; Hewitt-Taylor, 2002; Jones & Lyons, 2004; Zucker, 2001). Stake defines a case as an intrinsic or illustrative-bounded interactive system, with clear boundaries of where the case begins and ends. Intrinsic case studies are conducted to gain a better understanding of a particular phenomenon, whereas an illustrative case provides insight into an issue and facilitates understanding of something other than the case (Stake, 1995). Issues are identified to guide the study and the case is structured to reveal information, determine uniqueness, uncover shortcomings or merit, or facilitate planning for future inquiry (Stake, 1995). Yin begins by asking the question, "What is this case of?" It is necessary to predetermine what is to be studied and why, recognizing the study could be of individuals, organizations, processes, or policies (Yin, 2009).

Yin defines CSR as exploratory, descriptive, or explanatory and constructs cases as single or multiple with embedded multiple units of analysis or holistic with a single unit of analysis. According to Yin, a single case is similar to conducting a single experiment, and multiple cases represent multiple experiments and follow replication logic (Yin, 2009). Exploratory case studies answer "what" questions and are used to develop hypotheses and test propositions for further inquiry. Descriptive case studies are used to describe phenomena within their context, and explanatory case studies are used to answer "how" and "why" questions, as well as understand cause-and-effect relationships (Yin, 2009).

Whether using Yin's or Stake's approach to CSR, the researcher first clarifies and defines the case to be studied. For example, I wanted to study how NP role implementation occurred in a health authority. I wanted to understand why it was successfully implemented in some settings and not in others. As a result of my study, I wanted to ultimately explain the process used by health authority managers and those working in the setting in which new NPs were hired, to incorporate a new role into the mix of other health professionals who were often unfamiliar with the NP role and how the NP would function within the setting.

In my research, I made the decision to follow Yin's approach to CSR and the case I studied was the process of NP role implementation in primary care settings. I selected one provincial health authority for the study, thus a single case study. However, I selected multiple primary care settings within the health authority that had implemented the NP role. Consequently, I used a single case study with three embedded units of analysis (primary care settings). The use of three different settings contributed to the robustness of the study (Yin, 2009), and allowed me to explain more fully the complexity of the process than if I had selected one setting (Baxter & Jack, 2008). Had I selected one setting my intent would have been to explore how the process of role implementation occurred in that particular setting because perhaps something unusual occurred during or after the hiring of the NP. Stake might consider this an intrinsic case study.

Bounding of the Case

Bounding the case refers to limiting what the researcher will and will not study. Limitations may include the amount of time the researcher has to conduct the study and funding. Granting agencies usually expect research to be completed within a predetermined time frame. The funds available determine whether or not the researcher is available to travel and spend time in settings and pay research assistants and other administrative costs. In addition to these limitations, the clearer the researcher is on what is to be studied, the easier it is to bound or limit the case.

Again, referring to decisions I made, although the process of NP role implementation was occurring in other areas of the province, I limited my study to one regional health authority. It was further limited to those primary care settings that had implemented the NP role in the previous 6 months. Because each setting was situated within the same health authority, they were bounded as part of the health authority's organizational context and system. By purposively selecting those settings in which the role had been implemented a minimum of 6 months, I bound the case in time (minimum 6 months post-NP role implementation) and place (a health authority in the province; Miles & Huberman, 1994).

Reviewing the Literature

Previous research demonstrated that involvement and acceptance of managers, physicians, and other staff, and the intentions for the role influenced the process of NP role implementation (Sangster-Gormley, Martin-Misener, Downe-Wamboldt, & DiCenso, 2011). I used these concepts to develop the research questions, propositions, and conceptual framework that guided my study. I also used the concepts to structure my interview questions, and during the interviews I framed questions so that participants would describe how they were involved in the planning for an NP, their definition of the role, the fit of the NP with other providers, and so forth.

The health authority had implemented the NP role in a variety of different settings that served a wide variety of patient populations such as primarily community dwelling older adults, people who were homeless, or people with mental health and addiction issues. In all of these settings the organizational expectations for the NPs were the same. They were expected to provide primary health care services by increasing access to care, improving patient outcomes, and the functioning of multidisciplinary teams.

Case Selection

The implementation process was the case; to understand and explain the case I needed to locate settings where the process had occurred. The advantage of CSR is that the selection of cases is not blinded or controlled; instead all cases were purposively selected to demonstrate the phenomenon of study and permit in-depth investigation (Patton, 2002).

Prior to beginning my study I had been involved as a committee member in the health authority's NP implementation steering committee. My involvement gave me unique understanding of where NPs were being hired but not how managers and those in the primary care settings were going about hiring NPs. I also ask the health authority's chief nursing officer to serve as a decision-making partner for this research. The underlying intent of involving the steering committee and chief nursing officer in the beginning of the study was to enable the research to be relevant to the health authority and possibly influence knowledge translation and uptake (Lomas, 2000).

Together with the implementation steering committee, settings were identified that were of interest to the health authority. I sought maximum variability in the location, model of care provided in the setting, and patient population among the settings. Heterogeneity of settings helped to reduce bias and to explain how the concepts of involvement, acceptance, and intention influence the process of implementation (Sandelowski, 1993).

Sources of Data

Recruitment Strategy

Once the study received ethics approval, the selection of primary care settings was discussed with and approved by the health authority's implementation steering committee and the chief nursing officer. Previous involvement of decision-making partners facilitated identifying and gaining entry into the settings. Once the settings were identified, my next step was to contact the manager of a setting, or in some instances the current NP, to discuss the study and whether or not there was interest in participating. Participation was voluntary and all three settings I initially selected agreed to participate. Had one declined it would have been necessary to go back to the implementation steering committee to select another setting.

Sample Inclusion/Exclusion Criteria

As with any research method, the researcher must decide who and what to include and exclude. The decision is guided by identifying data sources expected to provide rich detail of the process under study. Again, I wanted to interview those people who were involved in the decision to hire the NP, the recruitment process, and those who had been working with the NP for at least 6 months. I knew from the literature that the first 6 months of employment for all new employees, including NPs, can be a time of learning organizational expectations. Inclusion of NPs, physicians, and other employees who had been in their positions for at least 6 months and were involved in the implementation process excluded participants who might not be able to contribute to the study (Brykczynski, 2009).

Data Collection

Yin (2009) lists six sources of data for case study research: (a) interviews, (b) documentation, (c) direct observation, (d) participant observation, (e) archival records, and (f) physical artifacts. Depending on the phenomenon of interest, a researcher may decide to use field notes, direct observation, or archival records. If so, data analysis would include all sources of data to explain the phenomenon. Early in the study, I made the decision not to observe participants in the settings because I did not believe this would assist me to explain the process of implementation.

The data sources I used were semi-structured interviews incorporating open-ended and focused questions and any available relevant documents. The research questions and conceptual framework guided the questions I asked during interviews. I asked participants to describe how they were involved in the implementation process, their understanding of the intention for the role, and their views on how the role was accepted. On completion of each interview, I summarized responses to the interview questions and asked participants if I captured their intent. All interviews were audio taped and transcribed verbatim for later review and analysis.

Data Analysis Strategy

The transcripts were imported into N-Vivo, data management software, for coding (Richards, 2005). Using N-Vivo for coding and managing data provided an electronic depository of data that could be easily retrieved and managed (Richards, 2005). How to manage data is another decision that had to be made early in the research process. Researchers familiar with analyzing qualitative data may have previously used N-Vivo. If not, it takes time to learn to use the software and there is an expense involved in purchasing it.

Ultimately, it is up to the researcher to decide how to analyze qualitative data. My original intent in developing the conceptual framework, propositions, and research questions was to use them to provide strategic direction for data analysis. Following these helped focus data analysis and reduced the temptation to analyze data outside the research questions (Bergen & While, 2000). Yin (2009) offers suggestions such as pattern matching, explanation building, or logic model. I used explanation building by iteratively interrogating the data to determine how participants were answering the research questions. As mentioned earlier, I used a single case study (one organization) with three embedded units of analysis (primary care settings). I began data analysis by first analyzing all of the data from each primary care setting individually. Once I completed my analysis of how NP implementation occurred in each primary care setting, I looked across the settings to look for similarities and differences in approaches to help me explain how it occurred within the organization as a whole. I expected the three primary care settings to be representative of all settings in the health authority where NPs had been hired, thus combining the findings contributed to the explanation of what occurred in the organization.

Rigor

Although some qualitative researchers use the terms trustworthiness, applicability, and dependability to describe rigor, Yin (2009) refers to this as construct validity, internal and external validity, and reliability. Regardless of terminology, the researcher must be clear when describing how the research was conducted so that the quality of the work can be judged by other researchers. Two strategies that helped me to maintain a detailed record of each step in the research process were the use of N-Vivo for memoing and record keeping and a decision-making partner involved in the research. Other researchers may have advisory boards as well as other team members who can assist to verify findings. Again, this needs to be considered early so that all aspects of the study are recorded from the beginning.

DISCUSSION

How Did CSR Contribute to Knowledge of New Role Implementation?

In total, I interviewed 16 participants, and reviewed a variety of documents. Depending on the number of interviews and types of data collected, a researcher can quickly become overwhelmed with the amount of data generated. Thus, another reason to pre-select the types of data sources to include.

Although there is a need to have adequate data, redundant data can over-whelm the researcher during data analysis. Using research questions and a conceptual framework assisted me in staying focused.

As a result of this study, I learned that implementing a new role is a complex process. The concepts of intention, acceptance, and involvement were interconnected and influenced the process. For instance, people in the setting wanted to know how the NP would function and how expectations of the NP were different from those of others. They wanted to be involved early in the planning process so that questions could be answered prior to an NP being hired. Prior knowledge of NP roles or previous working experiences with an NP helped others to more easily accept the NP as a new member of the team (Sangster-Gormley, Martin-Misener, & Burge, 2013).

Challenges

Learning CSR can be challenging. Researchers begin by deciding what to study and defining the case. The language can be confusing, such as how to differentiate between the case and CSR. The case is the phenomenon being studied including the locations where the study will be carried out, par-ticipants, and other data sources, whereas CSR refers to all components of the study or the overall method. Personally, I found it helpful to use Yin's approach. His texts provide step-by-step information about the research process despite seeming to lack instruction with data analysis. Fortunately, his 2009 text provided more clarity in how to approach data analysis. Once I began to build an explanation of how implementation unfolded in each of the settings, reading and coding the transcripts became easier. Researchers unfamiliar with qualitative research might consider collaborating with an experienced qualitative researcher to assist with getting started with data analysis and coding. As I began to record my findings, I found it helpful to think of how I would tell the story of what occurred in each setting, then combine individual stories to represent what happened in the organization. As with any skill or ability, after completing the first study using CSR, sub-sequent ones become easier to conduct.

SUMMARY

My first experience using CSR was for my dissertation. My PhD com-mittee was especially supportive in critiquing how I represented or doc-umented each case. Their feedback helped me clarify where more detail was required or explained differently. I also had access to a colleague who had experience using CSR with whom I could ask questions. This was tremendously valuable because my committee members had not previously used the method. Researchers or doctoral students contemplating using this method for the first time might consider where and how they will obtain guidance when determining how to structure the study, analyze, and document the findings.

REFERENCES

Baxter, P., & Jack, S. (2008). Qualitative case study methodology: Study design and implementation for novice researchers. *The Qualitative Report, 13*(4), 544–559.

Bergen, A., & While, A. (2000). A case for case studies: Exploring the use of case study design in community nursing research. *Journal of Advanced Nursing, 31*(4), 926–934.

Brykczynski, K. (2009). Role development of the advanced practice nurse. In A. Hamric, J. Spross & C. Hanson (Eds.), *Advanced practice nursing an integrative approach* (4th ed., pp. 95–120). St. Louis, MO: Saunders Elsevier.

Burns, N., & Grove, S. (2001). *The practice of nursing research: Conduct, critique, & utilization* (4th ed.). Philadelphia, PA: Saunders.

Creswell, J., & Miller, D. (2000). Determining validity in qualitative inquiry. *Theory Into Practice, 39*(3), 124–130.

Gangeness, J. E., & Yurkovich, E. (2006). Revisiting case study as a nursing research design. *Nurse Researcher, 13*(4), 7–18.

Guba, E., & Lincoln, Y. (1989). *Fourth generation evaluation.* Newbury Park, CA: Sage.

Hammersley, M. (1989). *The dilemma of qualitative method: Herbert Blumer and the Chicago tradition.* New York, NY: Routledge.

Hewitt-Taylor, J. (2002). Case study: An approach to qualitative inquiry. *Nursing Standard, 16*(20), 33–37.

Hutchinson, S. A. (2001). The development of qualitative health research: Taking stock. *Qualitative Health Research, 11*(4), 505–521.

Johnson, R., & Onwuegbuzie, A. (2004). Mixed methods research: A research paradigm whose time has come. *Educational Researcher, 33*(7), 14–26.

Jones, C., & Lyons, C. (2004). Case study: Design? Method? Or comprehensive strategy? *Nurse Researcher, 11*(3), 70–76.

Lomas, J. (2000). Connecting research and policy. *ISUMA: Canadian Journal of Policy Research, 1*(1), 140–144.

Miles, M., & Huberman, A. (1994). *An expanded sourcebook: Qualitative data analysis.* (2nd ed.). Thousand Oaks, CA: Sage.

Morse, J., & Richards, L. (2002). *Readme first for a user's guide to qualitative methods.* Thousand Oaks, CA: Sage.

Patton, M. (2002). *Qualitative research and evaluation methods* (3rd ed.). Thousand Oaks, CA: Sage.

Ragin, C. (1992). Introduction: Cases of "What is a case?" In C. Ragin & H. Becker (Eds.), *What is a Case? Exploring the Foundations of Social Inquiry* (pp. 1–18). Cambridge, UK: University Press.

Richards, L. (2005). *Handling qualitative data a practical guide.* Thousand Oaks, CA: Sage.

Sandelowski, M. (1993). Rigor or rigor mortis: The problem of rigor in qualitative research revisited. *Advances in Nursing Science, 16*(2), 1–8.

Sangster-Gormley, E., Martin-Misener, R., & Burge, F. (2013). A case study of nurse practitioner role implementation in primary care: What happens when new roles are introduced? *BMC Nursing, 12,* 1.

Sangster-Gormley, E., Martin-Misener, R., Downe-Wamboldt, B., & DiCenso, A. (2011). Factors affecting nurse practitioner role implementation in Canadian practice settings: An integrative review. *Journal of Advanced Nursing, 67*(6), 1178–1190.

Stake, R. (1995). *The art of case study research.* London, UK: Sage.

Twinn, S. (2003). Status of mixed methods research in nursing. In A. Tashakkori & C. Teddlie (Eds.), *Handbook of mixed methods in social and behavioral research* (pp. 541–556). Thousand Oaks, CA: Sage.

Yin, R. (2009). *Case study research: Design and methods* (4th ed.). Los Angeles, CA: Sage.

Zucker, D. (2001). Using case study methodology in nursing research [45 paragraphs]. *The Qualitative Report* [online serial], *6*(2). Retrieved from http://www.nova.edu.ezproxy.library.uvic.ca/ssss/QR/QR6–2/zucker.html

CHAPTER SEVEN

COMING HOME: VETERANS WITH PTSD ADAPTING TO LIFE AT HOME

Patricia Hentz

Only the dead have seen the end of war. I have seen the end of war, but the question is, Can I live again?

—From the film *Brothers* (2009)

This case study focuses on the experiences of veterans returning from war. It draws from a variety of sources including this author's clinical practice with veterans who were diagnosed with posttraumatic stress disorder (PTSD), historical accounts from literature, films, and research and theories in the areas of trauma and trauma treatment approaches. The focus of the study has been to examine, in depth, the challenges veterans face living with symptoms of PTSD and their process of reclaiming a "normal" life when returning home. The clinical sample for this study included veterans diagnosed with PTSD. However, the broader aim has been to explore and understand veterans' experiences beyond the diagnosis of PTSD and its list of symptoms.

Using two cross-case exemplars, the author hopes to provide the readers with an inside view of veterans' psychological challenges returning home from war. Several major themes emerged as relevant to the veterans' experiences that are presented within this chapter—these themes are reflected in two exemplar case examples. The major themes that were identified in this study included a heightened fear process, compensatory survival behaviors, social disengagement and attachment difficulties, and a shift in attachment bonds.

This case study aims at sensitizing the reader to the experience of veterans with PTSD and their challenges in recreating their lives after experiencing trauma during their military service in combat areas. Of specific interest was how trauma and military experiences impacted veterans' ability to recreate a sense of "normal" in their everyday lives. Utilizing a case study method framework, this study has sought to shift the focus from the abstract and conceptual list of symptomatology toward the personal and humanistic aspects connected to life experiences.

Case study research places emphasis on identifying the object of study within its social context and the importance of the bond between the object of study and the social context. To illustrate the object of study within its social context, this study has explored the experiences of veterans who have returned home and are experiencing combat-related PTSD. The object of study involved exploring their processes of adapting back to "life at home" and the attempts at coping with symptoms of PTSD. Foundational philosophical underpinnings for the case study research approach were adapted from ethnography and grounded theory research methods and the interviewing, data collection, and analysis involved an ongoing comparison of data and ongoing data analysis and the identification of major themes.

THE LITERATURE

The study of psychological trauma "means bearing witness to horrible events" (Herman, 1997, p. 7). For veterans, the process of healing is indeed a social process requiring a supportive social and political environment. As history has informed us, many veterans have not received the support needed to enable them to recover from their psychological trauma. As one Vietnam veteran shared with this researcher, "I have never told anyone outside of the military of my experiences in the Vietnam War ... you are the first person who was not in the military that I have told." I felt both privileged, and a sense of responsibility toward this veteran.

"To hold traumatic reality in consciousness requires a social context that affirms and protects.... For the larger society, the social context is created by political movements that give voice to the disempowered" (Herman, 1997, p. 9). In essence, the responsibility of this study has been to give voice to the experiences of veterans. The aforementioned veteran had been living with symptoms of PTSD for 40 years: fearful of crowds, trusted few except fellow veterans and family, and exhibited hypervigilance and exaggerated self-protection behaviors.

It was not until 1980 that the diagnosis of PTSD first made an appearance in the *Diagnostic and Statistical Manual of Mental Disorders* (3rd ed.; *DSM-III*; American Psychiatric Association [APA], 1980). The PTSD diagnosis was in direct response to the experiences of veterans who served in the Vietnam War. Before Vietnam War, terms such as "soldier's heart," "shell shock," and "war neurosis" were reflective of the psychological difficulties combat sol-diers experienced. It is unfortunate that soldiers in these earlier times were often viewed as "moral invalids" and many believed that these men should be court-martialed or dishonorably discharged. They were not offered medi-cal treatment (Herman, 1997). These war experiences were not unique to U.S. military. What we now describe as PTSD symptoms were similar to the *nev-rose de guerre* and *kriegsneurose* of the French and German scientific literature (Crocq & Crocq, 2000). During World War II, there was increased interest in *combat neurosis*, which was identified as a psychological problem. It was not seen as a moral deficit but rather was recognized that any man under fire could experience this break down. Appel and Beebe, two American psychi-atrists who studied war experiences, came to the conclusion that 200 to 240 days of combat seemed to be the limit of combat experience one could endure and beyond that the strain of combat was very likely. It was believed that the potential for breakdown was related to both the intensity and duration of the exposure to combat. Simply stated, "There is no such thing as getting used to combat" (Herman, 1997, p. 25). Cumulative research has supported the position that higher exposures to extreme stress are associated with greater symptomatology, what might be viewed as a dose–response relationship (King, King, Kean, Foy, & Fairbank, 1999, p. 164). These early ideas have been critical in the understanding of PTSD; both in understanding the risk factors as well as patterns of coping and resilience. What was identified as a protective factor against the development of PTSD symptoms was the strong emotional attachment created among soldiers. These attachments appeared to be grounded in an emotional dependence among peers and leaders and were directly related to both physical survival as well as soldiers' ability to cope. Veterans today speak about fellow "brothers and sisters" and how they trust them with their lives.

The reality of PTSD and its long-term effects has been very apparent among Vietnam veterans. An estimated 700,000 Vietnam veterans, almost a quarter of soldiers sent to Vietnam from 1964 to 1973, required some form of psychological help (Crocq & Crocq, 2000). PTSD presents as a chronic syndrome that causes significant psychological distress impacting on social, occupational, and relational aspects of the individual's life. Symptoms include "(i) recurrent and distressing re-experiencing of the event in the form of nightmares, intrusive thoughts or flashbacks; (ii) emotional numbing and avoidance of stimuli reminiscent of the trauma; (iii) and a persistent state of arousal or hypervigilance" (Crocq & Crocq, 2000, p. 53).

Our understanding and treatment of PTSD are still evolving. This researcher's work with Vietnam veterans, Iraq veterans, and veterans who served in Afghanistan has provided evidence that PTSD is chronic and persistent, impacting on the veterans social functioning and emotional well-being. As one veteran commented: "I have been in therapy 10 years and I was always told to try not to think about the trauma but that never worked." Many veterans from the Vietnam War have been living with PTSD symptoms for more than 40 years. Many described how they felt like they had become a different person after returning from war. Some spoke about how drugs or alcohol were a means of coping. Others described feeling isolated and out of place in society and a sense of guilt for having survived when so many had lost their lives.

CASE STUDY METHOD

As an advanced practice psychiatric nurse specializing in trauma and therapy approaches, it became evident that the many veterans were not adapting well after returning home from war. The veterans' symptoms met PTSD criteria and their means of adapting were often extreme and maladaptive. Their efforts to adapt in a nonmilitary environment seemed to defy logic and will. What became evident was that veterans had thoroughly honed their survival skills while in the military, and many of these overlearned skills had been incorporated into their daily lives. As one veteran who served in Iraq commented: "I learned from the Vietnam veterans, 'DNTA'." He explained that DNTA means, "do not trust anyone." Veterans with PTSD remain on high alert and are hypervigilant even in benign/safe situations.

Relevant to the study was how the social contexts, both in war and returning home, were critical to understanding the experiences of veterans. Two exemplar case examples included in this chapter focus attention on the social context highlighting the experience of the veteran and his trauma experience in the military and then after returning home. Direct quotes from veterans will also be presented as evidence to support the identified themes. Major themes within this study include a heightened fear process, compensatory survival behaviors, social disengagement, attachment difficulties, and a shift in attachment bonds.

Veterans go to great lengths to manage their PTSD symptoms through avoidance and compensatory coping mechanisms. Understanding the social context of war and the social context of being back home was key to understanding the broader issues related to how veterans were managing life with PTSD and their efforts to feel *normal*. Many of the veterans who engaged in trauma therapy experienced a significant decrease in PTSD symptoms and were able to regain a sense of who they were before war. Bessel Van der Kolk's research on trauma provides further insight into the understanding of veterans' experiences. "Being traumatized is not just being stuck in the past, it is just as much a problem of not being freely alive in the present" (Van der Kolk, 2014, p. 221).

"Case study research investigates contemporary phenomenon in its real-world context, especially when the boundaries between the phenomenon and the context may not be clearly evident" (Yin, 2014), p. 2). Thus, the focus of this study was to explore how veterans were managing their everyday lives after returning from combat. Data collection spanned 11 months and involved listening to veterans' trauma experiences as well as how they were adapting to life after returning home.

All veterans included in this study had been in active service in Vietnam, Iraq, or Afghanistan, and had been diagnosed with PTSD. The exclusion criterion for this study was not having a PTSD diagnosis. The veterans ranged in age from 28 to 70 years. Of the 15 veterans included in the case study, two were women. The participants included African Americans and Caucasian males. The two women included in the study were African American. The length and number of deployments varied and were not factors in the analysis. All of the veterans who had been included in this study were informed that information they shared could be used in publications or presentations and that they would not be individually identified in any of the presentations or publications. Direct quotes were used in the development of themes and for the case studies. However, the case studies represent a composite of examples and were not directly attributed to any one veteran.

A multiple case study approach was used using a comparison approach. This inductive approach to data collection involved a replication approach, by which patterns are identified and then compared with cases as the data collection progresses. For example, the DNTA theme was explored in each case reflecting a pattern of replication. This comparison approach helped to assure rigor and increase the reliability of the findings. Focus on the personal and social impacts of DNTA was explored in increased depth and complexity examining why, when, where, and how it occurred. To remain true to the data, this researcher maintained a research journal that included quotes and brief examples of veterans' experiences. Included were sections on reflections on the data, research memos, and research questions that were emerging from the data, patterns, and theoretical connections. Theoretical evidence and research were critical in the journaling process. The researcher reviewed major works in the areas of trauma and trauma treatment. None of the data included any personal identifying information about veterans. In addition to firsthand accounts from veterans, historical accounts, literature, and films were used to provide confirmatory evidence (Yin, 2014, p. 104). Yin (2014, p. 121) described the "use of multiple data sources as converging the lines of inquiry from different reference points."

As major themes were identified, data collection continued as a means of verifying the themes and testing out rival explanations.

ETHICAL ISSUES AND RESEARCH METHOD

A critical component in this case study research planning process was the attention to the ethical issues and most specifically, the protection of human subjects. The veterans included in this study were informed that their experiences with PTSD might be used in publications or presentations and that no identifying data would be used in the presentations or publications in order to protect their identity. They could choose to have their experiences included or choose not to have any of their experiences shared and were free to withdraw their consent at any time. As each of the veterans was already working with this researcher and had sought help with his PTSD symptoms, the actual research component added no additional risk in and of itself. The benefits for participants included the ability to share experiences related to PTSD in a safe and supportive environment.

An altruistic benefit for the veterans was in knowing that this information may play a role in helping other veterans in the future and may have an impact on services provided to veterans with PTSD. Participants were informed about the nature of the research and the researcher's intention to share information with professionals and the public about veterans' experiences adapting to life back home and dealing with PTSD symptoms in order to help others understand the challenges and the needs of veterans. This approach for maintaining anonymity was to present the multiple case studies as two cross-case analysis, thus not depicting any identifiers from a single case (Yin, 2014). Such case studies are reflective of the aggregate evidence. This approach maintains the integrity of the data and is presented in order to not reflect any single individual veteran's experience. Given the importance of protection of human subjects, and to some extent the challenges presented in the IRB process, presenting the data as using a cross-case approach and providing exemplary cases were chosen as a credible approach for reporting the significant findings while maintaining the highest level of protection for those participating in the research. Exemplary cross-case studies still adhere to the rigor of case study analysis and meet the general characteristics of case study research, including justifying the relevance and significance of the study, attending to the case and the social context, awareness of and exploring alternative perspectives that might challenge the findings, in-depth and sufficient evidence to support the findings, and presenting the findings in an engaging manner so that the reader is able to "arrive at an independent conclusion about the validity" (Yin, 2014, p. 205).

MAJOR THEMES

Research themes were gleaned from the following data: veterans' experiences related to combat trauma and veterans' experiences after returning home, historical accounts of veterans' war time experiences, research in the area of trauma and combat-related trauma, trauma theory, and films depicting combat trauma and veterans' lives after returning from war.

Theme One: Heightened Fear Response

The first theme that was universal among the veterans experiencing combat-related PTSD was "a heightened fear process." As discussed by Foa and Kozac (1986) and Foa, Hembree, and Rotherbaum (2007), fear in the presence of true danger is a normal protective response. However, the response becomes maladaptive or pathological when the individual experiences the following responses: (a) when the fear response does not accurately represent the world, (b) when avoidance behavior is employed in the presence of harmless stimuli, and (c) when nonharmful stimuli evoke a sense of threat and fear. The following examples illustrate veterans' experiences with heightened fear process.

Veterans could identify that their fear was not rational but at the same time they could not overcome it. Transitioning from a context of combat where danger was an everyday norm, the fear response for these veterans seemed "over learned." Benign situations in everyday living triggered their fear and avoidance. For many of the veterans, this exaggerated fear response had resulted in a narrowing of their social connections resulting in difficulties with relationships both at home and at work. Some coped by choosing occupations that were more dangerous in that these jobs literally required that they be "on guard." Examples included correctional officers and police officers. Others restricted their sphere of social interaction to manage their fear and anxiety by working in jobs that were more isolated.

Veteran Quotes: Heightened Fear Response

> When I got home from Afghanistan I got a job as a correctional officer. It was normal to be on guard and not trust anyone. It was part of my job to look for potentially dangerous situations.

> I never take a train or bus because you never know....it just is not safe.

> I only go to the movies if I can sit in the last row, last seat near the exit. If that seat is not available I just leave the theater. I could never sit in the middle of the theater, I would be looking around and would not be able to even watch the movie.

> If I go to a restaurant, I sit by the door and I have to face the entrance. I will not eat at a restaurant if I cannot sit near the exit and see the entrance.

> I cannot be in any crowds...I do not go to large department stores, the mall, sporting events or event home improvement stores. When I am in a room I take a mental inventory of everyone in the room. I look for any potential weapons that could be concealed. I watch everyone's behavior and try to determine who might pose a risk.

> I do not like to go too high.

> I am OK when I am sitting in a room with other veterans, then I feel safe.

> I can be with a small group of family but even a large family group makes me nervous. I cannot go to church and I am engaged to be married and I cannot imagine a big wedding.

> My wife wants me to go with her to the mall but I have to sit in the car. It is too stressful and I would never consider going into stores around the holidays.

> When I was in Iraq you never knew who the enemy was. It could even be a kid and you could not trust anyone. I have not been able to get over that feeling. I cannot work and I am home most of the time. You know, PTSD comes with its little friends, depression and anxiety.

Theme Two: Compensatory Survival Behaviors

Another overcompensating approach used by veterans was employing survival behaviors in everyday situations. Compensatory survival behaviors incorporate hypervigilance. Many of the veterans had created anticipatory protective systems aimed at survival, where they focused on surveillance of their surroundings and ever vigilant attention to detect any potential threat. Their survival instinct remained on high alert. A tremendous amount of time and energy was dedicated to survival behaviors depleting energy from creating a meaningful life. And, as noted by Ogden and Fisher (2015), survival is not living.

Veteran Quotes: Compensatory Survival Behaviors

I protect my home. I dug a fox hole in the backyard for protection.

When I sleep I have a knife under my pillow.

I never take the same route to or from work. You never know who is following you.

Whenever I see someone who is Asian walking down the street I make sure I cross the street. I do not trust "gooks."

I had a repair man come to the house the other day. I was in the living room with my 6 year old son. Before I let him into the house I frisked him.

When I take my son to the inside playground I look for all the exits. One playground had Plexiglas walls and only has one entrance/exit. I bring a glass cutter just in case I need to get out if the entrance is blocked.

Theme Three: Social Disengagement and Attachment Difficulties

Many veterans described how they had difficulty enjoying themselves and had a hard time being around people. They often stated that they felt awkward and were irritable. After returning from war they said that they saw the world differently. They had experienced the death of fellow soldiers and in some ways felt out of place back home. They had difficulty trusting others.

Veteran Quotes: Social Disengagement

My wife said she did not know me when I came home. She said to me that my husband did not come home. I don't feel close to her anymore. I can sit next to her on the couch and I feel nothing. She asked me for a divorce.

I learned from the Vietnam veterans: Do not trust anyone (DNTA). There are very few people I trust. I don't like to be around anyone I do not know. I just avoid those places.

(Quote from the movie *American Sniper* [Cooper, Eastwood, Lorenz, Lazar, & Morgan, 2014] wife speaking to her husband). "You have to make it back to us....You are not here....I need you to be human again."

I am on edge most of the time. I need to be aware of my anger. On a scale of 1–10, if my anger hits a 5 it goes straight to a 10 and I cannot control myself. This has been a big problem with work and family. I don't know how to be around people anymore.

Theme Four: Shift in Attachment Bonds

There are basic survival needs that include a need for safety and belonging. In healthy attachments, young children form attachment to caregivers to feel safe and secure. This process is referred to as the social engagement system. In times of war and danger, soldiers also search for attachments for security and protection. In the face of persistent danger, new attachments and bonds are often developed with fellow soldiers, brothers, and sisters creating a sense of loyalty and duty to protect. The phrase used, "I have your back" is reflective of the attachment bonds. Many veterans will even seek redeployment to be back with their fellow soldiers with whom they feel bonded and feel a duty to protect.

The opposite of these attachments has also been observed among veterans returning home who do not rekindle bonds with family or with other veterans but rather isolate themselves. Many of these veterans are represented in the homeless population.

Veteran Quotes: Shift in Attachment Bonds

I was leading a group of men and it was my responsibility to keep them safe. I watched two of my men blown up. I should have been able to prevent it. I still have nightmares of that day and it was 40 years ago.

My buddy was killed. He talked about going home. He was going to get married. He had a life ahead of him and was going to build a house and had a business to return to. I did not have any of these things. Why did he have to die? Why wasn't it me?

My buddy and I were on watch. We worked around the clock and each of us took turns sleeping. It was his turn to do watch and during his watch a truck passed a bit in the distance and they shot him in the head. I watched him die. I should never have gone to sleep. I should have been watching out for him. They understand the way no one else can.

I only share my experiences with other veterans. They know what it was like. No one else really understands or cares.

(From the movie *American Sniper* [Cooper et al., 2014], in response to thinking about his experience.) "The thing that haunts me is the guys I could not save."

From the move *Deer Hunter* (Cimino, 1978), the extreme form of severed attachments and psychological numbing was portrayed by the Vietnam veteran played by Christopher Walken. While in Southeast Asia, Walken's character is captured by the Vietcong. As prisoner of war (POW) he and his fellow POWs are forced to play a form of Russian roulette. A revolver with one bullet is passed back and forth between two prisoners and the spectators bet on which of the prisoners will blow his brains out: A terrifying experience. Walken is frozen in fear and unable to pull the trigger. However, after returning home he does not return to his home town, friends, or family but continues to engage in Russian roulette which eventually leads to his death.

Case Exemplars

The following examples have been constructed from the data using a cross-case approach. As discussed earlier, a cross-case approach uses data from multiple cases to construct a representative case. In doing so, it further protects the identity of participants. The names have been changed but the details depict actual experiences and common patterns. Both of the cases represent veterans who were in individual therapy to manage symptoms of chronic PTSD. The context of these cases includes the trauma experience while deployed and then living with PTSD after returning home.

Case One: Veteran Who Served in Iraq for 2 Years

John is a 39-year-old Iraq veteran. He described his time in Iraq as a time filled with anxiety and fear. John described experiences walking down the street seeing men, women, and children, and never knowing who might be the enemy. Being on guard was an everyday, sometimes every minute experience. "I never knew friend from foe." He stated that before his deployment he had learned from the older veterans, DNTA, meaning, "Do not trust anyone."

John has been home for 10 years. He thought things would be back to normal when he returned home, but that could not be further from the truth. At that time, he was married and had two sons who were 5 and 7 years of age. Within 2 years he experienced a divorce. Life was not "normal." He stated that his wife complained that her husband never came home. John had gravitated to work that used his military training. The year he returned he started a job as a correctional officer. He said:

> My work is a good fit, it feels comfortable because I know how to be "on guard" and how to keep the environment safe. All the skills I learned in the military seem to fit working in the jail but they don't fit well in the "world." In the jail you can yell at the inmates and show anger and be aggressive. What is hard is when I am not at work, I do not know how to feel safe.

John worked at the prison for 5 years until he suffered a back injury. He has now been unemployed for the past 5 years and spends most of his time at home. He lives with his girlfriend and he has joint custody of his two sons, now 15 and 17. John stated that he feels lucky to have an understanding girlfriend who understands his PTSD. "She knows I cannot go to the movies, sporting events, malls or stores." John avoids all crowds. John stated that his sons understand but also they wish he could do things with them. John's oldest is a varsity soccer player and John has never been able to attend any of his games because there are too many people around.

John has been in therapy at the veterans hospital on and off for the past 5 years. In our first meeting, John talked about how he felt bad that he cannot be the father he wants to be. He stated that he battles with depression and anxiety. In earlier therapies, he was told to try to distract himself and not think about the experiences in Iraq. But avoidance was only a short-term fix. John's son is graduating in May and John cannot imagine himself being able to attend. He would also like to get married in a year and cannot imagine being in a church filled with people.

Relearning How to Feel Safe: The Journey Back to "Normal"

Over the 10 years after Iraq, John's symptoms have actually gotten worse. He experiences extreme anxiety when he is any crowd except when he is with other veterans. He cannot go to the supermarket or a home improvement store and avoids public transportation. John shares that while he is well aware that his fears are not realistic, his overwhelming anxiety prevents him from normal life.

Ten years after returning from Iraq and 10 years living with PTSD symptoms, he engaged in a therapy that focused on processing the trauma memories along with progressive desensitization. The progressive desensitization began with experiences that he felt were the least threatening and ones where the anxiety and fear were manageable. For John, the first step was to go to the library with his sons where there were very few other people. On an anxiety scale of 1 to 100, John rated this experience a 20. Over a 2-week period, he went to the library six times. The first time he left after 10 minutes because his anxiety level was too intense. By the end of the second week he could look at magazines without constantly watching everyone around him. Over the next 6 months, the challenges increased. John went to the supermarket with his girlfriend and later was able to go to a home improvement store. Each new challenge was met with anxiety and with time that anxiety became more manageable. At 6 months, John was able to achieve one of his major goals; he attended his son's last soccer game of the season. Looking ahead John was working toward being able to go to his son's graduation.

John's progress continued but life was never back to how it was before he went to Iraq. Symptoms of PTSD lessened but the tendency to be overly vigilant and the hesitancy to be in large groups lingered. With the improvements, John was feeling optimistic that he was well on his way back.

Case Two: Vietnam Veteran

Bill is a 70-year-old Vietnam veteran who has had symptoms of PTSD for over 40 years. He was in the military for 10 years, 2 years in Vietnam as a sergeant. He described his close bond with the men in his unit. Although he feared for his life many times, what he found most distressing was when he lost two of his men on a search and surveillance mission while in Vietnam. This trauma has pledged Bill for 40 years with recurrent nightmares and flashbacks. He witnessed two of his men blown up and Bill still questions whether he could have prevented that tragedy. He stated that he has never forgiven himself.

Like other veterans with PTSD symptom, Bill works to suppress and avoid anything that might trigger memories of Vietnam. Avoidance and the use of alcohol have been Bill's approach to getting through the day. It is unfortunate that these have not helped ease the psychological pain or decrease the symptoms of PTSD. Bill was proud of his service in Vietnam and expressed sadness that his service was not appreciated by the American public. Bill stated that he was a different person when he came home. Before Vietnam, he was a down-to-earth, funny guy who loved having a good time and had lots of friends. Coming home was a different story. He described himself as having a short temper and much less tolerant. Like other veterans, he does not trust people. In any crowd, he watches and remains on "high alert." Bill shared that if he is on a bus, he knows how many people are on the bus, he watches who gets on and off. He looks at how they are dressed and whether they could have a concealed weapon. The idea of sleeping on a long bus ride is completely out of the question. Bill is married, has one son who is in the military, and has two grandsons.

One might say the PTSD manages Bill's life and he has learned to deal with it. He does so but avoids most crowds, does not go to the movies unless he can sit in the last row, last seat by the door, and he avoids parties or functions with a lot of people. Bill regrets that he cannot take his wife out to dinner unless they are able to sit at table by the door. He does not go inside the mall with his wife but rather he sits in the car and waits for her. He reluctantly goes to large family functions. Bill drives but is always on the alert. He varies his route home each day in case someone might be following him. He has nightmares two to three nights a week about Vietnam and has accidentally hit his wife once during the night when he had a nightmare. Bill is more at ease with other veterans and most of his close friends are veterans. A major area of avoidance for Bill is that he avoids all persons of Asian descent. Bill will cross the street rather than walk pass someone who is Asian. He will not go to a Chinese restaurant and avoids his neighbor who is Asian. On meeting Bill, he referred to all persons of Asian descent as "gooks." Bill has lived with PTSD symptoms for 40 years; he was seeking therapy again to see if he could manage it better. His grandchildren have asked "pop-pop" to take them to the movies, something that Bill has viewed as impossible.

From PTSD-Managed Life to Managing Life With PTSD

The first 3 months of therapy focused on the memory of the trauma and the feeling of guilt Bill was experiencing because he could not save his men. Bill started with 10 weeks of intense, prolonged exposure therapy, an approach that targets the pathological fear and avoidance. He was also given a homework assignment to start doing the things he had been avoiding for years. Over the weeks, Bill shifted from "I can never go to the movies if I cannot sit in the back by the door," to, "I was able to take my grandsons to the movies and sit toward the front." The constant surveillance of his surroundings lessened and Bill was able to go to the mall and to a restaurant with his wife without intense anxiety. However, Bill stated that first time he went to the restaurant and did not have the seat by the door he was unable to eat any of his meal. A major hurdle for Bill was to work on the fear and mistrust of persons of Asian descent. Bill faced this challenge and began with attempts to talk with his neighbor. He started with a wave and a hello. This progressed over several weeks to short conversations. During one of Bill's first interactions with his neighbor he asked, "Where are you from originally?" When his neighbor replied "New York," Bill was a bit surprised. Bill continued to make efforts to connect with the neighbor and admitted that the neighbor was a nice guy. After 4 months of work, Bill was able to go out to dinner weekly with his wife and not sit by the exit. Bill also went to stores but commented, "I never liked going to the mall...too bad my wife knows I can do it now."

SUMMARY

Like other veterans, Bill's and John's symptoms significantly impacted their social lives. When they sought out help in the past, the treatment focus had been on their symptoms of depression, anxiety, and substance use and not on how the symptoms of PTSD impacted on their daily life. It is unfortunate that too many veterans either do not seek treatment or drop out of treatment and many continue to have lives filled with fear and mistrust, guarded and on guard.

There are still limited resources for veterans. Many veterans are offered supportive therapy but the intense trauma therapy required to address the complex trauma symptoms is less available. In addition, there are fewer therapists specializing in trauma treatment. The aforementioned case examples briefly highlight the healing that is possible for veterans living with PTSD symptoms.

The hope is that this case study research has offered insights as well as spurred interest to understanding veterans' challenges returning home and the impact combat-related trauma has on their lives. It is also critical that treatment approaches continue to be developed to help veterans reclaim meaningful lives when they return. As stated by Herman (1997), trauma survivors need to feel safe, remember and mourn the losses associated with the trauma, and then reconnect to one's sense of self and community. The resolution of trauma and the psychological systems of PTSD for many veterans involves much more than supportive therapy. Veterans need to learn how to manage symptoms in a healthy way in order to create a future and a healthy self. They need to be able to manage the strong emotions associated with the traumatic memories and increase their control of memories. They need to not avoid the memories of the trauma but rather develop a meaningful memory of the trauma that is true to their feelings. And finally, they need to be able to reestablish healthy emotional attachments and be able to utilize their social supports after they rerun home from war.

Mental health care of veterans and their families will continue to be a priority concern as long as men and women in the military are being deployed. It is important to note that even veterans who have not suffered major trauma return with challenges readjusting to civilian life.

REFERENCES

American Psychiatric Association. (1980). *Diagnostic and statistical manual of mental disorders* (3rd ed.). Washington, DC: Author.

Cimino, M. (Producer), & Cimino, M. (Director). (1978). *Deer hunter* [Motion picture]. United States: Universal Studio.

Cooper, B., Eastwood, C., Lorenz, R., Lazar, A, & Morgan, P. (Producers), & Eastwood, C. (Director). (2014). *American sniper* [motion picture]. United States: Village Roadshow Pictures; Mad-Chance Productions.

Crocq, M., & Crocq, L. (2000). From shell shock and war neurosis to posttraumatic stress disorder: A history of psycho-traumatology. *Dialogues in Clinical Neuroscience, 2*(1), 47–55.

De Luca, M., Sighvatsson, S., & Kavanaugh, R. (Producers), & Sheridan, J. (Director). (2009). *Brothers* [Motion picture]. United States: Loinsgate.

Foa, E., Hembree, E. A., & Rotherbaum, B. O. (2007). *Prolonged exposure therapy for PTSD: Emotional processing of traumatic experiences.* New York, NY: Oxford University Press.

Foa, E., & Kozac, M. J. (1986). Emotional processing of fear: Exposure of corrective information. *Psychological Bulletin, 99,* 20–35.

Herman, J. (1997). *Trauma and recovery.* Jackson, TN: Basic Books.

King, D. W., King, La. A., Kean, T. M., Foy, D., W., & Fairbank, J. A. (1999). Posttraumatic stress disorder in a national sample of female and male Vietnam veterans: Risk factors, war-zone stressors and resilience-recovery variables. *Journal of Abnormal Psychology, 108*(1), 164–170.

Ogden, P., & Fisher, J. (2015). *Sensorimotor psychotherapy: Interventions for trauma and attachment.* New York, NY: W. W. Norton & Company.

Van der Kolk, B. (2014). *The body keeps score: Brain, mind and body in the healing of trauma.* New York, NY: Penguin Group.

Yin, R. K. (2014*). Case study research.* Thousand Oaks, CA: Sage.

CHAPTER EIGHT

ENABLING SYSTEMS RAISING AWARENESS OF BREAST CANCER AMONG MUSLIM OMANI WOMEN: A CASE STUDY EXEMPLAR

Esra Al Khasawneh and Michael C. Leocadio

THE NEED FOR A CASE STUDY

*B*reast cancer is the most common cancer among women and a major contributor to high rates of cancer-related morbidity and mortality in both developed and developing countries (WHO, 2015). Developing countries now bear a greater burden of the disease, as 62% of all breast-cancer–related deaths occur in these countries (International Agency for Research on Cancer [IARC], 2012) and cases are also diagnosed at later stages (Kumar, Burney, Al-Ajmi, & Al-Moundhri, 2011; WHO, 2015). Similarly, the burden of breast cancer is now growing and affecting women's health care in the Sultanate of Oman, as the disease presents itself among younger age groups and at more advanced stages than those in developed countries (Al-Moundhri, et al., 2004; Kumar et al., 2011). The age-adjusted annual incidences of breast cancer in Omani women from 1998 to 2008 had risen steadily from 13.4 per 100,000 in 1998 to 1999 to 22 per 100,000 in 2008 (Mehdi et al., 2014).

The Sultanate of Oman has developed and initiated different initiatives and programs to combat breast cancer. The Omani Ministry of Health (MoH) functions under the principle of universal health care, and to date has been successful in its commitment to the global Health For All (HFA) strategy (Alshishtawy, 2010; WHO, 2008). In 30 years, this program has managed to achieve enviable goals in improving Oman's health indicators: the under-five mortality has dropped 94%, and life expectancy at birth has improved from 60 years to 74 years (WHO, 2008). In addition, the MoH policies have significantly reduced the incidence of endemic communicable diseases such as malaria and tuberculosis.

Health planning is conducted by the MoH using a result-based approach to deliver evidence-based policies and practices (WHO, 2010). Policies are monitored and evaluated through performance indicators and updated on a 5-year basis (WHO, 2010). The ministry also supports research and development pursuant to its commitment to evidence-based practice in order to research and formulate policies. However, the WHO believes that the Omani health care system has room for improvement in the utilization of research results in the formulation of policies (WHO, 2010).

The health care system is based around a strong primary health care system, which serves the public on a *wilayat*, or district basis. As of 2013, the MoH was in charge of 49 hospitals, of which four are national referral hospitals in a certain governorate, and 10 are regional hospitals providing tertiary and secondary care (Alshishtawy, 2010). However, the frontline of national health care comprises 195 health centers divided among 61 **wilayat** (MoH, Oman, 2014). These include 23 "extended" health centers (with basic specialties), which provide a few secondary services and 69 health centers with beds. Overall, Oman is served by almost 20 physicians per 10,000 individuals and nearly 46 nurses per 10,000 individuals (WHO, 2014).

Each health center is essentially tasked with primary care, including family health, nutrition, and antenatal and neonatal care. Screening for infections, diabetes, and cardiovascular diseases is also conducted by primary health care facilities. Although minor infection management and long-term primary management of chronic illnesses, such as diabetes and cardiovascular diseases, is also conducted by the health centers, any secondary concerns are either referred to "extended" health centers or polyclinics, or specialized clinics in tertiary hospitals where inpatient treatment is managed.

GOVERNMENTAL BREAST HEALTH POLICY

Currently, Oman's national screening policy for breast cancer needs further development (WHO, 2014a, 2014b). Although the MoH provides mammography units in all regional and two specialist hospitals, these units are more utilized as diagnostic more than for their screening capacity. The MoH has developed operational guidelines for breast cancer early detection and screening program as of 2010 (MoH, Oman, 2010), the program is yet to be fully implemented. Furthermore, these guidelines are still focusing on the teaching of breast self-examination (BSE) to patients and instructing primary health centers to focus on clinical breast examinations (CBE; MoH, Oman, 2010). Current evidence on effective screening programs suggests that mammography as the primary modality of breast cancer screening (Nelson et al., 2009; NHSBSP, 2009). Further evidence gained from asset mapping shows that training for breast cancer screening programs is ongoing in one governorate and scheduled by the MoH for the last quarter of 2015.

As per current guidelines, potential breast cancer cases are referred by physicians at health centers to regional hospitals for mammography. In a certain governorate, the health centers refer to one of two tertiary hospitals, depending on the catchment area. This referral can take from 2 to 3 weeks for a mammography appointment, and mammography results can take several days. If mammography either confirms a cancer case or requires further investigation, all cases are referred to a government hospital with a specialized breast oncology clinic and manned by surgical oncologists. Alternatively, patients may choose to utilize a "one-stop" clinic run by a breast oncologist at a teaching hospital, where women can request a biopsy appointment if referred by their health center, and receive a diagnosis within the day.

NONGOVERNMENTAL BREAST HEALTH EFFORTS

A breast cancer education program was created in 2002 by a group of cancer survivors and their family members and friends; it was officially registered in April 2004 as the Oman National Association for Cancer Awareness (OCA). This program is dedicated to the promotion of cancer awareness in general (Nakhweh, 2014). So far, the OCA has played a significant role in the distribution of awareness materials and conducting accessible breast cancer awareness events in Oman. It also utilizes a mobile mammography unit, which visits every health center in *wilayat* in the capital area once annually and serves to educate catchment populations on the importance of screening and early detection for successful treatment of breast cancer.

Despite these efforts and initiatives, breast cancer remains to be poorly understood in terms of prevention and early detection and is missing from the population's health promotion practices. This is generally understood to be because of fear of cancer, shyness, poor health education, and difficult access to health care facilities (Kumar et al., 2011).

The situation in Oman prompted a group of researchers from different fields of medicine, nursing, and other allied health teams to conduct a study that determined the level of awareness of Omani women related to breast cancer and the intensity of the efforts of the different sectors of society to increase the public's awareness of the disease. The proposal was approved and funded under His Majesty Sultan Qaboos Strategic Budget, a government-initiated project. The team from nursing decided to pursue a case study that could be considered a baseline for further investigation and plan. The case study scanned the specific *wilayat*'s health centers on the services they offer to Muslim Omani women and how women respond to these services. It is worth mentioning that the case study is only a part of the bigger project intended to raise the awareness of Omani women to breast cancer and early detection practices.

THE PROCESS

Determining What We Know

An examination of existing literature related to breast cancer awareness and early detection led to the development of research questions that guided our inquiry. The necessity to conduct a study was founded on the increasing breast cancer cases in Oman and the limited literature on awareness and interventions to promote breast health in the country.

The literature search was conducted through different search engines (e.g., PubMed, Medline, CINAHL, Google Scholar). Relevant, peer-reviewed literature was identified, analyzed, appraised, and synthesized. The synthesis was then used to provide the researchers the best grounding to defend the project during the proposal. Using the keywords "breast cancer," "awareness," "early detection," "Arab," "Muslim," "incidence," and "beliefs," the literature search provided us significant themes, which were, and not limited to, the incidence of breast cancer in Arab countries, recent evidence on breast cancer, risk factors, awareness, early detection practices, and regional idiosyncrasies.

Although there is a substantial amount of literature and empirical evidence in the international arena, we encountered limitations for the Sultanate of Oman. Thus, the team decided to expand the study using terminologies that encompass not just Omanis, but Muslim women in general. Most of the literature specific to Muslim women was from studies conducted among Israeli, American, Iranian, Jordanian, and nonspecific Arab populations (e.g., Al Dasoqi, Zeilani, Abdalrahim, & Evans, 2013; Azaiza & Cohen, 2006; Azaiza, Cohen, Awad, & Daoud, 2010; Donnelly et al., 2013a; Donnelly et al., 2013b; El Saghir et al., 2007; Hatefnia et al., 2010; Kawar, 2013). The dearth of literature for Omani breast cancer early detection and awareness provided us the most valid and acceptable reasons to pursue the study.

The study objectives were focused primarily on the enabling systems of Omani Muslim women in increasing their awareness related to breast health and cancer. To place limits on the scope of the study and increase the feasibility of completing the project, case study propositions were made (Baxter & Jack, 2008). Based on the compiled literature, personal and/or professional experience, theories, and/or generalizations, this case study comprises the following propositions:

- To increase awareness, a holistic and comprehensive approach should be made (Donnelly & Hwang, 2015; Padela et al., 2015).
- Awareness and early detection are multifactorial phenomena and can be attributed to various information and motivational sources, and systems (Azaiza & Cohen, 2006; Kawar L. N., 2009; Padela et al., 2015; Vahabi, 2010).

Although not a requirement, the case study propositions were instrumental in providing focus and feasible results that informed further strategies in the study design and evolution. This focus was especially helpful in dismissing the many irrelevant propositions made during the early stages of our research, and guided us in developing our conceptual structure, framework, and scope. It is important to mention that this framework was modified with the themes and elements that were discovered during the course of the study. The propositions were also helpful in review during the synthesis and reporting of the results of the study. The initial framework utilized and shaped by the study is presented in Figure 8.1.

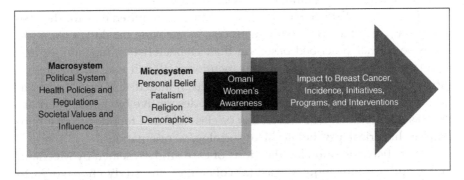

Figure 8.1 *Comprehensive and holistic systems affecting awareness on breast cancer.*

The review of the framework in Figure 8.1, grounded on the propositions mentioned, provided the organization of themes at the end of the study. Although the use of such a framework is apparently geared toward the quantitative paradigm and may delimit the inductive reasoning and nature of qualitative philosophy, we avoided this by employing strategies such as journaling in research diaries, consulting external experts, inclining to direct views on the personal stories of the informants, and supplementing with concurrent literature.

Selecting the Design

To achieve the objectives of the study, we utilized the case study design because: (a) we focused on individuals representing our phenomenon of interest; (b) it is studied in its natural context, bound by space and time; and (c) it facilitates a research description of the phenomenon because it is grounded in deep and varied sources of information (Hancock & Algozzine, 2006). In order to satisfy the criteria for case study research, we intended to focus on developing an in-depth understanding on how Omani women might be enabled to raise their awareness related to breast cancer.

Our study mostly employed the case study design proposed by Yin (2003). Our inquiry was relevant to such a design because: (a) we focus our study on determining *how* Omani women might be enabled, and *why* these enabling factors might influence the women's actions toward early detection practices for breast cancer; (b) we cannot manipulate the behavior of Omani women and other data sources; (c) we further explore holistic and contextual conditions where and when women can be made aware of breast cancer; and (d) we cannot delineate enabling systems because of their possible overlapping and encompassing influence on Omani women.

However, satisfaction of the aforementioned requirements for the case study was part of a larger iterative process in choosing the design. As such, it can be further described based on their characteristics, function, or disciplinary perspectives. Stake (1995) mentioned that it can be considered intrinsic, instrumental, or collective. Yin (2003) added that case study can be classified as exploratory, explanatory, or descriptive by nature. Merriam (2009) suggested that case studies can be classified and founded from ethnographic, historical, psychological, or sociological orientations.

To satisfy the said classifications of case study research by Merriam, Stake, and Yin, our inquiry was: (a) collective—the study endeavored to address issues of awareness that help us better conceptualize a theoretical outlook of the cases to facilitate theorizing for a larger collection of cases;

(b) descriptive—the study attempted to present an exhaustive description of enabling systems that increase the health awareness of women in Oman; (c) sociologically oriented—the study focuses on the examination of the structure, development, interaction, and collective behavior of different psychosocial systems linked with Omani women's breast health awareness.

Choosing the Cases

One of the most challenging experiences that we encountered in our case study was in the selection of the case, or determining the unit of analysis. Miles and Huberman (1994) defined a case as a phenomenon that occurs within a context; hence our "unit of analysis." In our study, an inquiry of enabling systems on how women might generate and/or increase awareness was the unit of analysis. Our initial tendency was to analyze the *wilayat* health centers at first, or utilize Omani women as our unit of analysis. However, our iterative process and discoveries provided us the shift from a data source–focused study to a more comprehensive but focused inquiry on the different systems affecting women's awareness. This happened chiefly because of the complex health care system in Oman and the propositions initially formulated for the study. First, the source of the data are health centers in the various *wilayat* of one of the main cities in Oman—owing to the centralized health care delivery system in Oman and their nearly immediate proximity of care to recipients. Second, in order to provide a more in-depth confirmation of the findings, we opted to interview the main recipients of the services—the Muslim Omani women. Five health centers in different *wilayats* were included, and 19 Muslim Omani women who were purposively selected aged 20 years or older and had not previously been diagnosed with breast cancer.

Aside from the selection of the most appropriate unit of analysis, cases should be circumscribed. Cases were bound based on the definition and context provided by the research questions, as established by Miles and Huberman (1994), and by time and place, as per Creswell's (2005) requirements. The women and the gatekeepers from each health center mentioned systems, groups, organizations, and individuals who might provide further information. However, because of resource limitations and established boundaries of the case study, the breadth and depth of the study was limited to the collection of information from the sampled Omani women, key informants in health centers, and published materials.

Gathering and Triangulating Data

One of the trademarks of case study research is the utilization of data from various sources, thus enhancing the trustworthiness of the findings (Patton, 2002; Yin, 2003). This also allows for qualitative as well as quantitative data to be collected; we converged these two types of data in order to help us understand the phenomenon as a whole, as well as the dynamics between the phenomenon and its factors—a distinct characteristic of case study research (Baxter & Jack, 2008).

Following the requirements of Russell et al. (2005), we ensured that data were collected and managed responsibly, ethically, and with confidentiality. To collect the data, the research was approved by the Research and Ethics Committee at Sultan Qaboos University, College of Nursing. After approval, extensive information was gathered using multiple forms of data collection (interviews, focus group discussions, review of documents and other relevant sources) from Omani women themselves and key health informants from different health centers in a governorate in Oman.

Interviews and focus group discussions were done using guided conversations and open-ended responses (Patton, 2002). However, even with the semi-structured questions provided, flexibility in the sequencing and wording were observed. After the initial interviews, transcripts were transformed into tables to facilitate cross-case analysis and to ensure that all data were collected and all the cases were equally attended. After the table was formed, interviews of key health informants were conducted with fixed responses for simplification and for further comparison.

Challenges were initially encountered during data collection, especially during interviews with Omani women. Local cultural and religious beliefs hindered us from collecting information from more data sources. We also faced difficulty collecting information for a topic, which is considered fearful and a bad omen for Omanis, and this aspect became part of our results through reflexive analysis. Breast cancer is an appalling matter for Omanis to talk about, and recruitment of informants was a hurdle. Women would refuse to participate as they believed that association with the study would put them at risk of contracting the disease, demonstrating another aspect of superstition in health behavior. Others refused because they did not deem themselves capable of "answering correctly." With various recruitment strategies, there were 19 women who were interviewed one by one and through focus group discussions. It is also important to note that interviews were conducted in Arabic and were translated to English afterwards. Interviewing key health informants from health centers was limited by time, availability, and logistical reasons. Five health center cases were included in the study, as represented by their respective key informant related to breast cancer-related initiatives and programs. Telephone interviews were conducted to augment and fill data gaps and for follow-ups.

The collection and follow-up of data from cases were aided by three trained research assistants who subscribed conscientiously to the research protocol (Mason, 2002) and used notepads and digital voice recorders. Consent and further protection of individual rights were provided to the research participants and their statements were presented anonymously and confidentially. Interviews and focus group discussions lasted 1.5 hours on average.

Public documents, collected through various means (e.g., MoH websites, health center breast cancer operational-guidelines booklet, among others), were validated and authenticated by the health center cases. Data from the public documents were considered authentic because publications are done either by the responsible agency for breast cancer or by the MoH.

Summarizing and Synthesizing Data

After translation and transcription and further refinement of study questions, data were reviewed to develop a holistic understanding of the cases. The information was summarized, first based on data sources and then further linked with each other for a more comprehensive view of the phenomenon under study. Other data not apparently relevant to the analysis was kept for further review and for future reference. Data were labeled and stored accordingly. Contact details of the key informants were stored confidentially for further information and follow-up. Mapping data from multiple sources was conducted to ensure adequate and efficient management of data.

As mentioned earlier, we utilized research diaries to promote reflexivity, in addition to noting important points during the interview, which were further counter-checked with the collected data. Experts were also consulted to scrutinize the documents to ensure data trustworthiness. After the inductive, iterative process and resynthesizing of the transcripts, themes were developed and cross-case analysis was conducted. Aside from triangulation, confirmation of the results was conducted mainly by sharing the results with the cases as an ethical obligation to the study participants. Further confirmation was done by involving expert reviewers and articulation and acknowledgment of the personal biases of the researchers through reflexivity (Creswell, 2005). With careful interpretation of the words, themes, characters, items, concepts, and semantics of the cases, the data were analyzed using the

Stage Model of Qualitative Content Analysis (Berg, 2004). The Stage Model of Qualitative Content Analysis is a systematic process of formulating criteria and categories from identifying the research question to developing beginning theory from the data.

The study protocol was developed based on the data analysis. It is important to note that the protocol will differ based on the design, purpose, and findings of the study. The protocol of the study is reflected as sections in this chapter.

Reporting Findings

Reporting the findings of the study is a challenge for the team because of the voluminous amount of data collected. There is no prescribed template to report a case study research. Reporting the findings were conducted using thematic analysis. The repetitive, ongoing review of the data collected led to the identification of recurrent patterns and themes. All themes mentioned are presented and supported with information, narrative excerpts from the informants, literature, and empirical evidence that directly address the research questions. These themes reflected the purpose of the paper, evolved from the data saturation, and are interconnected. Because of the interconnectedness of the themes, we decided to present the findings into three different levels. The results of the study were presented according to the primary data sources, which were (a) key health informants from health centers and documents; (b) Omani women; and (c) aggregated findings through the revised final conceptual framework. The conceptual framework synthesized the overlapping concepts of the findings and intensified the validation of the propositions initially presented.

To summarize the findings from the different cases, a table was presented together with the narrative to have a comprehensive and across-the-board analysis of the different facts related to the different *wilayat* health centers (see Table 8.1).

Direct statements from the various sources were also quoted to justify the existence of the significant themes. Table 8.2 includes examples of quotes that justify the themes of facts generated from the Muslim Omani women.

One way that we used to combine, integrate, and summarize findings from the wide array of data sources and to meet the propositions was to develop and refine the study's conceptual framework. In summary, we discovered that each of the cases presented similar and overarching themes encompassing the different enabling systems that they believe (will) enable(d) or inhibit(ed) them in increasing Muslim Omani women's

Table 8.1 *Excerpt From the Health Center Fact-Finding Results*

Category	Subcategory	Health Center 1	Health Center 2	Health Center 3	Health Center 4	Health Center 5
Staff numbers	No. of nurses	16	17	19	Unknown	19
	No. of doctors	14	13	13	Unknown	14
	No. of health educators	1	1	1	None	1
	No. of community health nurses	1	1	1	Unknown	≥1
	No. of school nurses	7	3	3–4	Unknown	4
	Existing community support group	No	No	Yes	Yes	Yes
Training for breast cancer screening	Staff trained in breast cancer screening	Yes	Yes	Yes	Yes	Yes
	No. of staff trained in breast cancer screening	2	2	4	2	2
	Frequency and length	Annually, 5 days	3× per annum, 4 days	Annually, 5 days	Annually, 5 days	Annually, 5 days
	Training of nontrained staff (by trained staff)	Yes	Yes	To be completed	Yes	To be completed

(continued)

Table 8.1 *Excerpt From the Health Center Fact-Finding Results*   *(continued)*

Category	Subcategory	Health Center 1	Health Center 2	Health Center 3	Health Center 4	Health Center 5
Enablers for breast cancer awareness and early detection		• Training of staff • In-house health educator • Health education activities in the community • Access to OCA's mobile mammogram unit	• Training of staff • In-house health educator • Health education activities in the community • Access to OCA's mobile mammogram unit	• Training of staff • In-house health educator • Community support group • Access to OCA's mobile mammogram unit • High levels of awareness in catchment population • Well-woman clinic • Data on women screened • Personal affiliations with senior oncologists • Contact tracing • Affiliation with Technical College	• Training of staff • Community support group • Access to OCA's mobile mammogram unit	• Training for staff • In-house health educator • Community support group • Access to OCA's mobile mammogram unit

Barriers to breast cancer awareness and early detection	Barriers to breast cancer early detection				
	• Lack of policy and breast cancer screening program • Less space in health center • Lack of access to the one-stop clinic at SQU-H • Time-consuming referral system • Limited days of service offered by OCA's mobile mammogram unit	• Lack of policy and breast cancer screening program • Huge travel distance between center and referral hospital • Time-consuming referral system • Less trained staff • Less education and awareness in the community • Lack of community support group	• Lack of policy and breast cancer screening program • Women unaware about breast cancer screening facilities • Mammography reports are sometimes incorrect • People from higher socioeconomic backgrounds get earlier appointments through personal connection or *wasta* • Passive health behaviors of men • Time-consuming referral system • Difficulty in sustaining young trained staff because of rotations	• Less space in health center • Passive health behaviors by men • Limited days of service offered by OCA's mobile mammogram unit	• Lack of policy and breast cancer screening program • Less education, awareness in the community • Men do not take responsibility of their women's health

(continued)

Table 8.1 *Excerpt From the Health Center Fact-Finding Results* (continued)

Category	Subcategory	Health Center 1	Health Center 2	Health Center 3	Health Center 4	Health Center 5
	Barriers in health education	• Lack of community support group • Less time available • Lack of budget for printing materials	• Less education and awareness in the community • Lack of community support group • Lack of leaflets or brochures • Lack of trained staff	• Lack of private space • Increased of burden, pressure on staff • Low quality training courses; lack focus on practical skills	• Absence of health educator	• Lack of male staff to spread awareness among men • Lack of leaflets or brochures
Requirements/ needs	Requirements for breast cancer screening	National screening program Screen all women with ages ≥ 40 Private space Special clinic so women do not wait in queue Expand size of center One-stop clinic for diagnosis; could be started in polyclinics as they have more space	• National screening program • Mammogram as standard for screening • Screen women every 5 years • Mammogram to be shifted to Seeb polyclinic • More space needed • More training courses	• National screening program • Mammogram as standard for screening • Screen all women with ages ≥ 20 years • Private building for screening • Better quality diagnosis, treatment	• Need a national breast cancer screening program • Mammogram as standard for screening • Increase awareness • Media campaign • Mobile mammography unit at girls' schools • Faster referral mechanism • Increase mammogram units	• National screening program • Private space • Increase training • Instructional videos and models to teach breast self-examination

| Requirements for breast health education | • Community support group
• Education materials | • Increase education and awareness
• Proper follow-up mechanisms
• Every woman should be registered for breast cancer screening
• A more complex information system, which alarms staff if a woman's breast screening is due | • More opportunities to access OCA mammogram unit
• Better designed breast cancer screening trainings
• Gap between implementation of national programs by MoH
• Increase staff for new programs | | • Need more staff to conduct extensive CBE |
| | | • Curriculum for health education
• More training courses
• Counseling training | • Community participation in health education events | • Increase staff | • Education materials
• Knowledge seminars in school |

(continued)

Table 8.1 *Excerpt From the Health Center Fact-Finding Results* *(continued)*

Category	Subcategory	Health Center 1	Health Center 2	Health Center 3	Health Center 4	Health Center 5
Additional information about current or potential initiatives in the pipeline		• Breast cancer clinic to be launched in all centers	• Breast cancer clinic to be launched in all centers	• Breast cancer clinic to be launched in all centers • New guidelines on breast cancer screening • New registers to record breast cancer screening data	• Objectives of 2015: all centers screen 50 females ages ≥ 40 • Pending updates to the 2010 manual on breast cancer screening	• None mentioned

CBE, clinical breast examination; MoH, Ministry of Health; OCÁ, Oman National Association for Cancer Awareness; SQU-H, Sultan Qaboos University and Hospital.

Table 8.2 *Themes Extracted From Discussions with Omani Women*

Theme	Description of Theme	Informant/ Data Source	Statement Excerpts
[I] don't even say "it"	The recognition of the Omani women that breast cancer is a fearful, ill-fate, cursed word. Talking about is almost the same thing with death and should be avoided to prevent having it.	F1, I9 F2, I7 F1, I2	This is how we feel. Glory for Allah! Cancer is associated with death, I mean. When I hear about cancer, it is death. Imagine *harim* (older married women). Anyone may tell her that she has cancer. She notices this but she does not want people to talk about it. [She] does not even want to say that she has cancer. They hide it. They don't like it if someone talks about it. If someone says that a person has this disease and that she is sick….she does not like it.
[I] knew/know "it"	The Omani women's existing awareness and need to know about breast cancer but still clouded with doubts, misinformation, fatalistic beliefs, powerlessness and inadequacy of information/support.	F2, I3 F2, I2 F1, I6	I mean most of what we eat these days [are] canned food we import from abroad. You know that canned food has preservatives and additives. We do not realize the harmful effects of such things, which may be a cause of this disease. This is a reminder to us of a topic/case to which we fail to pay attention yet it is too dangerous. Yet, it can be treated/is curable if discovered early. But if discovered late, it will not be easy to treat or cure so it may be incurable. A while ago there was an education campaign in the City Center to explain to women how to conduct the test daily at home by hand (manually) but I didn't know about it.

(continued)

131

Table 8.2 *Themes Extracted From Discussions with Omani Women* *(continued)*

Theme	Description of Theme	Informant/ Data Source	Statement Excerpts
[I] need help for "it"	The self-proclaimed urgent requirement of Omani women for themselves to be informed and made aware about breast cancer. This also pertains to the call for various key people or institutions (e.g., husbands, religious leaders, daughters, schools, health settings) to help women to be empowered about this health concern.	F2, I7 F1, I1 F1, I3	Our husbands, sons, and daughters should be given even with basic information. They should be warned and alarmed about the existence of a disease called breast cancer. It is necessary to have education to increase our awareness through SMS and others. This will encourage and promote awareness. This [awareness campaign] is very important [not just for breast cancer] for those who suffer or even those who do not. We need it now because many are suffering from it already.
[I] enable/inhibit to become aware of "it"	The acknowledgment of various factors that may facilitate or even prevented the women to gain awareness about breast cancer. This include enabling/inhibiting factors of cultural–religion– fatalistic system, personal– familial–environmental system, and health care–political–social system.	F1, I6 F1, I5 F2, I6	Yes, in the City Center (shopping mall), there was health education about the different tests on breast cancer but I was not able to attend the entire program. I have not received any SMS, seen an advertisement, or even heard any information about the program. Doctors themselves may educate the patients themselves during [women's] regular visit . . . or even to my husband who comes with me during my health center visit. If all will participate in this awareness campaign—our families, schools, mosques, and our older people—this will be a very effective health strategy. Also, make this accessible to everyone—especially in the villages— and implement different information dissemination techniques such as WhatsApp, SMS, TV advertisement, posters, mobile applications, and others.

F, focus group discussion; I, informant; SQU-H, Sultan Qaboos University and Hospital.

awareness. The systems mentioned, according to the increasing level of mod-ifiability, includes the personal (cultural–religion–fatalistic) system, inter-personal (familial–environmental) system, and health care–related system. Omani women shared their minimal yet necessary knowledge about breast cancer and provided different strategies to use the different systems to help Omani women gain more awareness and knowledge on breast cancer. The Enabling Systems Raising Awareness (ESRA) of Breast Cancer model was created to illustrate this interplay of systems (see Figure 8.2). The model highlights the all-embracing influence of external enabling systems on each other and particularly on Omani women through the "pouring-in process." However, the influence of Omani women to initiate interventions across the systems to increase awareness is an "outpouring process" that is considered an empowering internal enabling system. The model also highlights the role and recognition of each Omani woman to be an instrument or enabler of other women in the advocacy against breast cancer.

Addressing Trustworthiness Issues

The framework utilized to assess the trustworthiness of qualitative data is the Consolidated Criteria for Reporting Qualitative Research (COREQ) by Tong, Sainsbury, and Craig (2007) and the requirements for trustworthiness

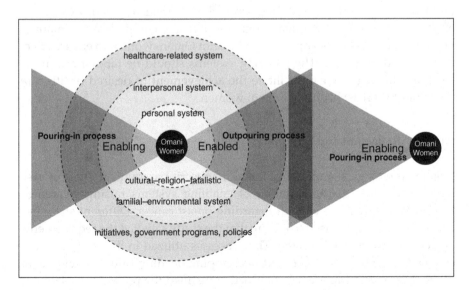

Figure 8.2 *The enabling systems to raise awareness of breast cancer model.*

as mentioned by Lincoln and Guba (1985). The framework focused on areas pertaining to the research team and reflexivity, study design (framework, participant selection, setting and data collection), analysis and findings (data analysis and reporting). Systematic strategies collecting data from purposively selected cases, data triangulation, constant comparison of data, achievement of saturation, expert consultation, member checks, use of reflexive notes, peer review and independent coding, and analysis of data are some of the procedures and tools utilized to ensure that trustworthiness is promoted throughout the study.

IMPACT OF THE STUDY

Cancer remains a challenge in Oman. Most people still refer to it as "that other disease" and remain afraid of mentioning it by name. Specific actions are needed to favor equitable access to breast screening for all women in Oman. Thus, a thorough understanding of the perceptions, attitudes, barriers, and facilitators in regard to breast cancer prevention perceived by Muslim Omani women is highly warranted. Collecting data on breast cancer is imperative for deciding the best ways to apply resources.

Culturally tailored breast cancer awareness and intervention can contribute to disseminating more knowledge and reducing the fear around breast cancer through education on symptoms, early screening and treatment, and promotion of systematic and programmed early detection. However, these efforts should only be implemented in a holistic, comprehensive manner using various strategies appealing to Muslim Omani women to ensure effectiveness and efficiency. The enabling systems should be tapped and must work together in order to facilitate the achievement of desired health care outcomes for breast health of Omani women.

Authors' Reflection and Summary

This methodological and instructional manuscript accounts the use of case study research in the exploration of enabling systems raising awareness among Muslim Omani women regarding breast cancer. Different strategies and approaches were used to ensure that the study satisfied the requirements of a case study research design. The processes utilized in the study are considered iterative, concurrent, and overlapping, leading to the development of the themes and framework that further justified the propositions laid out at the start of the inquiry.

The results are divided into three major syntheses and reflections. First, data from the different health centers and the documents yielded a summary table of the resources, services, facilities, and agencies that can be utilized to enhance the awareness of Omani women. Second, a more substantial incorporation of various systems that other data sources previously provided were specified by the Muslim Omani women. Lastly, the ESRA model or the realized framework was developed to unite all the enabling systems given in the previous levels of synthesis and reflections. The findings of the study intensified the need to unite efforts and therefore distribute activities and strategies to promote awareness about breast cancer among Muslim Omani women through various enabling systems. Inputs to health care policies and legislations will be communicated consequently as the result of the study.

Case study as a research design is a promising approach in acquiring an in-depth understanding of a global health issue. Use of this approach as a method of inquiry is expected to provide a more highly individualistic approach in answering health concerns. Researchers are highly encouraged to utilize this research tradition to generate new knowledge, health initiatives and programs, inform health policies, and conceptualize frameworks and models in a more all-inclusive way.

ACKNOWLEDGMENTS

We hereby acknowledge the following people and organizations for their contributions to this chapter: Sultan Qaboos University (SQU) and College of Nursing, Saad Siddiqui, Anum Khan, Ruby Natividad, Dr. Rasha Ahmad, Prof. Mansour Al-Moundhri, Dr. Yahya Al-Farsi, Dr. Vidya Seshan, and His Majesty's Strategic Research Fund.

REFERENCES

Al Dasoqi, K., Zeilani, R., Abdalrahim, M., & Evans, C. (2013). Screening for breast cancer among young Jordanian women: Ambiguity and apprehension. *International Nursing Review*, 60(3), 351–357.

Al-Moundhri, M., Al-Bahrani, B., Pervez, I., Ganguly, S. S., Nirmala, V., Al-Madhani, A., ...Grant, C. (2004). The outcome of treatment of breast cancer in a developing country—Oman. *Breast*, 13(2), 139–145.

Alshishtawy, M. M. (2010). Four decades of progress: Evolution of the health system in Oman. *Sultan Qaboos University Medical Journal*, 10(1), 12–22.

Azaiza, F., & Cohen, M. (2006). Health beliefs and rates of breast cancer screening among Arab women. *Journal of Women's Health (2002), 15*(5), 520–530.

Azaiza, F., Cohen, M., Awad, M., & Daoud, F. (2010). Factors associated with low screening for breast cancer in the Palestinian Authority: Relations of availability, environmental barriers, and cancer-related fatalism. *Cancer, 116*(19), 4646–4655.

Baxter, P., & Jack, S. (2008). Qualitative case study methodology: Study design and implementation for novice researchers. *The Qualitative Report*, 544–559.

Berg, B. L. (2004). *Qualitative research methods for the social sciences.* Boston, MA: Pearson.

Creswell, J. (2005). *Educational research: Planning, conducting, and evaluating quantitative and qualitative research.* Upper Saddle River, NJ: Prentice Hall.

Donnelly, T. T., Al Khater, A. H., Al-Bader, S. B., Al Kuwari, M. G., Al-Meer, N., Malik, M.,...Jong, F. C. (2013a). Arab women's breast cancer screening practices: A literature review. *Asian Pacific Journal of Cancer Prevention, 14*(8), 4519–4528.

Donnelly, T. T., Al Khater, A. H., Al-Bader, S. B., Al Kuwari, M. G., Al-Meer, N., Malik, M.,...Fung, T. (2013b). Beliefs and attitudes about breast cancer and screening practices among Arab women living in Qatar: A cross-sectional study. *BioMed Central Women's Health, 13,* 49.

Donnelly, T. T., & Hwang, J. (2015). Breast cancer screening interventions for Arabic women: A literature review. *Journal of Immigrant and Minority Health/Center for Minority Public Health, 17*(3), 925–939.

El Saghir, N. S., Khalil, M. K., Eid, T., El Kinge, A. R., Charafeddine, M., Geara, F.,...Shamseddine, A. I. (2007). Trends in epidemiology and management of breast cancer in developing Arab countries: A literature and registry analysis. *International Journal of Surgery, 5*(4), 225–233.

Hancock, D. R., & Algozzine, B. (2006). *Doing case study research.* New York, NY: Teachers College Press.

Hatefnia, E., Niknami, S., Bazargan, M., Mahmoodi, M., Lamyianm, M., & Alavi, N. (2010). Correlates of mammography utilization among working Muslim Iranian women. *Health Care for Women International, 31*(6), 499–514.

International Agency for Research on Cancer (IARC). (2012). Retrieved from GLOBOCAN: http://globocan.iarc.fr/Pages/fact_sheets_cancer.aspx

Kawar, L. N. (2009). Jordanian and Palestinian immigrant women's knowledge, affect, cultural attitudes, health habits, and participation in breast cancer screening. *Health Care for Women International, 30*(9), 768–782.

Kawar, L. N. (2013). Barriers to breast cancer screening participation among Jordanian and Palestinian American women. *European Journal of Oncology Nursing: The Official Journal of European Oncology Nursing Society, 17*(1), 88–94.

Kumar, S., Burney, I. A., Al-Ajmi, A., & Al-Moundhri, M. S. (2011). Changing trends of breast cancer survival in sultanate of Oman. *Journal of Oncology, 2011,* 316243.

Lincoln, Y., & Guba, E. (1985). *Naturalistic inquiry.* Newbury Park, CA: Sage.

Mason, J. (2002). *Qualitative researching* (2nd ed.). Thousand Oaks, CA: Sage.

Mehdi, I., Monem, E. A., Al Bahrani, B. J., Al Kharusi, S., Nada, A. M., Al Lawati, J., & Al Lawati, N. (2014). Age at diagnosis of female breast cancer in Oman: Issues and implications. *South Asian Journal of Cancer, 3*(2), 101–106.

Merriam, S. B. (2009). *Qualitative research: A guide to design and implementation.* San Francisco, CA: Jossey-Bass.

Miles, M. B., & Huberman, M. A. (1994). *Qualitative data analysis.* Thousand Oaks, CA: Sage.

Ministry of Health, Oman (MoH, Oman). (2010). *Early detection & screening for breast cancer: Operational guidelines* (1st ed.). Muscat: Ministry of Health.

Ministry of Health, Oman (MoH, Oman). (2014). *Health vision 2050.* Muscat: Ministry of Health.

Nakhweh. (2014). *National association for cancer awareness.* Retrieved from http://www.nakhweh.org/en/organizations/788-National-Association-for-Cancer-Awareness

National Health Service Breast Screening Programme (NHSBSP). (2009). *Clinical guidelines for breast cancer screening assessment.* Sheffield: NHS Cancer Screening Programs.

Nelson, H. D., Tyne, K., Naik, A., Bougatsos, C., Chan, B. K., & Humphrey, L.; U.S. Preventive Services Task Force. (2009). Screening for breast cancer: An update for the U.S. Preventive Services Task Force. *Annals of Internal Medicine, 151*(10), 727–37, W237.

Padela, A. I., Murrar, S., Adviento, B., Liao, C., Hosseinian, Z., Peek, M., & Curlin, F. (2015). Associations between religion-related factors and breast cancer screening among American Muslims. *Journal of Immigrant and Minority Health / Center for Minority Public Health, 17*(3), 660–669.

Patton, M. Q. (2002). *Qualitative evaluation and research methods.* Newbury Park, CA: Sage.

Russell, C., Gregory, M., Ciliska, D., Ploeg, J., Guyatt, G., Cohen, M.,...Newman, M. (2005). Qualitative research. In A. DiCenso, N. Cullum, D. Ciliska, & G. Guyatt, *Evidence-based nursing: A guide to clinical practice* (pp. 120–136). Philadelphia, PA: Mosby.

Stake, R. E. (1995). *The Art of Case Study Research.* Thousand Oaks, CA: Sage.

Tong, A, Sainsbury, P., & Craig, J. (2007). Consolidated criteria for reporting qualitative research (COREQ): A 32-item checklist for interviews and focus groups. *International Journal of Qualitative Healthcare, 19*(6), 349–357.

Vahabi, M. (2010). Iranian women's perception and beliefs about breast cancer. *Health Care for Women International, 31*(9), 817–830.

World Health Organization. (2008). *Primary health care in action: Oman.* Retrieved from http://www.who.int/whr/2008/media_centre/country_profiles/en/index9.html

World Health Organization. (2010). *Country cooperation strategies for WHO and Oman.* Geneva, Switzerland: Author.

World Health Organization. (2014a). *Cancer country profile: Oman.* Geneva, Switzerland: Author.

World Health Organization. (2014b). *Eastern Mediterranean region: Framework for health information systems and core indicators for monitoring health situation and health system performance, 2014.* Geneva, Switzerland: Author.

World Health Organization. (2015). *Breast cancer: Prevention and control.* Retrieved from http://www.who.int/cancer/detection/breastcancer/en/index1.html

Yin, R. K. (2003). *Case study research: Design and methods: Applied social research methods* (Vol. 5). Thousand Oaks, CA: Sage.

CHAPTER NINE

CASE STUDY METHODS FOR GRADUATE STUDENTS

Mary de Chesnay and Genie E. Dorman

Research courses for nurse practitioner (NP) students are generally not appreciated by these high-functioning clinicians—at least until they graduate and see what evidence-based practice really means. The authors have taught research and health policy for many years (de Chesnay) and served as the administrator of a master's degree program and certification reviewer (Dorman), and they regularly receive feedback that the students would prefer to spend more time on clinical skills and little to no time on theory and research courses. NP programs do not include a thesis requirement and many allow for exercises in research rather than full-scale studies or even replication studies. Even doctor of nursing practice programs (DNP) might accept a nonresearch dissertation such as a business plan or a program evaluation plan in lieu of a research project with the rigor of a research doctorate dissertation.

However, if students are to understand and practice from an evidence base, they should have some research content—that means doing something that involves collecting and analyzing data. We can make this process less painless if we encourage case study research as their research competency outcome. Case studies not only teach the research process, but also have the benefit of helping students develop intensive listening skills they can use when confronted with 15-minute patient visit requirements in their future busy practice settings.

CLINICAL CASE STUDIES VERSUS RESEARCH CASE STUDIES

Clinical case studies are a traditional learning activity in medical practice and nursing baccalaureate programs (Eftekhari & Darlison, 2014; Winkelman, Kelley, & Savrin, 2012). The usual model is for a clinician to write up a report on a person of interest or "case" and then present the history, disease progression, and response to treatment to a team of health care professionals who might or might not be on the same unit. Often these presentations are offered as "Grand Rounds," in which many staff are invited, not just the staff caring for the patient presented.

Eftekhari and Darlison (2014) presented the progression of atrial flutter and mesothelioma in a 69-year-old carpenter. They describe the process of "overshadowing," which is a term used to describe how cancer diagnosis overshadows comorbid diagnoses, such as heart failure. When the cardiac and oncology specialists reviewed the case together, they redefined the sequence of atrial flutter and decided on a treatment option that was optimal for the patient.

Klepping (2012) presented the case of "Jack," a 16-year-old male with nasopharyngeal carcinoma who was admitted to a hospice as he was approaching the end of life. She describes a multimethod treatment approach including drug therapy and anxiety alleviation within the context of palliative team care.

It is not a major leap to conduct a research case study on a clinical topic of interest to the student. In this chapter, the author presents the model of teaching research to NPs with the case study approach and to health policy doctoral students, some of whom are NPs earning a research doctorate. The rest of the book consists of examples from the master's degree and doctoral students themselves.

CURRICULUM

Master's Degree Sequence

Non-NP students in our program conduct thesis research, but the NPs have a heavy curriculum for the clinical courses and the faculty determined that the best fit for them is a two-semester, two-credit-each sequence beginning in the spring of the first year and ending in the fall of the second year. They write the proposal and go through institutional review board (IRB) during the spring semester and present the study results in the fall, allowing them to graduate on time in December. This allows them to use the summer to collect data if they wish, as the summer is a lighter semester for them. However, the sequence is designed for them to collect data early in the fall. They take the theory course in the spring concurrent with the first research course so they have the theoretical support for whatever study they plan to conduct.

Emphasis in the first course is on reviewing basic quantitative and qualitative designs and methods, data analysis for each type of design, systematically reviewing the literature, linking research with evidence for practice, and theoretical support for research questions. The course is comprehensive and all students complete exercises in both quantitative and qualitative methods as well as a systematic review of the literature on their topics. They have lectures on statistical analysis and content analysis. All prepare an IRB protocol. In the second course, students present their research including how they collected and analyzed data, challenges they faced, and how these were addressed, and develop plans to disseminate results.

At the beginning of the sequence, students are asked whether they are more interested in working with large numbers of subjects, such as in surveys or experiments, or in listening to people tell their stories about various diseases and health issues. When almost all students chose the latter and it was apparent they would choose qualitative designs, they were encouraged to use the case study approach or the life history approach (a life history or even ethnography can be viewed as a case study.) Examples of both are included in this book.

Students were allowed to work in teams of two and all but one student who lived far from campus chose to do so. They could divide the work any way they wished but each would receive the same grade, so they were encouraged to make sure they had a fair distribution of effort. There were no complaints on the final evaluation forms for the sequence. Many commented that they had dreaded the course but came to appreciate what they learned and how they could use what they learned in practice.

The teams whose work is published in this book studied a variety of "cases" that were of interest to themselves and that gave access to appropriate people to interview about their experiences. Tatroe and Elledge traveled to another state to interview a combat veteran who had posttraumatic stress disorder (PTSD) and traumatic brain injury (TBI) from his tours of duty in Afghanistan. He returned home to be trained in how to use a therapy dog and is now a national spokesperson for other combat veterans. Anderson and Chambers interviewed a young woman with Hodgkin's lymphoma. Kigundu and Sairo were profoundly touched by the story of fellow African immigrants' loss of a child. Couse and Heard conducted a life history of an older woman living with HIV.

All the students used semistructured interviews and some used limited participant observation. Those who conducted life histories also collected genogram and timeline information, but these were not published in order to protect the privacy of the participants because too much information would identify them.

Doctoral Course in Health Policy

The two chapters written by Kathy Barnett and Amy Pope are based on a fieldwork assignment completed as a requirement for a doctoral-level health policy course. This course provides an orientation to various analytical and substantive components fundamental to health policy. Students develop skills in analysis, application, evaluation, and development of policies related to public health with a focus on issues related to inequalities in health services such as access, costs, utilization, and rationing. Health care policies, methods, and delivery systems are compared within developed and developing countries. Real situations are examined in which specific policy decisions are made by public and private health officials.

Course content includes:

- Historical, political, economic, and cultural context of health policy
- Politics and policy in the context of health disparities
- Principles and consequences of health policy making
- Examination of health policy in local and global contexts
- Formulation of solutions to specific health policy problems

Course objectives include:

- Understand historical, political, economic, and cultural contexts of policy making in health
- Describe how politics and public health policies affect health disparity in both local and global populations
- Explicate the principles that can be used to make reasonable policy choices
- Evaluate the major consequences of a specific health services policy problem
- Apply principles in health policy to a specific substantive area of public health or health care services
- Formulate and justify a solution to a specific health services policy problem

Students accomplish these objectives using a participatory action research (PAR) approach conducting a literature review and appropriate fieldwork in an area of interest resulting in a potentially publishable paper. Human trafficking, herbal supplements, childhood obesity, aging in place, prevention of youth violence with firearms, funding for immigrants and refugees, homelessness programs, and the promotion of collegiate civility are previously selected topics.

This fieldwork assignment accounted for 30% of the final course grade and was designed to enable the student to conduct an in-depth exploration of a selected area of interest in health policy.

These two students chose to approach the assignment by conducting case study research and they did so in different ways. Both of the students selected areas related to their experiences as practicing nurses. Barnett, a labor and delivery nurse, chose to investigate the health consequences and legal implications resulting from maternal drug use. She interviewed people associated with a program for mothers who enter the criminal justice system. In this study, the case is the program, and the interviews were designed to elicit information about the program and how it works. Barnett obtained IRB approval as she interviewed human subjects.

Pope, who worked as critical care nurse caring for adult heart transplant patients, focused on the established policies and resulting ethical dilemmas surrounding pediatric lung transplantation by investigating a legal case that had received wide news coverage. This case was based on the Pediatric Lung Allocation Policy, in which Sarah Murnaghan, a 10-year-old girl with cystic fibrosis was given only weeks to live, and yet, was denied a lung because of the rule of not giving lungs to patients younger than 12 years. Pope content analyzed news accounts and chatted informally about the issue with people who were experts in the field. Using fieldwork in examining complex real-life situations like these and then summarizing their findings as case studies provided these students with the opportunity to further hone their skills in critical analysis, evaluation, and reflective judgment.

SUMMARY

This chapter has been an explanation of how case study research can be an effective tool for NP students to meet research competency objectives and for doctoral students to examine cases of health policy from a critical perspective. Although there remains a role for clinical case studies, the authors suggest that research case studies are cost-effective and easy to manage for students in accelerated NP programs and will help them to appreciate research as a way to improve practice.

REFERENCES

Eftekhari, H., & Darlison, L. (2014). Treatment for atrial flutter in a patient with heart failure and mesothelioma: A case study. *British Journal of Cardiac Nursing, 9*(12), 599–602.

Klepping, L. (2012). Total pain: A reflective case study addressing the experience of a terminally ill adolescent. *International Journal of Palliative Nursing, 18*(3), 115–123.

Winkelman, C., Kelley, C., & Savrin, C. (2012). Case histories in the education of advanced practice nurses. *Critical Care Nurse, 32*(4), 1–17.

CHAPTER TEN

CANINE PARTNERS IN HEALTH CARE

Leslie Himot, Tanya Gordon, Rhonda L. Harrison, and Mary de Chesnay

PURPOSE

The purpose of the following case studies is to explain the process of employing animals in therapy and to document the health and mental health benefits of animal-assisted therapy (AAT). Two animals and their handlers were participants as well as an orthopedic surgeon who brings his dog comfort patients in his waiting room. With a lack of literature describing the use of therapy dogs in rehabilitation facilities and physician's offices, these qualitative data lend insight into how beneficial AAT can be and what it means to nursing. The results may relate to outpatient settings and clinics where advanced practice nurses or clinic nurses may use animals as a part of therapy.

LITERATURE REVIEW

AAT or "pet therapy" has had an increased presence in literature with a surge in recent research methodologies exploring this complementary alternative medicine (CAM) intervention; however, the use of therapy dogs with patients undergoing rehabilitation and in other therapeutic milieu's (physician offices) is mostly anecdotal and lacking in rigorous research. The American Veterinary Medical Association (AVMA, 2012) estimates that 69.9 million U.S. households own a pet dog, and 74.4 million own a pet cat. Veterinary researchers have found that benefits to pet ownership include an increase in social interactions and attention, improvement in mood, and extended life expectancy (O'Haire, 2010). According to Horowitz (2010), AAT has a vast array of benefits for patients including relaxation, reduction in pain, improved hemodynamic measures, reduced anxiety and agitation, and reported improvement of overall quality of life by patients. Studies carried out in nursing care facilities have shown a decrease in loneliness (Banks & Banks, 2002; Chu et al., 2009). Therapy dogs have been shown to reduce anxiety scores in patients waiting for appointments (Kelly et al., 2011; Ruchman, Ruchman, Jaeger, Durand, & Kelly, 2011). Other literature reports that AAT enhances socialization and has been used with child victims of sexual abuse, and used to enhance the general well-being in adults with mental health diagnoses, such as dementia and with the elderly (Himot & deChesnay, 2016; Wilson & Netting, 1983).

Facility dogs are trained to work with a handler in health care and educational settings (Facility Dogs, 2015). These dogs may simply provide comfort measures for patients or may actively participate in physical therapy sessions. Therapy dogs often participate in therapy sessions or perform episodic visits, and many of their handlers are either therapists or volunteers. Nurses as therapy dog handlers is an under-researched role within current literature as is the use of animals in other therapeutic milieus. With the use of facility therapy dogs becoming more abundant, the experience of a facility dog and his nurse-handler at a rehabilitation facility is worthy of exploration.

The perspective of studying AAT from the point of view of owners who use their dogs in their own practice was inspired by one of the author's (de Chesnay) experiences as a psychotherapist treating child sexual abuse during the 1970s (Himot & de Chesnay, 2016).

The mother of a young child requested my help because she was sure her estranged husband had molested their daughter during one of his custody weekends. In working with the child to elicit her story of what the father had done to her, nothing worked to get her to talk. I decided to terminate therapy and to take my Airedale with me to the last session because the child told me she wanted to be a veterinarian and loved animals. We went for a walk and I asked her to tell the dog what happened. To her mother's and my amazement, she did! And, indeed, the father had molested her.

Although the aforementioned story was not part of the case study, it documents a long tradition of an alternative therapy.

METHODOLOGY

Design

The design is case study. Case study research is generally considered a qualitative design but may involve mixed methods, either qualitative or quantitative. In this study, qualitative methods were used. A semi-structured interview guide was combined with participant observation to document how AAT works. Interviews and observation sessions were conducted at the nurse's, physician's, and dog's workplace to observe the team on duty.

Sample

A purposive sample of one nurse-handler and her facility dog was chosen for this case study. In addition, an orthopedic surgeon and his dog were also chosen by a separate investigator. Pseudonyms are used for the nurse, the physician, and the dogs. Grace, the nurse-handler, is employed at a rehabilitation facility. Travis, the dog, has been in her care for more than 3 years, and has served as a certified facility dog for more than 3 years. This team has worked together since he was obtained from an organization that trains and places therapy and service dogs. The expertise achieved by this team is adequate to provide detailed information regarding facility dogs and other stated areas of interest. The orthopedic surgeon has been in practice for more than 15 years and has taken his dog, Chips, to work with him for 4 of those years. Written informed consent was obtained, and the Kennesaw State University Institutional Review Board provided approval for this case study.

Settings

The interviews occurred in both a rehabilitation facility while the team was on duty and in the physician's office while the canine was present. See the interview guide in Table 10.1. The interview for the rehabilitation facility was conducted in a private area away from patients by request and for the comfort of the participants. The rehabilitation facility is a large spinal cord injury and traumatic brain injury hospital located in the southeastern United States. The interview was also conducted in a private environment to facilitate the observation of the dog's behavior while in an off-duty stance. The physician's office is located in a suburb of Atlanta, Georgia, and sees approximately 18 patients per day as orthopedic follow-up.

Table 10.1 *Semi-Structured Interview Guide*

1. Tell me about how you came to do this work.
2. How did you acquire this animal?
3. Tell me about the animals training and how you work with the animal with a patient.
4. Tell me a story about the animal interacting with a patient.
5. What kinds of patients would not work well with this animal?
6. What challenges have you faced in doing this work?
7. What else would you like me to know about your work?

Instruments and Data Analysis

Semi-structured interviews and participant observation comprise the methods used for the study. In case study research, content analysis was used to develop a typology of key concepts, which are then analyzed for themes. The primary tool is a semi-structured interview guide consisting of a short set of questions designed to elicit stories about what they do in practice. The secondary tool is a period or periods of participant observation; that is, seeing the animal in action.

Both investigators participated in the interview and observation processes. Time was maximized by preparing known inquiries before our interview. The researchers are nursing professionals; one is employed at the same facility as the nurse-handler, enabling the investigators to connect with the participant on a professional level, establishing a rapport that allowed for information to flow freely without hindrance because of a lack of trust between the interviewee and interviewers. The interviewer for the physician's office canine is a certified nurse educator and senior lecturer at a metropolitan Atlanta University.

RESULTS

Structure—Physician's Office

Dr. Jennings, a practicing orthopedic surgeon in Marietta, Georgia, takes his dog, Chips, to work every Wednesday. What began as a way to get his Labrador retriever out of the house one day a week, changed the way this physician looked at AAT in his own practice. The physician noticed that his patients and families were less anxious when his dog, Chips, was present in the waiting room and in the exam room.

The investigator was interested in qualitative data with participant observation to document how AAT was used in a physician's office. Through a period of two separate Wednesdays, the investigator, observed the canine in action.

Dr. Jennings did not start out thinking his dog, Chips, would be any more than a companion to his office staff during the day. His desire was to get his dog out of the house, which generally consisted of long hours alone. What transpired was a different way of building a sense of rapport with his patients. Dr. Jennings now feels Chips has become an "extension" in his ability to make patients feel at ease and serve as a distraction to those who often come in with a great deal of pain from orthopedic fractures and other disabling conditions.

One patient in his late seventies, who was accompanied by his son, was obviously in a great deal of pain following an open reduction, internal fixation of the right forearm, which had been fractured in a fall 1 week previously with the resultant surgery. The patient was in the office for his first follow-up visit. The son did all the talking for his father, stating that he was "withdrawn and not his usual self" acknowledging that the surgery had taken a lot out of him. As Dr. Jennings was explaining the role of anesthesia in the elderly and its effects in delayed clearing of the sensorium, Chips made his appearance in the cubicle where the elderly man had not said one word. At that moment, the patient spoke and asked, "What kind of dog is that?" Dr. Jennings stated later that at this moment he realized he should be engaging the patient rather than the son in conversation. Chips was a transitional object facilitating the relationship between the physician and his elderly patient.

The physician also noted a change in his staff's mood on Wednesdays when Chips came to work.

> Staff morale was improved when Chips was around. The staff would perform their routine tasks but often with a greater positive behaviors such as smiling and giving physical contact to the dog. Staff often strived to be the one to take Chips for a walk.

Dr. Jennings noted that a few patients might not be as "into" Chips as most patients, and he and the staff took particular note of those who seemed uncomfortable and kept Chips in the back office for the duration of the visit. Anecdotal responses from those patients that did not seem to want interaction with Chips included patients who had "had a bad experience with a dog" or had allergies.

Emerging themes noted by this researcher/observer included statements from patients and families that, "the animal provided a distraction, pleasure, and entertainment" to the patients waiting for their orthopedic appointments. In addition, "the animal reminded me of home and my own dog." Several patients noted that the animal "provided company" as many came alone. Many of the patients reported to the physician that the presence of the dog eased their pain.

Structure—Rehabilitation Unit

Grace is a registered nurse with more than 8 years of rehabilitation nursing experience. She was paired with now 5-year-old Labrador, Travis, a professionally trained therapy dog, about 3 years ago. This team is considered full time at the facility which for Travis means working three 12-hour shifts per week. The success of this team hinges greatly on the commitment of the handler, which starts even before acquiring a dog.

Grace's interest for therapy dogs was sparked early in her career during an experience with a patient and his wife. The wife was involved with a pet therapy organization and shared many stories with Grace about the benefits these dogs can provide. At this point, Grace knew she somehow wanted to be involved with these dogs but wanted more nursing experience before making this commitment. A few years later, a puppy raiser for a therapy dog organization brought a Labrador puppy to the facility for training purposes and reignited Grace's interest in this field. This time, more confident in her experience level and feeling ready to take on the commitment, Grace began pursuing avenues that would lead to her acquiring a facility dog.

Before receiving Travis, Grace was required to participate in an intensive training program. She spent many hours reading and testing over information regarding the care qualities, such as the dog's temperament, trainability, health, and physical attributes, are all important when it comes to facility dogs. According to Grace, Travis is calm, kind, patient, and loving, which are common qualities among the Labrador breed. She believes that these qualities cannot be taught but are qualities necessary for an effective facility dog. She was also required to attend a week of intensive instruction at the therapy dog training facility to learn how to give commands and work with these dogs. Grace and Travis developed a strategy to deliver care to their patients. Grace's responsibilities as a nurse did not change after acquiring Travis. She still had to care for her assigned patients while developing a plan on how to care for Travis' needs at work and allowing him to perform his duties as a facility dog. Initially, Travis accompanied Grace on her rounds of distributing medications. This was a huge success and loved by the patients. Travis spends time independently in the ICU because it is a closed unit. According to Grace, in the ICU:

The staff is very familiar and comfortable with Travis so they are very well aware of where he is and he loves code rapids...he loves to be in the mix and he loves the excitement of everybody doing this and that...so the nurses on the other side, where I work...know that if there is a code rapid and Travis is in ICU that we have to go get him, so he is right there in the mix, loving it!

According to Grace, when he is in the ICU, the patient's family members

talk about Travis and they talk about how much it means to them that he comes in, he just walks in without even being called, it is like he is checking on them and he will go to the members of the family and just sit next to them and just wait and just sit and be petted or talked to or he will just lay there.

Also according to Grace, Travis was not taught to do this, but figured it out on his own. She also attributes a self-led awareness of surroundings stating:

He is a big dog, he is, but he is extremely gentle and it is, again, not being taught, he can get into the bed with a patient on a ventilator and IVs and know exactly where to lay down next to that person and he will use his paw to tap around or to feel around and make sure that he can lay there and that he is not laying on anything, such as tubings or a shoulder or a hip or something. He knows and he was not taught that.

While working with adolescent spinal cord injury (SCI) patients, Grace observes "an interesting process" with these patients.

When they first arrive to the rehabilitation hospital, on ventilators, scared and anxious, they hear about Travis and want him to visit. Initially, I do make a point to have Travis spend a lot of time with them so that they can get through the anxiety so that they can go on to therapy and do what they need to do so that they can eventually [wean from the ventilator].

As they get stronger, more comfortable, wean from the ventilator, and become more mobile, the teens need Travis less. She has also observed an effect on the family: "The family is more engaged. The family is more hands on." As the patient progresses through rehab the patients still love Travis, but his job is done and he moves to the next patient.

Grace also recognizes Travis's ability to provide care to the family members who are coping with the traumatic life change of their loved ones. Grace describes his effect on the patient's family members:

Travis is great for the kids because the kids are also thrown into this chaotic mess, ordeal that has happened with the family and they are crying and they are lashing out or acting out and you bring Travis in there and he's a huge, great distraction. So the kid calms down and is happy and smiling so the family can concentrate on something else for a while or they get that break from the child or the children being upset and crying.

Travis is able to spend time with family members and patients, offering the kind of support that nurses would love to give, but do not always have the time.

Travis also participates in end of life care. Grace describes:

End of life care is very tragic, it usually means that they have already been through a really tough, long road of the unknown and just a lot of tragedy so Travis going in the room, the family, the stress isn't there like it was before, the anxiety, the fear. Travis just brings that calm with him, again, being the nurse's dog he nurses people. He loves them, he comforts them. He is very patient and he will lay there for a very long time and just let the family pet on him, love him.

Themes

Nurse-handler-therapy dog teams are not represented in current literature; this finding is further corroborated by Grace stating that she was the first nurse the organization working with her facility has ever teamed with a therapy dog. Instead of focused and episodic encounters with patients during therapy sessions, the nurse's dog has the benefit of spending a much longer amount of time with a single patient. The dog in this case has helped patients manage their anxiety, decreasing the need for pharmacological intervention. This has benefited nurses because anxious patients tend to call for the nurse more frequently and require more nursing time. The nurse's dog works as an extender for nursing care. In addition to this role, it has been identified that a nurse's dog provides a huge service to the family members of patients. Simply the presence of a nurse's dog seems to bring about a comfort or security that leads to positive outcomes for the patients. These patients experience an improvement in anxiety and have an increased motivation to participate in therapy enabling them to attain rehabilitation goals. Therapy dogs' ability to increase motivation for therapy sessions is documented in several studies (Abate et al., 2011; Bode, Costa, & Frey, 2007; Macauley, 2006). The presence of the dog encourages rest, healing, better nutrition, and calmness during a period of coping with traumatic injury. The nurse's dog role extends beyond meeting functional therapy driven goals. Throughout the interview, the participant described multiple examples of how Travis had a positive impact on family members as they are coping with supporting their family member through traumatic injury.

DISCUSSION

Commonalities between the two research facilities include a noted reduction in anxiety of patients and families. Throughout both interviews, the participants described multiple examples of how the animals had a positive impact on family members as they are coping with supporting their family member through traumatic injury or recovery. Both investigators noted an increased engagement of both patient and family when the animal was present. Morale of both staff and patients increased when the animals made their rounds.

SUMMARY

Grace's and Travis's, as well as Dr. Jennings's and Chips's, contribution to pet therapy and this emerging concept is paramount in providing an exemplar for all nurses to the benefits that a nurse-handler with a facility or therapy dog can provide. The use of a canine in a physician's office can transcend the anxiety of such follow-up visits. These benefits go far beyond only participating in therapy sessions and meeting functional goals. These teams can provide benefits within inpatient, outpatient, and private practice settings for patients, their family members, and even for staff members. With the nurse's dog becoming an extension of the nurse or physician and having the ability to self-guide treatments according to patient and family needs, these teams have the potential to change the future of nursing.

REFERENCES

Abate, S., Zucconi, M., & Boxer, B. (2011). Impact of canine-assisted ambulation on hospitalized chronic heart failure patients' ambulation outcomes and satisfaction. *The Journal of Cardiovascular Nursing, 26*(3), 224–230. Retrieved from http://dx.doi.org.proxy.kennesaw.edu/10.1097/JCN.0b013e3182010bd6

American Veterinary Medical Association. (2012). *U.S. pet ownership and demographics sourcebook.* Schaumburg, IL: Author

Banks, M. R., & Banks, W. A. (2002). The effects of animal-assisted therapy on loneliness in an elderly population in long-term care facilities. *The Journals of Gerontology, Series A. Biological Sciences and Medical Sciences, 57*(7), M428–M432.

Bode, R., Costa, B., & Frey, J. (2007). The impact of animal-assisted therapy on patient ambulation: A feasibility study. *American Journal of Health Promotion, 6*(3), 7–19.

Chu, C. I., Liu, C. Y., Sun, C. T., & Lin, J. (2009). The effect of animal-assisted activity on inpatients with schizophrenia. *Journal of Psychosocial Nursing and Mental Health Services, 47*(12), 42–48.

Facility Dogs. (2015). Retrieved from http://www.cci.org/site/c.cdKGIRNqEmG/b.4011121

Himot, L., & de Chesnay, M. (2016). Pet therapy in nursing. In M. de Chesnay & B. Anderson (Eds.), *Caring for the vulnerable* (pp. 311–320). Burlington, MA: Jones and Bartlett.

Horowitz, S. (2010). Animal-assisted therapy for inpatients: Tapping the unique healing power of the human–animal bond. *Alternative and Complementary Therapies, 16*(6), 339–343. doi:10.1089/act.2010.16603

Kelly, E., Anderson, C., Garma, S., Russell, H., Klaas, S., Gorzkowski, J., & Vogel, L. (2011). Relationships between the psychological characteristics of youth with spinal cord injury and their primary caregivers. *Spinal Cord, 49*(2), 200–205.

Macauley, B. (2006). Animal-assisted therapy for persons with aphasia. *Journal of Rehabilitation Research and Development, 43*(3), 357–366.

O'Haire, M. (2010). Companion animals and human health: Benefits, challenges, and the road ahead. *Journal of Veterinary Behavior: Clinical Applications and Research, 5*, 226–234.

Ruchman, R., Ruchman, A., Jaeger, J., Durand, D., & Kelly, P. (2011). Animal-assisted anxiolysis prior to MRI. *American Journal of Roentgenology, 196*, A120–A134.

Wilson, C., & Netting, F. (1983). Companion animals and the elderly: A state of the art summary. *Journal of the American Veterinary Medical Association, 183*(12), 425–429.

CHAPTER ELEVEN

FROM THE HORSE'S MOUTH: CASE STUDY OF A HANDLER'S PERSPECTIVE OF EQUINE-FACILITATED THERAPY

Christopher Hayes and Christopher R. Walker

*A*nimal-assisted therapy (AAT) is a growing field and is quickly becoming an alternative to traditional therapies for cerebral palsy, postural impairment, language disabilities, multiple sclerosis, spinal cord injuries, and psychiatric disorders with varying rates of success. The efficacy of equine-facilitated therapy (EFT), also known as hippotherapy, is subjective in nature. Why it should be used and the outcomes expected differ from person to person prescribing the therapy. The purpose of this chapter is to elicit the perspective from an equine therapist who conducts EFT. Few research studies have documented the perspective of the equine therapist on the success of EFT, or what constitutes a successful application of equine-assisted therapy. A relatively new treatment for the aforementioned therapies, EFT has little research involving the equine therapist in general and fewer still with case study research involved.

PROBLEM STATEMENT

This research includes an extensive literature review of EFT for both the patients and the horse handlers. It also illustrates the theoretical background of the therapy including different references to the psychological perspective of different researchers. The chapter presents a discussion of the state of research using the available empirical studies and the reports on the topic. Finally, the literature presents reviews of the alternate application of the therapy in different situations.

There appears to be a deficiency in research focusing on the perspective and contributions of the handler. This research aims to identify what parameters and situations are helpful to conclude in successful application of EFT. The handler's perspective is an often overlooked and a critical aspect of the success of EFT with patients selected for this type of therapy. Handlers are tasked with the responsibility to train the animal and match the animal with the participant. However, there is little history or research on how this relationship between the animal and the handler is established and maintained over the course of the animal's time as a therapy companion. This research is significant because it can further help clinicians to appropriately identify, refer, and prescribe the correct patients for this type of therapy.

LITERATURE REVIEW

EFT represents a type of AAT. Notably, EFT describes the application of horses as an important part of the physiological and psychological therapy method. There are different methods that are applied in equine therapy including mounted, unmounted, and vaulting activities. Mounting activities include riding the animal itself or using a horse and carriage. The horse and carriage give EFT an option to those who otherwise may not be able to mount a horse because of weight, balance, fatigue, fear of heights, or the ability to sit astride. Unmounted activities use techniques such as teaching individuals how to interact with the horse and the equine environment. These behaviors entail safety, grooming, leading, and stall- and barn-related tasks. Unmounted activities also include experiences of handling and lunging a horse. This teaches the horse to walk in an enclosed circular pen that helps the horse to learn its correct bend. This helps the horse to understand that when carrying a rider, it learns to bend into the curves when turning so that the horse itself does not lose balance. Interactive vaulting is an activity in which the patients perform movements on and around the horse. These movements can be very simple such as sitting without holding onto the surcingle or a more elaborate compulsory move such as kneeling or standing on the horse (Gardiner & Frewin, 2005).

EFT presents literature that has a huge reliance on theoretical propositions leading to uncertainty of the results of the initial application. Many therapists are unwilling to try out the experimental therapies, instead relying on established protocols and treatments (Gardiner & Frewin, 2005). The longitudinal studies that apply biofeedback such as the varying heart rate, skin conductance, and alpha and beta brain activity could serve to provide viable results to measure the outcome of EFT. There are numerous propositions of biofeedback in different studies that propose the association of biofeedback to psychological parameters (Brandt, 2013; Drinkhouse, Birmingham, Fillman & Jedlicka, 2015). Physiological parameters could be applied in the measurement of the variables after the application of EFT to patients.

Within the review of literature, all authors agree that their studies had only a small number of participants and that their work needs to be conducted on a large-scale population to see if the results would be replicated. The authors strongly agree that EFT should involve a minimum of two experts and the participant (handler, therapist, and participant/subject). There appears to be an agreement among the authors about the training the handler and therapist must have prior to becoming involved with equine-assisted therapy to include, partnership with Equine Assisted Growth and Learning Association (EAGALA), and North American Riding for the Handicapped Association (NARHA).

There also appears to be an agreement that AAT in general and equine-assisted therapy in particular can be conducted across a wide spectrum of conditions and can have positive outcomes for all of the subjects that are exposed to this particular therapy. They all agree that EFT should be further explored in large-scale research studies and followed over time to see if the effects of the therapy are long term in nature or only short term. There is also consensus among the literature that a particular goal should be set for each participant and the therapy should be geared toward achieving that goal.

Points of interest where the literature is not in agreement seem to be how long therapies should be introduced to the subjects. Some researchers felt that short therapy sessions with exposure as little as one to two times could make an impact on conditions. Others disagree and claim that the therapies should be for a continued period of time for weeks to months to have a true understanding if the therapy is beneficial. A short duration of exposure to the experimental treatment was mentioned as a limitation in several of the reviewed articles. Varying sample sizes were also mentioned as a limitation, whereas other researchers did not see this necessarily as a limitation or drawback to their research.

There is a gap in the literature from the perspective of the handler and their involvement with the research and day-to-day work with the animals. There does not appear to be any insight in the literature review to address this perspective and how the handler's involvement shapes the therapy toward individualized participants. Because of this gap in the literature surrounding these aspects of EFT, this research is needed to provide this unique perspective related to research for EFT and addresses some steps necessary for patient-focused care.

METHODOLOGY

Design

A single case study was used to elicit answers to our research question: What parameters and situations are helpful to conclude in successful application of EFT? An interview was conducted with a single cultural participant, a horse handler that works in equine-assisted therapy. A participant was found who was willing to share her experience. Contact with the handler was made and she was interviewed over the summer.

Sample

Only one participant was interviewed. The participant was recruited by an informal referral from a known associate. The participant was selected because of her profession of being a handler of horses for a company that provides EFT. Asking the participant to use an alias, instead of using her real name, protected her identity. Informed consent was obtained with a written contract with the participant. Although conducting research, all measures were taken to maintain the privacy of the participant. Data were stored on a personal computer that was password protected.

Setting

The interviews were conducted at a small equine therapy facility located in a large metropolitan area in the southeastern United States and has been participating in and providing equine-assisted therapy for more than 15 years. The program has over 45 participants involved in therapy each week. There are six staff members and over 30 volunteers that help out each week on a rotational basis to help serve as many clients as possible. The handler was comfortable with conducting the interview at her place of employment so no other venue was necessary to conduct the research.

Instruments

The data collected were in the form of answers to the questions regarding the perspective of the handler in relation to AAT in general and equine therapy in particular. The procedure for eliciting the answers in the case study was a question and answer semi-structured interview with a single cultural participant. We asked each question and gave the participant the opportunity to interpret the question and answer each question with no time limits. This provided time for impromptu questions and answers. The following questions were used during the interview:

1. How did the handler get involved with EFT?
2. What does certification entail?
3. How is the horse chosen for EFT and specifically for each subject/patient?
4. How are patients selected for EFT versus other AAT?
5. What is the process for a subject to get involved with EFT?
6. What challenges have you faced in doing this work?
7. Tell me a story about a great patient experience.
8. What else would you like us to know about your work?

Data Analysis

The interview of the handler helped to elicit insight into the gaps of information. It was anticipated that two interviews would take place. The first interview was to go through the primary questions and receive feedback. A second interview was scheduled and conducted to answer questions that emerged from the analysis of the first interview. There was also use of participant observation and observation with patients during the first interview. The researchers met to analyze the data together to verify that they both agreed on the understanding of what was said during the interview. This was done to come up with a consensus and to help identify ongoing themes and concepts.

Rigor

The data were content analyzed and the answers were accepted as true and honest answers as the researchers had no reason to believe that the participant lied during the interviews. If another researcher asked the same questions, it is anticipated that the answers would be the same.

RESULTS

Handler

Our handler, "Margaret" (pseudonym), is a Professional Association of Therapeutic Horsemanship (PATH)-international certified therapeutic riding instructor. Margaret has been around horses all of her life and has been riding horses for 19 years. She has a bachelor's degree in psychology. She currently owns a horse ranch, where she offers riding lessons. She also works at a facility that offers EFT to all patient types. She has been working at this facility since she became certified in November of 2014, but has been teaching riding lessons as a subcontractor for about 10 years. Margaret tells us, "Horses are my life." PATH International is the certifying organization. PATH is the leading organization, around the world, for certifying and supporting these types of therapeutic riding instructors. In 1969, PATH was founded by the NARHA to help promote horsemanship and riding, as an alternative avenue of therapy for people with special needs (PATH International, 2015).

Equines

The horses implemented at this site are chosen and applied after careful consideration. Choosing the correct horses is critical to creating bonds and relationships with the individual participants. Quarter horses and Welsh ponies are the two breeds that are usually selected at Margaret's facility because of their calm nature. She told us that they "typically don't have thoroughbreds or warm bloods, they are too hot headed." These breeds typically need someone like a trained professional who knows how to handle them. Per the interview, mild-mannered horses are the best. She describes a good horse as, "where sirens could go off and the horse could care less. It's really the horse's personality more so that's most important." The normal process of selecting a horse has different avenues. Ads are placed in search of a therapy horse and ads are responded to if a compatible breed is up for sale. Many times older, retired horses are bought because of availability. She told us that "purchasing retired horses could benefit the horses as well as the patients." Usually, they "can no longer jump or do competition, but they need to keep moving and keep some level of fitness." Some people are willing to donate horses as well. The trainers and handlers evaluate the horses to determine their compatibility and demeanor. Based on the evaluation, the determination is made to see whether to purchase the horse and implement into therapy sessions or if the horse does not meet the criteria. Once purchased, the handler trains the horses to learn the possible maneuvers and typical strategies used during therapy. If all criteria and training are met, the horse interacts with patients.

Observations

Observing clients during their session was the validating factor for all the information obtained during the interview. On the day of the interview, we had an opportunity to observe participants and their interaction with the horse, the handler, and her two assistants. Each participant had a different condition and a couple had multiple conditions. The different diagnoses observed were numerous. Autism, cerebral palsy, attention deficit hyperactivity disorder (ADHD), and others were being treated. EFT is not only limited to treating patients with physical or mental disorders. Psychological and emotional disabilities can be treated with EFT as well. Although each session had very different conditions/disorders, many of the therapy sessions started similar and became more specific moving forward in the session, as to individualize toward the strengths and likes of the participant. The main focus of each session was to ensure that all parties were involved. The parent(s), volunteers, and patient are all part of the session and need to be included to help create a cohesive and happy environment for the participant to maximize the benefits from the therapeutic session. Mounting, vaulting, the motion of the horse, communication, and other aspects of riding allowed for improvement in most of the impairments that brought the patient into therapy initially.

One observation, in particular, was an overwhelming success each time the participant had a session. He is a 25-year-old patient with cerebral palsy (CP) and mitochondria disorder. He weighed about 20 pounds and was only 26 inches tall with no verbal speech and very limited movement at the beginning of the session. When we first met him, we had no idea how the handler was going to be able to put him on a horse. His body was stiff and his legs were unable to separate. It was a challenge, but the handler put him on a bareback pad (a pad that lies on the horse's back and straps under the belly of the horse to secure) and laid him on his back. The motion of the horse's back and hind end was so soothing for him that his muscles eventually relaxed. After his muscle relaxed enough, they were able to put him into a chair position. As the session progressed, the handler and her assistants started to introduce stuffed animals and played music that he enjoyed. He became more responsive to voice and he would point and say "go" to get the pony to walk forward. Margaret would later tell us:

> It is those kind of responses to riding a horse that are amazing. Those are the days that I enjoy the most! His mother would later tell us, this was the only type of therapy that has ever helped her child to this magnitude. She explained that, "His flexibility will last for 1 to 2 days, which is a great improvement in my opinion."

The observations reflected the literature that studied effects of EFT. Bertoti (1988) performed a study on the effects of horseback riding on posture in children with CP. The study concluded that there was much improvement in posture, muscle tone, and balance post sessions. In 2011, Granados and Agis conducted a study to review the concept of feeling better after an EFT session in children with special needs. They found that hippotherapy, which affects multiple body systems, leads to psychological relief and improved social interaction (Granados & Agis, 2011). These findings amplify the information gained from these observations.

Challenges

The interview with Margaret and the observations helped to provide insight into how bonds are formed and ongoing themes of the sessions, but also the challenges met with this type of therapy. All types of therapies have some degree of challenges. Margaret explained to us that the most obvious challenge is the manual labor put into the lessons, the care of the horses, and the farm itself.

> The daily work of a horse handler can be very physically demanding on the body of the handler.

Caring for the horses and the farm are daily grinds. Adding lessons to the daily agenda does offer some nonphysical benefits, such as emotional reward, buts add to the physical toll. It is worth being noted that through previous experiences, it was found that if horses are not in good shape, good health, or are overworked, it will affect the therapy session and ultimately affect the children. Grooming, feeding, and exercising the horses are all typical daily tasks done prior to sessions. Another challenge adding to the physical demands is the hours accrued during the workweek. A typical week demands 65 to 70 hours. A therapeutic riding instructor is not usually paid on an hourly basis, but by session. This career choice is not typically chosen for its financial rewards; it has to be a passionate choice. This field rarely yields monetary benefits and security. Margaret said,

> For those who are interested in getting into this career, you must have the passion to help those with disabilities as well as the love for horses. This is not a get rich kind of career. However, this is an extremely rewarding one.

A prevailing challenge is the demeanor that the patient arrives in. There may be days that the student is not having a good day and that affects how the horse reacts, which does not make for a beneficial lesson. The bond between the participant and the horse would be altered and would affect the entire session.

Margaret also mentioned the challenge that insurance doesn't typically cover this type of therapy. The financial impact of having a child with a special condition or special need is already heavily felt by the parent(s). Adding a type of therapy, which most likely isn't covered by insurance, can increase the financial burden. Margaret says,

> We have a lot of kids that come from community health. Those that don't have insurance and can't afford to have other means to get therapy can go through community health. So, we do get a lot of those kids. Some insurances do cover sessions. Here the sessions are not covered by insurance because there are no hippotherapists licensed. We do have the community outreach programs that will help pay for it or it is self-pay. This type of therapy is often over looked. There is not much information given to the public about it. It is a great form of therapy for all types of disabilities. It is slowly emerging from the other forms of pet therapy.

DISCUSSION

After conducting interviews and observing patients with Margaret, the following typology of themes and concepts was developed. There were several themes that emerged from the research including, but not limited to, self-confidence, acceptance and inclusion, increased motivation, and improved verbal communication skills.

As so often is the case, many of the patients that Margaret works with and who choose EFT as their therapy of choice have experienced exclusion in many day-to-day activities that their peers take for granted. EFT offers its clients the ability to feel included in activities that otherwise may seem limited to only those who have no physical or mental limitations.

Inclusion and acceptance were overriding concepts that emerged during the interviews with Margaret and during the observation with the therapy patients. Each patient at some point felt that they were accepted for themselves without being singled out because of their condition or excluded from participation because of it. They found that no matter how debilitating their condition might be, the therapist and handler were able to work around the limitations and find a way for the therapy to benefit each of them in some capacity. The setting and one-on-one therapy cultivates acceptance and a nonjudgmental atmosphere for the patient to thrive.

Other than fostering acceptance in the patient, the use of horses in EFT is observed to be effective in enhancing patients' confidence and serenity while enabling him or her to cultivate trust in the people around them. Bachi, Terkel, and Teichman (2012) identified distinctive attributes of horses that facilitate the acquisition of these values. For example, the power possessed by the horses is known to be effective in stimulating or persuading an otherwise defiant patient to see a psychologist and to collaborate. The idea behind EFT is that being nonjudgmental animals, horses are best suited to project love, together with acceptance to therapy patients. Gradually, allowing the client to ride on the horse enables him or her to develop self-confidence and a positive self-worth.

In addition to providing therapeutic assistance to persons with mental and emotional problems, EFT is also applied in treating children suffering from chronic dysfunctions. According to Hakanson (2008), the use of horses when administering hippotherapy treatment has been noted to help improve balance, muscle tone, and posture. An important point to note regarding this theme is that people with mobility issues find significant help from EFT in that the therapy is provided in the form of leisurely and pleasurable activities versus typical regimented physical therapy sessions. Similar views are expressed by a number of researchers whose findings are compiled by Hallberg (2008). For example, the physiological benefit of horses was first realized in 1780 following the finding that riding with a leg on each side of a horse was the best way of maintaining one's gait.

The finding discussed earlier inspired numerous experiments, leading to the emergence of the concept of hippotherapy that postulates that horse riding helps in normalizing one's muscle tone, as well as enhancing body control and coordination. At the same time, experiments have confirmed that horse riding is an effective technique of improving spasticity, body symmetry, and head, as well as postural, control. Other documented benefits of EFT include enhanced sensorimotor perceptions, normal automatic responses, and the suppression of "pathological movement patterns" (Hallberg, 2008).

A vital observation has been made concerning the effectiveness of hippotherapy in restoring or improving muscle symmetry to children suffering from spasticity conditions such as CP. According to Hallberg (2008), therapeutic riding is so effective that notable reductions in spasticity can be achieved within a period as short as 8 minutes of riding. Because of this observation, therapeutic riding is viewed to be a more desirable therapeutic intervention when compared with invasive neurosurgery or botulinum injection; two methods used to treat CP.

Hallberg (2008) also reports the findings of a study conducted in 1988 in which 27 children with CP were offered horse riding twice every week as a part of their therapy. At the end of the study, it was found that the children that had taken part in the horse-riding activity had made substantial improvements in terms of balance, rotational skills, postural control, spasticity, and muscle rigidity. From these outcomes, it was concluded that horse riding has physiological as well as psychological benefits. The psychological benefits that apply to children take the form of enhanced self-confidence and self-esteem, which enable them to move or change their posture without fear.

Adults, too, have been observed to benefit considerably from EFT. Using therapeutic riding to treat adults with physical disabilities has been established to have considerable therapeutic benefits. Like children, adults enjoy significant postural gains and decreased spasticity when they take part in therapeutic riding. More specifically, therapeutic riding strengthens the necks and backs of adults with physical disabilities, especially when the person rides astride the horse (Hallberg, 2008).

Worms (2009) conducted a study with the purpose of exploring the overall benefits that EFT generates to patients and practitioners. The study results revealed a number of useful themes. An important observation made about EFT is that it facilitates immediate feedback, which is associated with themes such as increased honesty and self-awareness on the part of the patient. Moreover, it was found that EFT is an effective technique of minimizing the fear along with feelings of intimidation commonly exhibited by patients undergoing trauma treatment. Accordingly, EFT is a good technique of motivating patients to speak about their experiences, thereby improving the way in which they engage with others.

EFT boosts a client's willingness to share his or her experiences in that the client is given freedom to groom the horse, hence finding himself or herself able to open up albeit unconsciously. As Bachi et al. (2012) report, horse grooming contains substantial therapeutic effects that not only motivates the client to open up, but also improves his or her interpersonal (verbal) skills. Jake, another therapy client, has a speech impediment and stutters quite a bit while trying to speak and express himself. Margaret not only uses riding techniques to help with these troubles, but also employs horse groomers. During the grooming session, Jake stands to one side of the horse and Margaret strategically stands on the other using the horse as a barrier or partition between the two of them. Margaret has noticed significant improvement in his stuttering when Jake is grooming the horse and talking to Margaret about a topic. The distraction of the activity in addition to the calming affect the grooming has on Jake helps him to relax, instead of concentrating on his speech; he relaxes and engages more easily with the handler and therapist.

Riding horses for therapeutic purposes has psychological benefits that include improved self-confidence, enhanced empathy, and an ability to develop trust in other people. Similarly, EFT has been proven to help boost one's verbal skills. With regard to physiological benefits, EFT is associated with notable outcomes such as improved muscle symmetry and posture control. Accordingly, EFT is strongly recommended for young and elderly patients who have mobility or spasticity issues.

However, there are some distinct negative results that have been identified including decreased self-esteem and aggression (Corring, Lunderberg, & Rudnick, 2013). These results have been attributed to the attachment and subsequent loss of the animal once therapy sessions end. There are no long-term studies that address this common concern.

Research to include patient and family testimonials should be included in future research to conclude additional themes and validate the ones that have been garnered from this research. The current research allows insight into a new area of research that has not yet been tapped by taking into account the insight that the handler and therapist have about outcomes.

The researchers sought to determine what parameters and situations are helpful to conclude in successful application of EFT. Based on the cultural participants' responses, this research has found that making sure of a sound relationship between the horse and patient, as well as the handler and horse, was necessary to have successful therapy sessions. Also, the client had to be willing and able to engage in EFT. This was critical to its success or failure. A safe physical environment was also necessary for successful application.

Future research can benefit from this research by expanding on the themes that were represented in the handler's testimony. In addition, future studies should include a large multicentered study that should be controlled, longitudinal, and standardized.

IMPLICATIONS

This type of therapy would be beneficial to a multitude of patients. After our literature review, interview, and observations, we highly recommend that all nurse practitioners (NPs), and providers in general, become familiar with EFT and its benefits. Having this resource can open up doors for many patients that are not responding to traditional therapy treatments. With patient-centered care emerging as the best practice, EFT should become more popular as a mainstream therapy for patients with certain conditions. NPs can also help to advocate for change with insurance industries to cover this practice as a suitable therapy. As the therapy gains more exposure and the results are shown to be effective, the Centers for Medicare and Medicaid are likely to approve payment for the services. NPs can also help to shape the use of EFT by becoming familiar with local charities that help pay for these resources in lieu of insurance. Margaret mentioned that several charities help pay for EFT at her particular site and this might be an option in other EFT facilities as well.

SUMMARY

EFT has been a treatment option for several conditions for more than 45 years. There is a high rate of satisfaction among patients, therapists, and practitioners. The results from the observations clearly show benefits being obtained through this type of therapy. Though we were limited in the amount of observations conducted, each individual observed was able to progress to some degree with their conditions. More often than not, each parent verbalized that the sessions were a valuable resource for his or her child or children. It is still considered an alternative treatment to traditional therapy but with high rates of success, it could become a standard treatment offered to thousands of patients each year. It is recommended that additional research be conducted to examine the effectiveness of this treatment for those suffering from conditions such as CP, postural impairment, language disabilities, multiple sclerosis, spinal cord injuries, and psychiatric disorders. As more Americans are open to alternative treatments, such as EFT, it is a possibility that more clients will see this therapy as a viable option as an adjunct to traditional therapy or as a stand-alone therapy. Moreover, it is imperative that health insurance plans, as well as Medicare and Medicaid, adopt EFT and other AATs as alternatives to traditional therapy, which will allow NPs and other providers to better serve their patient populations. The point of view from the handler is of value and helps provide firsthand insight into the benefits of EFT. The handler's opinion should be used in assisting to evaluate effectiveness of therapy in future research.

REFERENCES

Bachi, K., Terkel, J., & Teichman, M. (2012). Equine-facilitated psychotherapy for at-risk adolescents: The influence on self-image, self-control and trust. *Clinical Child Psychology and Psychiatry, 17*(2), 1–15.

Bertoti, B. D. (1988). Effect of therapeutic horseback riding on posture in children with cerebral palsy. *Journal of the American Physical Therapy Association, 68*(10), 1505–1512.

Brandt, C. (2013). Equine-facilitated psychotherapy as a complementary treatment intervention. *Journal of Counselling and Professional Psychology, 2*, 23–42.

Corring, D., Lundberg, E., & Rudnick, A. (2013). Therapeutic horseback riding for ACT patients with schizophrenia. *Community Mental Health Journal, 49*(1), 121–126.

Drinkhouse, M., Birmingham, S., Fillman, R., & Jedlicka, H. (2015). Correlation of human and horse heart rates during equine-assisted therapy sessions with at-risk youths: A pilot study. *Journal of Student Research, 1*(3), 22–25.

Gardiner, B., & Frewin, K. (2005). New age or old sage? A review of equine assisted psychotherapy. *The Australian Journal of Counselling and Psychotherapy, 6*, 13–17.

Granados, C. A., & Agis, F. I. (2011). Why children with special needs feel better with hippo-therapy sessions: A conceptual review. *The Journal of Alternative and Complementary Medicine, 17*(3), 191–197.

Hakanson, M. (2008). *Equine assisted therapy in physiotherapy.* Retrieved from http://halsansnatur.se/images/stories/MHakanssonarticle.pdf

Hallberg, L. (2008). *Walking the way of the horse: Exploring the power of the horse-human relationship.* New York, NY: iUniverse.

PATH International. (2015). *Professional association of therapeutic horsemanship international.* Retrieved from http://www.pathintl.org

Worms, K. (2009). *Why horses? Why not horses! Equine-facilitated therapy for mental health treatment.* Retrieved from https://dspace.smith.edu/bitstream/handle/11020/10178/FINAL-THESIS-K.WORMS.pdf?sequence=1

CHAPTER TWELVE

"I'm the Guy With the Dog": Life History of a Combat Veteran Suffering From PTSD and TBI

Stacey Tatroe and Laura D. Elledge

"War and its personal outcome are phenomena different from anything known in civilian life" (Tick, 2005, as cited in Dillon, 2013, p. 13). As our soldiers continue to serve and protect our interest and freedoms, there are increasing numbers of veterans that have specific medical needs. Current medical practice is not effectively meeting these needs using traditional therapies and medications. Veterans have a significantly high rate of posttraumatic stress disorder (PTSD) and traumatic brain injury (TBI) diagnosis as well as an increased risk of suicide. "According to the U.S. Department of Veterans Affairs [2012], approximately 300,000 veterans of the Iraq and Afghanistan wars, nearly 20% of the returning forces are likely to suffer from either PTSD or major depression" (as cited in Dillon, 2013, p. 4). Although these numbers are staggering, they continue to rise as our soldiers are deployed to active theaters of war. McCarl (2013) states that increased suicidal behavior and higher suicide attempts are directly linked to PTSD and TBI. In 2010, the U.S. Department of Veterans Affairs (VA) estimated a loss of 18 veterans per day to suicide (as cited in McCarl, 2013). That number is also estimated to be higher today. The *Suicide Data Report, 2012* published by the VA Mental Health Services estimated 22.2 veterans commit suicide each day (Kemp & Bossart, 2012). The purpose of this study is to examine the life history of one such veteran and discover how he has dealt with his diagnosis and treatment of PTSD and TBI since his return from multiple deployments.

Problem Statement

What is one combat veteran's experience with PTSD and TBI and how did the use of a service dog impact his success in overcoming these diagnoses?

"Since September 11, 2001, more than 1.5 million troops have been deployed in support of the war in Iraq and Afghanistan" (Dillon, 2013, p. 1). In health care practice today, there are increased interactions with veterans who are products of the VA health system. This exposes the dysfunction and lack of managing both physical and psychological conditions and highlights an urgent need for civilian health care to be more involved and more cognizant of all aspects of the care needed by veterans. "To understand what troubles those who go to war, it is vital to understand the nature of trauma and post-traumatic stress reaction" (McGuire, 2010, as cited in Dillon, 2013, p. 13). Although the VA is making strides to renovate the programs available to treat veterans with PTSD with evidence-based psychotherapies, veterans are still struggling and suicide rates continue to rise (Finley, 2014). According to Yount, Olmert, and Lee (2012) returning veterans diagnosed with PTSD or other mental health conditions, 60% of those still meet criteria for PTSD after treatment with empirically supported interventions. The multitude of veterans spilling over into civilian health care demands a better understanding of these veterans, their experiences, their specific diagnoses, and successful treatments.

After a thorough review of the literature on the topic of combat veterans with PTSD and TBI and the use of service dog therapy, there are extremely limited research studies in this specific field of study. It is concluded that not only is the literature extremely limited and cannot be categorized as research, but also the majority of all of the literature pertaining to this subject are in agreement that more research is desperately needed. The current published articles contain anecdotal evidence and background information on separate aspects of the topics. Dillon's (2013) efforts were not without the same difficulties locating and identifying current research. "While little difficulty was experienced finding literature regarding outcomes of PTSD treatment, the effects of service animals and PTSD seemed to be lacking within the literature" (Dillon, 2013, p. 48). Dillon's thesis (2013) concludes the following: states the obvious problem with the incidence of PTSD and suicide among combat veterans; acknowledges the failures of current treatments; recognizes the benefits of animal-assisted therapies (AAT); praises the efforts of current programs using service dogs in treating veterans with PTSD; and tirelessly attempts to initiate a local program of such with the VA to benefit veterans with PTSD. Dillon's thesis and area of study is social work. "From a social work perspective, this gap in literature is alarming when attending to the needs of clients from a holistic, bio–psycho–social systems approach" (Dillon, 2013, p. 48). These concerns from a primary health care perspective are equivocal.

Assumptions

This life history will be conducted with the assumption that this combat veteran will be relaying the truth as he sees it.

Definitions

It is important to note there are specific differences between a veteran and a combat veteran. A veteran is anyone who has ever served in the military. A combat veteran is defined as a military person, including reservist and National Guard, who served on active duty in a theater of combat operations, otherwise known as war. War "pushes soldiers to go beyond what is thought to be humanly possible" (Dillon, 2013, p. 14). Although there are many illnesses, psychiatric and medical, that plagued veterans, the combat veteran in this life history study leads the focus to PTSD and TBI.

PTSD is defined by the American Psychiatric Association (APA, 2000) as numbed emotions, hyperarousal, reliving the traumatic event(s), and avoiding stimuli associated with the trauma(s) (as cited in Dillon, 2013, p. 15). Although PTSD can affect anyone following a trauma, Shay (1994) suggests there are essential manifestations in postwar veterans following combat trauma (as cited in Dillon, 2013, p. 15). These include loss of authority over mental functioning (especially memory and perception); persistent mobilization for lethal danger; potential for violence; chronic health problems; expectation of betrayal and exploitation; lack of trust; and substance abuse (Shay, 1994, as cited in Dillon, 2013).

TBI is defined as an injury to the brain caused by trauma. It can be graded as mild, moderate, or severe. Symptoms included for TBI are photophobia, hyperacusis, anxiety, chronic depression, detachment, stoicism, malaise, delayed thought processes, recurrent headaches, fatigue, difficulty with concentration, and simple organizational difficulties (as cited in Dillon, 2013).

Today, the VA (2015) states, "Clinically, there is not enough research yet to know if dogs actually help treat PTSD and its symptoms. Evidenced-based therapies and medications for PTSD are supported by research" (VA, 2015, para 2). According to the VA and U.S. Department of Defense (DOD), current recommended or traditional treatments for PTSD and TBI include a combination of psychosocial or cognitive behavioral therapies and pharmacologic interventions. Dillon (2013) reports that first-line therapies used by the VA and DOD are prolonged exposure (PE) therapy and cognitive processing therapy (CPT). The PE therapy includes four main therapy components: psychoevaluation, in vivo exposure, imaginal exposure, and emotional processing (Dillon, 2013). CPT therapy includes both cognitive and exposure components (Dillon, 2013). Currently, these are the only VA financially covered therapies provided for veterans with PTSD. Psychotropic medications are also commonly used in the treatment of PTSD. Pharmacotherapy is easier than talk therapy, is less time-intensive, and can be administered by nonmental health professionals (Dillon, 2013). Despite the fact that research has found insufficient evidence supporting the efficacy of medications for PTSD, it continues to be included in the current recommended treatment guidelines (Sharpless & Barber, 2011, as cited in Dillon, 2013).

The key feature in this combat veteran's recovery is the introduction of a trained service dog. Service dog is defined as "any dog that is individually trained to do work or perform tasks for the benefit of an individual with a disability, including a physical, sensory, psychiatric, intellectual, or other mental disability" (as cited by Shubert, 2012, p. 21). Yount et al. (2012) find that there is a void in rigorous scientific evidence needed to gain the support from the VA and DOD to fund programs in the placement of service dogs with veterans suffering from psychiatric disabilities. "Successful programs such as animal assisted therapy remain unknown to the medical community at large and, consequently, underutilized, despite their demonstrated efficacy and the rehabilitative milieu" (Yeager & Irwin, 2012, p. 57).

LITERATURE REVIEW

It is significant to point out the lack of existing research studies that are focused on veterans suffering with PTSD and/or TBI and the utilization of service dog therapy in their treatment. The gaps in said research are glaringly evident and potentiate the lack of financing of alternative therapy programs for veterans.

Service Dog Training Program for Treatment of Posttraumatic Stress in Service Members

This is a cumulative review of Yount's research projects involving service dogs and veterans with PTSD (Yount et al., 2012). Yount developed a program for the treatment of veterans suffering from PTSD using service dogs. The service dog program he established was designed to be a safe alternative to drug therapy in traumatic brain injury patients (Yount et al., 2012). The program consists of veterans suffering from PTSD being given the opportunity to participate in the training of dogs that are destined to be the service dogs of other veterans with disabilities. The review covers findings discovered through multiple project sites with varying numbers of participants. All were conducted at military treatment facilities. Yount found throughout the research sites that his program was cost-effective by "providing dog-assisted therapeutic relief to the largest number of PTSD patients with a limited number of service dogs" (Yount et al., 2012, p. 64).

Yount et al. (2012) found that both the warrior trainer and the service dog recipient were provided the opportunity to benefit from powerful relief of PTSD symptoms that bonding with the dog provides. Not only was the program found to be cost-effective, but also clinically impactful. Yount et al. (2012) found that the clinicians and instructors from the program recorded many improvements based on a collection of their anecdotal reports.

The theory on why this works is thought to have a medical basis having to do with the neurochemistry of the brain, specifically oxytocin. Handlin et al. (2011) found that after 15 minutes of interaction both dog and owner displayed a decrease in their heart rate along with a significant increase in their serum oxytocin level (as cited in Yount et al., 2012). Yount et al. (2012) hypothesize that this therapy of human–animal bonding works because of increased levels of the neurochemical oxytocin, which is an antistress agent in humans, caused by the interaction with dogs. The goal was not only to advance the understanding of animals and their healing power, but also "provide the rigorous science that the Department of Defense and the Department of Veterans Affairs need to support animal-assisted therapy programs and the placement of service dogs with service members and Veterans with psychiatric and physical disabilities" (Yount et al., 2012, p. 67).

Potential Benefits of Canine Companionship for Military Veterans with PTSD

Let it be noted that this study was not discovered in the original search based on the keywords specific to this study: combat veterans, PTSD, TBI, service dog, veterans. Dates included in the original search went back to 1972. The decision was made to attempt to find and include at least one loosely related research study. It was found that the study does not pertain specifically to service dogs and therefore was not inclusive of the original search criteria. The researchers recognize the study may have limited application (Stern et al., 2013).

The study was a retrospective survey of 30 veterans with a diagnosis of PTSD. The selection for inclusion in the study was based on their participation in treatment at VA outpatient clinics and voluntary admissions made by the veterans to their primary clinicians that they had been helped by their dogs. After obtaining written informed consents, participants were given a packet that contained a series of different questionnaires:

- The Beck Depression Inventory (DBI-II): A survey in which respondants reflect on the previous 2 weeks and scale their depressive symptoms in 21 different statement groups. The survey uses a Likert scale of 0 to 3, 0 being no disturbance and 3 being maximal disturbances.
- The Dog Information Sheet: An 18-item questionnaire specific to this study. Used to gather details about the canine. Questions inquired about length of ownership, any training classes, the veteran's caretaking role, hours of interaction, and so forth.
- The Dog Relationship Questionnaire: A Likert scale survey developed specifically for this study. It included 18 statements, which were rated 1 to 5 with 1 meaning strongly disagree and 5 meaning strongly agree. Statements included pertained to common PTSD symptoms and statements that had been quoted from patients, such as "Since I got my dog, I've...felt calmer, felt less lonely, felt less worried that someone might harm me or my family, felt less depressed, felt less angry or irritable."
- Lexington Attachment to Pets Scale (LAPS): "This is a validated Likert scale that contains 23 statements about respondants' beliefs about their non-human companion, to which they are asked if they strongly agree, somewhat agree, somewhat disagree, or strongly agree" (Stern et al., 2013, p. 573).
- PTSD Checklist–Military Version (PCL-M): A Likert scale with 17 measures that evaluate the severity of PTSD symptoms for the previous month. Scored on a 5-point scale, 1 being "not at all" and 5 being "extremely." This scale is "psychometrically sound and is the instrument recommended to assess PTSD in military members by the VA/DOD clinical practice guideline for the Management of Post-Traumatic Stress" (Stern et al., 2013, p. 573).
- Veterans 36-item Short Form Health Survey and Health Behaviors Questionnaire: This tool assesses the quality of life in veterans related to their health. This provides scores for mental- and physical-health–related quality of life.

Results reported that these veterans experienced improvement in several areas by having a relationship with a dog. These improvements included feeling less depressed, calmer, less lonely, decreased worry about their family's safety, as well as their own safety, and they had improved self-worth. The study also found that these veterans enjoyed nature and exercised more and reported a very close and supportive relationship with their dog.

A few additional findings were that the veterans, although they still experienced harmful memories, they sensed their dogs tried to cheer them up when this occurred. This suggests that the dog, in some way, decreases the negative impact of reliving their trauma. About 86% of the participants felt that their dogs made attempts to comfort them during nightmares.

METHODOLOGY

The method for this life history was based on de Chesnay's ethnographic life history design (de Chesnay, 2005). The sample consists of one person who was recruited because he was a graduate of a service dog program catering to veterans with PTSD and TBI. Three methods of data collection were used to complete the study: semi-structured interviews, genogram, and timeline, although in qualitative research, the primary tool is the researchers and their ability to establish rapport. A basic foundation of rapport was established through multiple e-mails and messages about the prospect of conducting the study. Once institutional review board (IRB) approval was obtained, the researchers traveled to the study subject's home to conduct the interviews and to observe him in his own surroundings, his home life, and his interactions with his service dog. The study subject has a vested interest in the accurate depiction of his story and the success of this therapy being reported. Immediately following the interview, the researchers debriefed their experience and recorded their initial thoughts and findings. The interview was audio recorded and transcribed. Each researcher independently read the transcript looking for key concepts to emerge. Replicability was insured by the researchers following the written proposal and using specific written interview questions. In an unusual twist after data were collected, the participant requested that we use his real name so an amendment to the IRB was solicited in order to accommodate his wishes.

RESULTS

Retired Captain Jason Haag served 14 years in the United States Marine Corps and completed three deployments to active theaters of war, two tours of duty to Iraq and one to Afghanistan. As a result of his service, he was highly decorated to include the Purple Heart and the Navy and Marine Corps Commendation Medal of Valor Device and Gold Star, among many others. His military career ended in a medical retirement because of the diagnosis of PTSD and TBI. Jason suffered through multiple-failed treatments until finally being provided his service dog, Axel. He received Axel from an organization that rescues canines and specifically trains them to assist combat veterans with the unique needs of those suffering with PTSD and/or TBI. Jason states that his "mission is to be a living representative of an active combat veteran who has overcome the debilitating effects of PTSD and TBI with the help of my service dog, Axel."

He is currently the national director of Military Affairs for the American Humane Association. As a public speaker he works now with military veterans, press, public, and policy makers, to give a voice to the community of veterans who suffer in silence, and to serve as a beacon of hope that combat veterans can live a life "that is whole and free of fear."

Five concepts emerged from the interviews: protector, sacrifice, darkness, fortitude, and redemption. All of these concepts weave themselves throughout Jason's life with the exception of darkness. Darkness encompasses a period of time that he passed through and then emerged from.

Jason has been a protector since he joined the marines. His desire has been to protect his country, his fellow soldiers, his family, and fellow veterans. In talking about the marines, he shared that he quickly knew he was where he was supposed to be and doing what he was meant to do. Following 9/11, he willingly heeded the call to war fulfilling the duty to protect his country. After his first deployment, which was traumatic in many ways for him, he returned with the need to protect the new soldiers from seeing and experiencing what he had already lived through. Jason said, "If I could take the place of somebody else that had never been through it, I'd rather be that guy." He consistently referred to his fellow soldiers as "my guys." He protected his family by not divulging the extent of his injuries in battle as well as the depth of his suffering following his return. He isolated himself from his family in order to keep himself from harming them by living in his own basement for close to a year. He commented that he would emerge from the basement only after the kids had gone to bed. His life now is driven by the hope that his story will reach "even one" veteran suffering from PTSD.

The second concept to emerge was sacrifice. Jason has suffered personal, physical, and emotional sacrifice in his life. Sacrifice is to surrender or give up, or permit injury, or disadvantage to, for the sake of something else. Most notably, Jason sacrificed something that no human being should ever have to sacrifice, his humanity. War is the thing nightmares are made of. The innocence of the human mind and psyche are lost to bloodshed and lives taken. What is seen and experienced can never be unseen. Much like the tattoos that adorn many parts of his body and serve as personal memorials for all he has experienced and lost, this forever resides within him as the thing that broke him, the thing that scares him, and one of the things that drives him to save others. What follows is a poem written by Jason and displayed as one of his most prominent tattoos:

> There has been so much sorrow
> sowed from this War
> It has brought tears, chaos
> tragedy and death.
> Friendships forged with the
> destruction, charred wreckage
> littered all over the desolate land.
> So many friends and enemies blood
> spilled on the scorched earth.
> Our souls linked as the screams of death
> echo through this War. Forever coupled by the
> devastation, until the last breath…
> Your pain has washed away, though flooded into
> ours to stay. The torment of emptiness by the loss
> from this War.

Personally, he gave up a life with his family during the years of his deployment and the period of darkness that he lived through following those deployments. He went months without communication with his wife. She laughed that an entire box of her letters and care packages she sent to him on his first deployment were returned to her after Jason was already home from that 6-month deployment. Physically, Jason recalls being awake for 48 hours at a time and going for almost 6 months without actually showering. He received a Purple Heart for the injuries he suffered in Iraq. Emotionally, in essence, he has sacrificed himself. As a marine, he feels the need to display strength in all things and he has had to sacrifice those ideals in order to admit publically that he is not "indestructible." Even with successful treatment of PTSD and TBI, he acknowledges that he will never be himself again.

Darkness is the next concept. The term darkness was first used by Jason's wife in describing Jason's worst days of struggling with PTSD and TBI and his journey of seeking treatment. Through many subsequent analyses of the interview transcripts, it was found to be a critical concept in this life history. This darkness began during Jason's first deployment. Jason attributes this first deployment as a major defining moment in his life and the most likely cause of his PTSD and TBI. He cites the many firsts that occurred there: the first time he was shot at; the first time he was shot; and the first time he shot someone. He also admits it was "the first time I killed someone and saw others being killed." He described his frustration with multiple-failed attempts with the therapies offered by the military. He was overcome with worry about soldiers still deployed; he was having nightmares and was unable to sleep; he developed what he called the "fucking shakes," and he could not reintegrate into his normal family routine. He was so emotionally unstable during episodes of flashbacks that he feared for the safety of his family. He sequestered himself to living in the basement apart from his family. He slept with a gun under his pillow and spiraled to the point that his only communication with his wife was through text message. He was effectively a prisoner in his own home. He was concerned he would succumb to his hopelessness and commit suicide. At his worst and during his darkest days, he was faced with an ultimatum to either find effective treatment and get it together, or lose his family.

How Jason responded to this ultimatum exemplified the fourth concept, fortitude. Fortitude is courage in pain or adversity. On deeper reflection of Jason's life, this concept is evident throughout. His fortitude is an indelible component of his character that drives him to adapt and overcome adversity. His formidable years were overshadowed by his parents' struggle with alcoholism. As a teenager, his own behavior and choices found him facing legal consequences that lost him first, a college scholarship and then later, a chance at the possibility of professional sports. In fact, he chose to join the marines when a judge presented it as an option in lieu of jail. When he was in battle, he refused to be medically evacuated after being shot and suffering the close impact of rocket-propelled grenade. He recalls that the medic "bandaged my legs up and I just walked off back to my squad. I took some antibiotics and we pushed on." Being an ethos of the marines, his fortitude was recognized and garnered him battlefield rank and the opportunity to become an officer. The discretionary power of Jason's fortitude carried him through the early days of his undiagnosed PTSD and TBI, poor coping mechanisms, multiple-failed attempts at formal treatment, resisting the temptation of suicide, and ultimately discovering effective treatment.

This courage in pain or in adversity bridged him into rehabilitation leading to the final concept of redemption. Redemption verses recovery was chosen because recovery suggests a return to normal, whereas redemption is a deliverance or rescue from the pain and adversity he has overcome. In this case, redemption came in the form of a dog, Axel, that was also in need of being rescued. Jason turned to an organization that specializes in rescuing dogs from kill shelters and training them to become service dogs to wounded veterans suffering from PTSD and/or TBI. Although skeptical of both dogs and this form of treatment, Jason was awarded and then accepted a slot in this organization's program. The dogs are chosen, trained, and paired specifically with the veterans. Jason and Axel were put together and spent 3 weeks at this organization's facility where they participated in daily training and bonding. They learned to use this partnership to be able to function together. Quickly, Jason realized the potential of this treatment when Axel woke him from multiple nightmares during their stay. They graduated the program and flew home together. Just after landing, Jason took Axel to his son's lacrosse game, something he had been incapable of prior to Axel. That night, for the first time in more than a year, he slept in his bedroom with his wife. He did not return to the basement. Four months later, Jason and Axel traveled to Colorado to go snowboarding. Jason says once they got to their hotel room, they stopped and looked at each other and he said to Axel, "Holy shit, we just got on a plane and flew to Colorado." That is when he knew it worked. This occurred two-and-half years ago. Jason is not back to normal. By his own admission he will never be who he was before war. With Axel, he has adapted and overcome to create a new normal. This new normal is Jason with Axel, two inseparable parts of a whole. Jason's wife describes Axel as "the missing piece Jason didn't know he was searching for." In his words, "I've gone from I to we." Although his road to redemption has never been straight, with Axel he has reinvented himself and has taken on a new mission with new goals that go above and beyond a personal rehabilitation. They did not stop with just fixing Jason. Together they are driven to speak out and raise awareness of the suffering of other veterans and the availability of this formidable, effective treatment. In doing so, paired with Axel, Jason once again exemplifies the aforementioned concepts of this life history: protector, sacrifice, and fortitude.

DISCUSSION

What is one combat veteran's experience with PTSD and TBI and how did the use of a service dog impact his success in overcoming these diagnoses?

This life history answers the research questions posed in this study. Jason's use of his service dog, Axel, unquestionably impacted his success in overcoming the diagnoses of PTSD and TBI. It was proven to be the most viable treatment option used by this combat veteran suffering from a very unique version of PTSD and TBI caused by the atrocities of war, one that is not responsive to the typical, accepted therapies or treatments offered by the military and/or traditional medicine.

The DOD and the VA currently only recommend and financially cover a combination of psychosocial or cognitive behavioral therapies and pharmacological interventions. Jason reports previously being on upwards of 20 different medications at one time, with no improvement. The psychosocial and cognitive behavioral therapies approved and recommended by the DOD and VA are basically types of talk therapies that are based on reexperiencing and desensitization techniques. When Jason was asked if he felt these types of talk therapies actually go against the mentality of a marine, he simply nodded his head and said, "Absolutely, yes." Nonetheless, Jason participated fully in the options provided to him. He attempted these therapies at multiple levels on multiple occasions. Jason's wife who was a firsthand observer during many of these treatment sessions, explains,

> Jason tried, he definitely did. I sat through some pretty painful sessions. And it just, no matter which way he went at it or how he talked about it. We do marriage therapy and it is difficult for us, but he is able to do that. But talking about his Marine Corp stuff, it just does not work.

Jason, himself, on discussing talk therapy for the treatment of PTSD feels that it is probably a valuable option for a typical case of PTSD stemming from a single traumatic event, but for a combat veteran who has experienced multiple traumas over extended periods of time, it is not effective at all. "There are not enough minutes of time for me to talk through, over and over, all of the traumatic events that I experienced, it is just not possible," states Jason.

"Coming home doesn't mean their war is over; for some veterans, it means a new battle begins" (The Battle Buddy Foundation, 2014). Messinger (2013), in studying vigilance and attention among veterans, found that military service has profound effects on shaping identity, it is a set of practices that contrasts with civilian life and its perceptions. These individuals are bound together to form a community, and

> This community is distinguished from the civilian world in that collectively it takes an oath that binds members to each other and to their

country. This community demands that individuals place their trust, indeed their life, in one another's hands. (Messinger, 2013, p. 204)

Although these attributes do not dissipate at the end of service for the individual soldier, this sense of community is depleted as they are reintegrated in to a civilian life. On his return home, Jason was no longer surrounded by his community of like-minded and trained battle buddies. His adaptation was further hindered by his PTSD and TBI. Axel has assumed the role of his battle buddy and his constant community. As a specially trained service dog, Axel, performs tasks specific to this combat veteran's needs, such tasks include, but are not limited to:

Guarding doors

Remaining vigilantly by his side at all times, acting as a second set of eyes and remembering everything

Sensing an increased pulse or increased blood pressure during times of escalating anxiety and leaning into Jason's thigh to comfort and calm him

Separating Jason from situations that may trigger his PTSD, many times to the point of opening doors and physically pulling him away

Turning and covering Jason's back or watching his six (military way of saying watching his back), anytime he has to have his back turned to activity going on behind him, such as stepping to a counter to pay for items.

Axel wakes Jason from nightmares and leads him out of flashbacks. When Jason's memory fails him because of his TBI, Axel can also remember necessary items and bring them to Jason and he can always locate where they parked the car.

In this life history, it is glaringly evident that this service dog helps mitigate the symptoms that make civilian life difficult for Jason. Axel allows Jason to live in the present and participate fully in his life and the lives of his family, whereas, all other available treatment options dwell on the past. Jason may never be capable of entirely dealing with all of his experiences, they are a part of him and will always be with him, much like his tattoos.

There is not an area of clinical practice that does not or will not be exposed to a veteran or veterans. In medicine, in general, there is a lack of awareness, interest, understanding, and acceptance of things thought of as alternative medicine or therapies. In fact, Shubert (2012) states that analysis of service dogs and veteran therapy are "frequently met with skepticism largely because of the relative paucity of scientific documentation (i.e., randomized control trials) and the heavy reliance on anecdotal accounts" (p. 24). Evidence-based practice is only as good as the breadth of the subjects that have been studied. It is the study of existing clinical practice. There is no room for successful therapies or treatments without the scientific data to support it and there will be no scientific data to support it if it is not currently in practice. Metaphorically, health care and the practice of medicine are restricted to this box of only what is known. There is no scientific evidence, as of yet, to implicate the success of this alternative therapy into evidence-based practice. Until more is published on this alternative therapy, there will be no advancement of its inclusion by medical professionals as a viable treatment option for those who suffer from PTSD and TBI. Current knowledge levels of this therapy genre reflect that only 34% of therapists surveyed were familiar with service dogs and only 27% had considered a service dog for their patients (Zapft and Rough, 2002, as cited in Dillon, 2013). It is imperative that not only nurse practitioners, but all disciplines of health care are informed and educated about veterans, PTSD, the risk of suicide, and alternative treatments with an emphasis of thinking outside the box of evidence-based practice.

"Life histories are unique in creating the possibilities for going beyond the conventional notions of what constitutes useful knowledge, for brushing with the muted subjectivities of those we research, and for revealing the transmutation of unobservable experience" (Kouritzin, 2000, p. 30). Current medical practice is typically based on quantitative research and evidence-based practice. Although limited research currently exists on the usage of service dogs as treatment for combat veterans with PTSD and/or TBI and it is not a prescribed/accepted clinical practice, this life history definitively demonstrates its success. Credence must be placed on the value of this type of research for this area of study. The implications of this life history reflect that the military and medical communities need to look beyond traditional treatment options for combat veterans with PTSD and/or TBI. Service dogs are an effective alternative treatment that should be added as a viable option to the currently approved psychosocial and cognitive behavioral therapies.

SUMMARY

We had driven to Jason and Axel's hometown and were in the midst of making the final arrangements for our first face-to-face meeting with them. Our phones buzzed with a new text message, "I'll be the guy with the dog" says Jason. That is pretty profound. After meeting them, it is hard to imagine Jason before Axel as the "shell of a man" he described himself to be. At first, you notice Jason because of Axel. Then his presence and personality start to fill the room and Axel becomes the constant quiet shadow, the glue, which is effortlessly and indiscriminately holding it all together. It is hard to explain, obviously it is a guy and a dog, but it is so much more than that. There is an unspoken language and bond between them and an aura of energy emitting from them that connects them and makes them stronger as a pair than they could ever be separately. Jason is inarguably an American hero, but he calls Axel his hero and credits him with saving his life. It is a circle of life, per se. Jason has gone from being a protector to being protected, and that protection is allowing him to protect others once again. It is kismet that Axel's birthday happens to fall on the anniversary of the events that awarded Jason the Purple Heart.

More money, more time, and more effort needs to be invested into studying what is proven to be a successful treatment option for our veterans suffering from PTSD and/or TBI. The organization that trained and provided Axel to Jason, among many like it have multiple success stories that can contribute to the evolution of this form of treatment into evidence-based practice. In addition, the numbers of success stories from these organizations could support a quantitative study. This therapy is in practice, it is being proven every day, and just needs to be documented.

The United States military has perfected the art of war. We do it better than anyone else in the world. But we have not figured out how to bring those warriors home and make them whole again. (Jason, 2015)

REFERENCES

American Psychiatric Association (APA). (2000). *Diagnostic and statistical manual of mental disorders* (4th ed., text rev.). Washington, DC: Author.

de Chesnay, M. (2005). "Can't keep me down": Life histories of successful African American adults. In M. de Chesnay (Ed.), *Caring for the vulnerable* (pp. 221–232). Sudbury, MA: Jones and Bartlett.

Dillon, J. (2013). *A supplementary intervention of service dogs utilized with veterans diagnosed with PTSD: A grand proposal.* Master's thesis. California State University, Long Beach. Retrieved from http://gradworks.umi.com/15/24/1524192 .html

Finley, E. (2014). Empowering veterans with PTSD in the recovery era: Advancing dialogue and integrating services. *Annals of Anthropological Practice, 37*(2), 75–91.

Kemp, J., & Bossart, R. (2012). *Suicide data report, 2012.* Retrieved from http://www .va.gov/opa/docs/suicide-data-report-2012-final.pdf

Kouritzin, S. (2000). Bringing life to research: Life history research and ESL. *TESL Canada Journal, 17*(2), 1–35.

McCarl, L. I. (2013). "To have no yesterday": The rise of suicide rates in the military and among veterans. *Creighton Law Review, 46*(3), 393–432.

Messinger, S. (2013). Vigilance and attention among U.S. service members and veterans after combat. *Anthropology of Consciousness, 24*(2), 191–207.

Shubert, J. (2012). Therapy dogs and stress management assistance during disasters. *U.S. Army Medical Department Journal, 4,* 74–78.

Stern, S. L., Donahue, D. A., Allison, S., Hatch, J. P., Lancaster, C. L., Benson, T. A., & Peterson, A. L. (2013). Potential benefits of canine companionship for military veterans with posttraumatic stress disorder (PTSD). *Society & Animals, 21*(6), 568–581.

The Battle Buddy Foundation. (2014, August 12). Retrieved from http://www.tbbf .org/22-veterans-commit-suicide-daily/08-2014

U.S. Department of Veterans Affairs (VA). (n.d.). *PTSD.* http://www.va.gov/opa/ issues/ptsd.asp

Yeager, A. F., & Irwin, J. (2012). Rehabilitative canine interactions at the Walter Reed National Military Medical Center. *US Army Medical Department Journal,* 57–61.

Yount, R. A., Olmert, M. D., & Lee, M. R. (2012). Service dog training program for treatment of posttraumatic stress in service members. *U.S. Army Medical Department Journal, 4,* 63–69.

CHAPTER THIRTEEN

"CHEERING MYSELF ON": BELLA'S STORY

Melissa Anderson and Nancy Chambers

U nderstanding the life history of an exceptional young adult female, as a Hodgkin's lymphoma survivor, is the purpose of this study. Researchers conducted an ethnographic life-history study exploring the participant's events in her life, from childhood to present day, with the goal of examining the adversity she has overcome. The rationale for choosing a life-history format was to permit the participant to guide the interview, allowing for her culture and personal reflections to be explored. Using the life-history framework, researchers seek to tell the story of a person through their own eyes, and within the context of their culture (deChesney & Batson, 2016). Additionally, the life-history approach can teach researchers about how an individual views his or her illness and the problems he or she faces (de Chesnay, 2005, 2015). This style differs from an autobiography in that the researchers are interpreting the story as it relates to a research question, not just relaying the facts (de Chesnay & Batson, 2016). The life-history approach allows the participant to take the lead, while the researcher follows, permitting for the purist form of exploration. Researchers chose this topic because of the limited amount of research on young adult survivorship, and the unique challenges this population faces following a diagnosis of Hodgkin's lymphoma.

RESEARCH QUESTION

What are the influences, both internal and external, that can help a young adult female overcome the adversity of a cancer diagnosis?

Significance

Hodgkin's lymphoma is a cancer of the bone and blood marrow affecting the white blood cells having a significant immunological impact on a patient (Leukemia and Lymphoma Society, 2015). Most commonly diagnosed in young adults in their twenties, the 5-year survival rate is 85% (The American Cancer Society, 2015). Although the survival rate is high, the long-term effects can be widespread. Listening to the words of a young adult cancer survivor provided the nurse practitioner researchers with an in-depth understanding of what it means to be a survivor during this stage of life.

Conceptual Definitions

Young adult: Male or female between the ages 18 and 40 years
Survivorship: Living beyond remission or cure from cancer
Health-related quality of life (HRQOL): A subjective evaluation of positive and negative aspects of life as they relate to physical and mental health
Quality of life (QOL): A subjective evaluation of positive and negative aspects of life

SUMMARY OF CURRENT LITERATURE

Before beginning the research, a systematic literature review was conducted using the following key words: Hodgkin's lymphoma, survivorship, female, young adult, and quality of life. Out of 261 articles that met the criteria, 244 articles were excluded, and 17 were chosen for review. Four common concepts emerged: physical activity, QOL indicators, social support, and fertility needs. For space purposes, only a summary of the literature review is included in this chapter.

Physical Activity

There is consensus among researchers that physical activity increases QOL for cancer patients and survivors (Badr et al., 2013; Belanger, Plotnikoff, Clark, & Courneya, 2012; Gjerset, Fosså, Courneya, Skovlund, & Thorsen, 2011). Research by Gjerset et al. (2011) showed that cancer survivors often have low participation in organized sports and physical activity. No studies were able to make causation as to why few survivors are physically active, and how inactivity affects long-term survival and QOL.

QOL Indicators

Social support, emotional support, and attitude contribute to QOL in a cancer survivor (Bellizzi et al., 2012; Monteiro, Torres, Morgadinho, & Pereira, 2013). Research by Calaminus et al. (2014) showed lower emotional and social functioning in cancer survivors, with higher symptom levels in women. Cancer survivors younger than 30 years of age reported lower levels of social functioning, higher levels of financial difficulties, increased tobacco usage, and more sexual concerns (Hall et al., 2012).

Social Support

Social networking and social support measures are favorably associated with improved physical functioning and HRQOL (Roper, Cooley, McDermott, & Fawcett, 2013; Soares et al., 2013). Levels of stress for the cancer survivor are inversely related to perceived social support, support group involvement, and physical activity (Brunet, Love, Ramphal, & Sabiston, 2014). A study by McLaughlin et al. (2012) suggested that survivors with weak social connections, and little support from friends and family, could benefit from social media interaction and interventions.

Fertility

A study by Eeltink et al. (2013) concluded that 30% of cancer survivors do not know their fertility status. Gorman, Bailey, Pierce, and Su (2012) found that there is value for young adult cancer survivors to have access to information regarding fertility, parenting options, and support navigating these issues. A review of literature found that one of the largest knowledge deficits for young adult cancer survivors is related to fertility needs (Eeiltink et al., 2013; Gorman et al., 2012).

METHODOLOGY

Sample

The research sample consisted of one informant, a 27-year-old Caucasian female diagnosed at the age of 22 years. This was a purposive sampling looking for a young adult female cancer survivor, between the ages of 18 and

40 years, who had overcome the adversity of cancer. The participant was chosen because of her positive outlook on her survivorship. She wears it as a badge of honor and continues to tell her story hoping to inspire others. The informant was enthusiastic, and provided an informative reflection of surviving beyond a cancer diagnosis. Confidentiality was maintained to preserve the participant's identity, and the pseudonym Bella was chosen.

Procedures

Researchers began by recruiting the participant via telephone. Researchers then reviewed the consent document, obtaining both verbal and written consent from the participant. "The Consent to Perform Research Form," as created by Mary de Chesnay, was used, and all questions were answered. The location, time, and setting for the interview was chosen by the participant. The researchers and participant met at a coffee shop near the participant's home. Rapport was quickly attained, and the interview was completed within 2 hours. Researchers ensured comfort and privacy, and the interaction lent itself to a free flow of information.

Instrumentation

Instrumentation used for this study included a semi-structured interview, tape recordings, transcriptions of recordings, a genogram, and a chronological timeline of life events. For the semi-structured interview, both researchers were present and used the format first described by de Chesnay (2005). Changes were made to questions to allow for specificity of participant and her survivorship of cancer. A list of these questions is included in Table 13.1. Both a genogram and timeline were created with the participant to better understand her lineage and perceived important life events. These are excluded from this paper to maintain the privacy of the participant.

Rigor and Data Analysis

The accuracy of this single life history relied on the participant herself, her feelings, and the words she chose to relay her story. Replicability was maintained by following the detailed proposal and using standard interview questions from Table 13.1.

After the interview, verbatim transcriptions of the interview recordings were completed. The transcripts were evaluated by both researchers.

Table 13.1 *Semi-Structured Interview Guide*

1. As we explained when we asked you to allow us to interview you, we understand that you were diagnosed with Hodgkin's lymphoma about 5 years ago and that you are in remission. Tell us how you learned you had cancer.
2. What was your reaction at the time you learned you had cancer? For example, What thoughts and feelings did you have and what did you do?
3. How did your family learn you had cancer?
4. What were their reactions?
5. What support did you have from family, friends, health care professionals, and so on?
6. What were the primary ways you coped with your illness?
7. You mentioned that being physically active helped you become a survivor, can you tell us how that helped you?
8. Tell us about how you have used your survivorship to help others.
9. What is the single most powerful force in your life that helps you cope, not just with the diagnosis of Hodgkin's lymphoma, but also the problems of daily life?
10. What have we not asked that you think we should have asked?

Emerging concepts were extracted from the transcripts, and organized into themes.

RESULTS

Emerging from the interviews were four prominent themes: learned coping mechanisms, physical fitness, employment, and social support. Learned coping mechanisms evolved because of Bella's difficult childhood. Bella grew up in a home with her mother, father, and sister, who was 10 years older. Bella's mother was an alcoholic, which had a significant impact on her father's ability to care for her older sister. His perceived failure in parenting changed the way he cared for Bella. "Dad's way of fixing our home was not to fix my mom, because he couldn't do that, but was just to help me."

Bella described her childhood as busy, always out of the home, constantly being active and distracted. Activities such as sports, music, and community involvement were her father's way of keeping her out of the house. As she got older, she also made choices to spend her free time with other families.

It's so easy to be insecure and not want to be a burden on others, and it's scary to ask people to join them and their family.

She felt that it was important to create a family outside of her own, and sought out friends who could fill that role.

Bella's elementary school recognized that her mother suffered from alcoholism. The school system stepped in to create a foundation of support throughout her childhood. She was cared for by social workers, teachers, and administrative staff, who intervened on her behalf. She was enrolled in Al-Anon, Alateen (two programs for alcoholism), and continuous counseling. The coping skills she acquired from these interventions would drive her future outcomes. She actively pursued gymnastics and music throughout her childhood. Her high school principal supported her at school activities, and even spoke about her at graduation. Bella received continuous support from people in the school and community. "I made a choice to succeed, which was different than my family."

The second theme is physical fitness. Being physically active has always been an important part of Bella's life. Bella became a skilled gymnast in elementary school, and continued to be active throughout college as a competitive cheerleader. She did not allow cancer or its treatment to keep her from cheerleading. Her oncologist would give her blood transfusions on Friday so that she could be strong for weekend cheer competitions. During treatment, her coaches gave her the option of not competing. She refused to sit out and stated, "I just won't do two backflips, I'll only do one." During her treatment, she was featured on a television sports channel and in a cheerleading magazine as a competitive cheerleader fighting cancer.

During her treatment, she continued to stay active, and was encouraged by her oncologist to take the pain medications so that it was possible. Posttreatment and post-cheerleading career, she attributes her positive attitude to her constant physical activity. She is the captain of her Ultimate Frisbee team and continues to train at the gym four to five times per week. Bella's belief is that "exercise is a natural painkiller." She also believes that exercise puts you around positive people. "Athletes are positive people. If I am around high energy, then I am high energy."

The third theme is employment. Bella got her diagnosis of Hodgkin's lymphoma 4 months after starting her first job as a nurse. Her diagnosis was delayed by 3 months because of her employer's required probationary time for insurance eligibility. By the time she saw the oncologist, she had an orange-size tumor under her axilla. Her diagnosis presented enormous challenges for her at work. Bella did not expect special treatment, but struggled to balance treatment with such a physical job. She needed 16 weeks of chemotherapy, but only could get 12 weeks of medical leave from work. For the last 4 weeks, she would receive chemotherapy at the beginning of the week, allowing for work hours at the end of the week. This left little time for recovery.

When radiation treatment began, she had used all of her leave, and had no choice but to work during treatment.

> When I was doing radiation, I would work all night and get radiation during the day. If I didn't, I would have no home and no insurance.

Bella tried to work part time, but was refused because of seniority. She also tried to move to a day shift, and was denied again.

> I was competing against a bunch of young, healthy women, and I was not able to keep up.

Bella chose to take a job as an oncology nurse in hopes that there would be greater understanding of her medical needs. She was forthright in her interview, and discussed her attendance issues.

> I told them, that in return for their patience, they will get someone who really wanted to be there and would stay for my career.

Bella has found support in her new position, and has been offered multiple schedule options to accommodate her. This new position has provided her with day shift hours, sterile working conditions, and an understanding of her needs as a cancer survivor. Since starting this position in early 2015, she has been a patient for 32 days on this floor and they continue their support of her as a coworker and a patient. Bella dreams of being financially and physically able to go back to school to get her master's degree in nursing education.

The fourth theme is social support. Because Bella's homelife was disrupted by her mother's alcoholism, her support system consisted of strong outside influences. This community focus that was so important to her in her childhood set the tone for how she manages her life today. During cancer treatment, she continued to meet with her cheer teammates and compete as much as possible. Even when she could not cheer, she would attend practices to be supportive of her teammates to maintain that connection that provided her emotional support. She recalls the extensive encouragement and love from her friends, and how they brought her gifts and cried with her on the day she was diagnosed.

Social media has had a significant impact on how she gains and gives support. When Bella posted her diagnosis on Facebook, she was overwhelmed by the response stating, "I got 300 comments on Facebook!" She uses Facebook as a resource to connect with other people who understand her circumstances. She uses social media as a source of overall motivation in survivorship, and rejoices in seeing survivors having families and thriving. Social media provides her an instantaneous feeling of love and support, even by people she has never met.

Social media also allows Bella to give and get information about medications, side effects, and treatments. "I think technology is really important for survivors." She feels that knowledge is power, and the more information you have, the more you can advocate for yourself. She is proud to be involved in multiple cancer support groups. "I'm wearing one of my shirts from my groups tonight. This group gives makeovers to cancer patients not feeling good about themselves." She volunteers as a cheer coach for a special needs team, and accredits helping others as a way to keep her positive attitude.

So I keep telling myself, this is only temporary. I am going to help someone someday, this is going to be a great story someday.

DISCUSSION

The following interrelates the four themes described earlier with current literature. In a literature review conducted by Masten and Coatsworth (1998), it was found that process-oriented approaches can have a positive effect on children who have been raised in unfavorable environments. These processes include teachers who build self-efficacy, develop talents, and who help to open doors to opportunities for success. These processes were repeatedly used in Bella's early childhood. Her teachers and counselors helped to keep her involved in extracurricular activities and alcohol counseling, all which gave her confidence that she could be successful. Additionally, the authors found that children's success and protection can be impacted by multiple organizations outside the family unit. Much of Bella's childhood experiences were focused outside of the home. Both she and her father sought out opportunities for protection and growth.

In a research study by Short and Ayers (1989), findings showed that young children of alcoholics were interested in getting help. By seeking help, they learned positive coping skills for use both inside and outside the home. Bella was taught these strategies by attending Alonon and Alateen. She learned the importance of asking people for help, eliminating fear of rejection as an obstacle.

In a study by Belanger et al. (2012), researchers found that participating in organized sports resulted in better psychosocial health and QOL outcomes for cancer survivors. However, Blanchard et al. (2003) reported that only 30% to 60% of survivors ever return to pre-cancer level of activity. Bella attributes physical activity and being on a team as part of her success in childhood, and her recovery from cancer. Keats, Courneya, Danielsen, and Whitsett (1999) supported this with evidence that survivors who maintained organized sports participation throughout the cancer experiences reported positive self-concept and greater physical abilities. Going to the gym and being a part of a Frisbee team are key components in helping to maintain Bella's positive attitude. Though she continues to have issues with recurrent infections, she maintains that physical activity, which keeps her strong.

Employment and cancer survivorship is a well-researched topic. A study by Fobair et al. (1986) reported that 42% of Hodgkin's survivors have difficulties when they return to work. Reasons for these difficulties include changes in roles, discrimination, and need for accommodations (Alfano & Rowland, 2006; Morrison & Thomas, 2014). Bella faced all three of these issues. Maintaining her night schedule with her decreased energy continually put her in the position of having to choose between job security and her health. Her employer could not provide accommodations, and the demands of the hospital were placed over her medical needs.

Bella continues to have health concerns and hospitalizations. Her immunocompromised state and recurrent infections are an everyday struggle even 5 years after diagnosis. Being in remission from cancer does not mean you are out of the woods (Alfano & Rowland, 2006). Roper et al. (2013) addressed the issue of the financial and occupational damage that even minor illnesses can cause survivors.

Social support is critical for young adult survivors. In a study by Rosenberg, Yi-Frazier, Wharton, Gordon, and Jones (2014), researchers found that 100% of adolescent and young adult participants placed meeting other cancer survivors as a priority. These researchers clarified that support received from similar age peers with a cancer history could be more advantageous than support from family and friends. Bella uses social media to connect with other cancer survivors. For her, it provides access to resources, as well as promotes relationships with other cancer survivors. In a study on survivorship in the age of social networking, Bender, O'Grady, and Jadad (2008) corroborated with Bella's experience that peer networking allows for self-management, and a forum to share emotional concerns. Similar to Bella's circumstances, a study by McLaughlin et al. (2012) found that social networking was more critical for cancer patients with less family communication.

CONCLUSION

Implications for Nurse Practitioners

Understanding influences, both internal and external, that can increase HRQOL for young adult cancer survivors, is valuable information for the discipline of health care. This is especially true for primary care nurse practitioners. Although cancer patients are cared for during treatment by several specialties, nurse practitioners can play an important role in survivorship. This involves managing acute illness, vaccination maintenance, family planning, dermatological concerns, and psychosocial needs. Nurse practitioners can develop anticipatory care, interventions, and services that can help young adult cancer survivors navigate the journey from patient to survivor and beyond.

A priority for the nurse practitioner is health promotion. Hodgkin's lymphoma survivors continually live in an immunocompromised state. Ensuring these patients are revaccinated is critical. Additionally, the nurse practitioner must encourage a healthy lifestyle, which includes a nutritious diet and physical activity. The nurse practitioner must assess the patient's level of activity and encourage involvement in organized sports or physical exercise. Providing education on health promotion at each visit is critical in preventing future illness.

Employment for Hodgkin's lymphoma patients can be a difficult path to navigate. Providing anticipatory guidance for challenges regarding frequent illness, continued medical follow-up, and discrimination that can occur in the workplace can assist patients with successful reentry into the workplace. It is the responsibility of the nurse practitioner to provide employer documentation on current and future health needs, allowing for, and encouraging necessary workplace accommodations.

Although not discussed in this interview, the nurse practitioner must educate the survivor on the importance of health maintenance. This includes serial labs, procedures, and office visits to evaluate the patient's health status. Bella uses social media to gather information on issues such as medications, treatments, and screenings. Although online support can be a valuable resource, there can be concerns with accuracy and applicability to individual survivors. The nurse practitioner must provide guidance on appropriate use of this information, directing these survivors toward reliable Internet resources.

An important concept that emerged from this interview with Bella was her learned ability to seek support. An effective strategy for the nurse practitioner can be assessing the survivor's current coping skills, and how these skills will assist with his or her survivorship. Some of the coping mechanisms include the survivor's acknowledgment of the problem, expression of needs, availability of resources, and the willingness to seek help. Depending on where the survivor is in this process, the nurse practitioner can identify obstacles and help to move the patient through these stages. The goal is to improve the survivor's self-efficacy to identify and seek support. As Bella explained in her interview, survivors can be both on the giving and receiving end of support, and both are therapeutic.

Recommendations for Further Research

With a high survival rate, there is a new generation of young adults surviving a diagnosis of Hodgkin's lymphoma. In our society, we are often defined by our occupation, and managing work with medical needs can impede earning potential, career advancement, respect in the workplace and self-esteem. Young adult survivors are often just beginning their career, and future research is needed to identify work environments that are supportive to their needs. With an immunocompromised status, these patients have difficulty maintaining employment. Research is needed to identify interventions and accommodations to help maintain employment. Financial implications of this disease can be profound, and research is needed on support and services that can be provided.

Self-care is an important part of survivorship. There is a lack of research on lifestyle interventions for Hodgkin's lymphoma survivors. More information is needed on what type of physical activity promotes a high QOL. Future research is needed to identify the most effective activities, how often survivors should be active, and what restrictions need to be placed on these young adults. Additionally, research would be beneficial on dietary recommendations to promote long term immunity and optimal health.

Social support plays integral role in overcoming and surviving cancer and the literature reviewed supported this concept. However, the research did not assess what type of social support services would be most effective. Future research is needed on social media and how support in survivorship can be given or gotten online. In this age of technology, how support services are administered can be as instrumental as the services themselves.

SUMMARY

This life-history study examined survivorship of Hodgkin's lymphoma in the young adult population. The study participant's past circumstances provided her with the skills and attitude to help overcome her cancer diagnosis and achieve a high QOL. The findings of her life story helped to identify concepts that can be instrumental in resilience over adversity. During the study, four common themes emerged including learned coping mechanisms, physical fitness, employment, and social support. Researchers evaluated how these relate to current literature and explored directions for future research. The intention of this study was to provide information to the medical community to assist this unique population through the journey of survivorship after a diagnosis of Hodgkin's lymphoma.

REFERENCES

Alfano, C., & Rowland, J. (2006). Recovery issues in cancer survivorship: A new challenge for supportive care. *The Cancer Journal, 12*(5), 1–12.

American Cancer Society. (2015). *Survival rates for Hodgkin's disease by stage.* Retrieved from http://www.cancer.org/cancer/hodgkindisease/index

Badr, H., Chandra, J., Paxton, R. J., Ater, J. L., Urbauer, D., Cruz, C. S., & Demark-Wahnefried, W. (2013). Health-related quality of life, lifestyle behaviors, and intervention preferences of survivors of childhood cancer. *Journal of Cancer Survivorship: Research and Practice, 7*(4), 523–534.

Belanger, L., Plotnikoff, R., Clark, A., & Courneya, K. (2012). Prevalence, correlates, and psychosocial outcomes of sport participation in young adult cancer survivors. *Psychology of Sport and Exercise, 14*, 298–304.

Bellizzi, K. M., Smith, A., Schmidt, S., Keegan, T. H., Zebrack, B., Lynch, C. F., ... Simon, M.; Adolescent and Young Adult Health Outcomes and Patient Experience (AYA HOPE) Study Collaborative Group. (2012). Positive and negative psychosocial impact of being diagnosed with cancer as an adolescent or young adult. *Cancer, 118*(20), 5155–5162.

Bender, J. L., O'Grady, L., & Jadad, A. R. (2008). Supporting cancer patients through the continuum of care: A view from the age of social networks and computer-mediated communication. *Current Oncology (Toronto, Ont.), 15*(Suppl. 2), s107. es42–s107.es47.

Blanchard, C., Denniston, M., Baker, F., Ainsworth, S., Courneya, K., Hann, D., ... Kennedy, J. (2003). Do adults change their lifestyle behaviors after a cancer diagnosis? *American Journal of Health Behaviors, 27*, 246–256.

Brunet, J., Love, C., Ramphal, R., & Sabiston, C. M. (2014). Stress and physical activity in young adults treated for cancer: The moderating role of social support. *Supportive Care in Cancer: Official Journal of the Multinational Association of Supportive Care in Cancer, 22*(3), 689–695.

Calaminus, G., Dörffel, W., Baust, K., Teske, C., Riepenhausen, M., Brämswig, J., ... Schellong, G. (2014). Quality of life in long-term survivors following treatment for Hodgkin's disease during childhood and adolescence in the German multicentre studies between 1978 and 2002. *Supportive Care in Cancer:*

Official Journal of the Multinational Association of Supportive Care in Cancer, 22(6), 1519–1529.

de Chesnay, M. (2005). "Can't keep me down": Life histories of successful African American adults. In M. de Chesnay (Ed.), *Caring for the vulnerable* (pp. 221–232). Sudbury, MA: Jones & Bartlett.

de Chesnay, M. (2015). *Nursing research using life history: Qualitative designs and methods in nursing.* New York, NY: Springer Publishing Company.

de Chesnay, M., & Batson, A. (2016). Life history of Jim: "I am not broken." In M. de Chesnay & B. Anderson (Eds.).*Caring for the vulnerable* (pp. 235–242). Burlington, MA: Jones & Bartlett.

Eeltink, C. M., Incrocci, L., Witte, B. I., Meurs, S., Visser, O., Huijgens, P., & Verdonck-de Leeuw, I. M. (2013). Fertility and sexual function in female Hodgkin lymphoma survivors of reproductive age. *Journal of Clinical Nursing, 22*(23–24), 3513–3521.

Fobair, P., Hoppe, R. T., Bloom, J., Cox, R., Varghese, A., & Spiegel, D. (1986). Psychosocial problems among survivors of Hodgkin's disease. *Journal of Clinical Oncology: Official Journal of the American Society of Clinical Oncology, 4*(5), 805–814.

Gjerset, G. M., Fosså, S. D., Courneya, K. S., Skovlund, E., & Thorsen, L. (2011). Exercise behavior in cancer survivors and associated factors. *Journal of Cancer Survivorship: Research and Practice, 5*(1), 35–43.

Gorman, J. R., Bailey, S., Pierce, J. P., & Su, H. I. (2012). How do you feel about fertility and parenthood? The voices of young female cancer survivors. *Journal of Cancer Survivorship: Research and Practice, 6*(2), 200–209.

Hall, A. E., Boyes, A. W., Bowman, J., Walsh, R. A., James, E. L., & Girgis, A. (2012). Young adult cancer survivors' psychosocial well-being: A cross-sectional study assessing quality of life, unmet needs, and health behaviors. *Supportive Care in Cancer: Official Journal of the Multinational Association of Supportive Care in Cancer, 20*(6), 1333–1341.

Keats, M. R., Courneya, K. S., Danielsen, S., & Whitsett, S. F. (1999). Leisure-time physical activity and psychosocial well-being in adolescents after cancer diagnosis. *Journal of Pediatric Oncology Nursing: Official Journal of the Association of Pediatric Oncology Nurses, 16*(4), 180–188.

Leukemia and Lymphoma Society. (2015). *Facts and statistics.* Retrieved from https://www.lls.org/http%3A/llsorg.prod.acquia-sites.com/facts-and-statistics/facts-and-statistics-overview/facts-and-statistics/childhood-blood-cancer-facts-and-statistics

Masten, A. S., & Coatsworth, J. D. (1998). The development of competence in favorable and unfavorable environments. Lessons from research on successful children. *The American psychologist Psychologist, 53*(2), 205–220.

McLaughlin, M., Nam, Y., Gould, J., Pade, C., Meeske, K., Ruccione, K., & Fulk, J. (2012). A videosharing social networking intervention for young adult cancer survivors. *Computers in Human Behavior, 28*, 631–641.

Monteiro, S., Torres, A., Morgadinho, R., & Pereira, A. (2013). Psychosocial outcomes in young adults with cancer: Emotional distress, quality of life and personal growth. *Archives of Psychiatric Nursing, 27*(6), 299–305.

Morrison, T. L., & Thomas, R. L. (2014). Survivors' experiences of return to work following cancer: A photovoice study. *Canadian Journal of Occupational Therapy. Revue Canadienne D'ergothe´Rapie, 81*(3), 163–172.

Roper, K., Cooley, M. E., McDermott, K., & Fawcett, J. (2013). Health-related quality of life after treatment of Hodgkin lymphoma in young adults. *Oncology Nursing Forum, 40*(4), 349–360.

Rosenberg, A. R., Yi-Frazier, J. P., Wharton, C., Gordon, K., & Jones, B. (2014). Contributors and inhibitors of resilience among adolescents and young adults with cancer. *Journal of Adolescent and Young Adult Oncology, 3*(4), 185–193.

Short, J., & Ayers, T. (1989). A preventative intervention for children in alcoholic families: Results of a pilot study. *Family Relations, 38*(3), 295–300.

Soares, A., Biasoli, I., Scheliga, A., Baptista, R. L., Brabo, E. P., Morais, J. C.,…Spector, N. (2013). Association of social network and social support with health-related quality of life and fatigue in long-term survivors of Hodgkin lymphoma. *Supportive Care in Cancer: Official Journal of the Multinational Association of Supportive Care in Cancer, 21*(8), 2153–2159.

CHAPTER FOURTEEN

LOSS OF A CHILD TO AN AFRICAN FAMILY: A PHENOMENOLOGICAL CASE STUDY

Jacqueline Kigundu and Titus Sairo

This study investigates the effects of grief on one family system and how the family was able to cope with the loss of a family member. This is accomplished by following a qualitative research case study design with a phenomenological approach. The researcher interviews an African immigrant couple to determine how the family has handled grief and mourning. The rationale for undertaking this study is to find out if we can discover ways of helping grieving parents following the loss of a child or any significant loss. Several concepts are evaluated for applicability.

REVIEW OF THE LITERATURE

Elisabeth Kübler-Ross (1969) first described the five stages of grief. These stages are part of the Kübler-Ross model inspired by working with terminally ill patients. The five stages do not occur in a linear fashion but can occur in any order according to the person or persons dealing with grief. The five stages include denial, anger, bargaining, depression, and acceptance. Denial is the stage wherein the survivor imagines a false preferable reality. Survivors do not believe that their loved ones are gone forever, but instead have an unrealistic view of the death. Anger is referred to as the stage where a person's anger is directed at the person who died and at oneself for being unable to prevent the loved one's death. Bargaining is the stage where the individuals who are grieving believe that they may have been able to control and prevent the loss of their family member, and depression is the stage where the individual becomes saddened by the certainty of death, and the individual becomes silent, refuses visitors, and spends much of the time being mournful and sullen. This stage is necessary for the process of healing to begin. Lastly, acceptance is the stage when the individuals are at a point where they recognize the current state of their lives, without their loved one, as a reality and can live with that understanding.

According to Bolden (2007), Kübler-Ross and Kessler noted multiple roles that individuals hold in life and the need to mourn those losses. There is a general expectation by many that people should live for a long time. Therefore, the death of a child is considered to be exceptionally shocking. This shows that grief does not end with the loss of a loved one but that it extends to all the aspects of the grieving person's life. For example, planning the holidays and anniversary events bring back the memory of the loved ones. Changes in the bereaved sexual life, as well as personal self-care habits, were also noted in those involved in grief. Also, details surrounding one's death can significantly affect the way in which individuals grieve. The shame associated with suicide affects how one grieves, and grieving and coping with death as a result of a disaster, chronic disease, such as Alzheimer's, and sudden death are different in each case. Lastly, failure to grieve a loss has also been noted to leave a void when the loss has not been effectively addressed (Bolden, 2007).

Holtslander and McMillan (2011), define bereavement as the objective loss of someone significant, and grief as a reaction. It is important to observe and assess the effects of grief and bereavement on an individual and the family. One theory that facilitates the understanding of the family function and role is the family systems theory. The family systems theory is based on the belief that the family is an interconnected unit or system wherein the actions of one family member affect all members in the family system. The theory examines the organization, structure, and complexity of families and familial relationships. Bowen, a family systems theorist, discusses family therapy patterns in families over generations. These patterns are also known as the multigenerational transmission processes. For example, one death in a family will affect several generations in different ways leading to reorganization of the family. The death of an adult child will affect the biological parents and siblings, but it may also affect the grandparents. If the great grandparents of the adult child are alive, they may also grieve for the loss as well. The grandparents will not only grieve for their great-grandchild but also the great-grandchild's children (Bowen, 2004).

Most family theorists also explore family members' emotional, social, and psychological boundaries with one another. Minuchin, another family systems theorist, discusses concepts that are focused on familial boundaries. These boundaries are defined as respectful limits or social rules that govern the development and maintenance of interpersonal relationships. In family systems theory, healthy interpersonal boundaries permit appropriate degrees of emotional intimacy between two people. Families with few boundaries may be considered enmeshed or so deeply involved with one another that individual family members have difficulty establishing individual identities separate from their families. Family therapists often examine healthy and unhealthy boundaries within a family system (Bowen, 2004).

RELEVANCE TO NURSING

Nurses deal with patients during all stages of life that span from birth to death. The literature review reveals that research is lacking on the effect of grief on family systems. Much research has been done relating to the loss of neonates, infants, and children, but not much research has been done regarding the loss of adult children and the effects of the loss on the family systems. Ineffective coping with loss has been associated with negative emotions that can lead to disease. Effective coping, on the other hand, has been found to improve family relations. The aim of this research is to establish the effects that grief has on family systems and if there are lessons nurse practitioners (NPs) can learn from this study about overcoming grief. NPs can then apply the findings to assist other individuals or families that find themselves in similar situations. The findings of this research can generate evidence-based knowledge for the family nurse practitioner (FNP) profession.

Grief Related to the Family Systems Theory

The loss of a loved one through death can have many effects on the bereaved. Death and grieving can prove to be an intense undertaking for affected families. Some of the effects of grief and dying on family members can include feelings of despair, sadness, depression, and conflict among family members. Coping with the loss of a loved one effectively can prove to be beneficial for the bereaved, whereas ineffective coping can lead to mental illness, marital problems, and behavioral disorders (Carmon, Western, Miller, Pearson, & Fowler, 2010).

It is important to understand the family systems theory to better understand the effects of grief on the family. The family systems theory is a conceptual framework theory that tackles the concepts of looking at the family as one entity that is made up of many parts. Therefore, using the family systems theory, it is theorized that grief will not only affect the individual that is bereaved, but the family as a whole. This point of view can enable the researcher to observe the conceptual effects of grieving on the role and function of the family. Looking at a family as a unit enables the researcher to observe the processes of the family as well. These grieving processes of overcoming grief include mourning rituals, teamwork toward overcoming grief, social and emotional support among family members, and therapeutic conversation among family members.

According to the systems view of the family, effects of grief of one family member have been theorized to have an effect on the other family members. The associated reactions of grief of an individual are also associated with the relationships among family members. There are two types of major constructs to consider when looking at grief related to the family: structural forms and general constructs. Structural forms of family systems theory will help the researcher understand any gaps in the structure in the family following the death of a loved one. General concepts, on the other hand, will help the researcher understand any multigenerational processes in which similar themes of dealing with grief may be seen emerging among generations (Rosenblatt, 2013). Observing both can be beneficial for the researcher in the assessment of the effects of grief on the family.

To gain more understanding of the effects of grief on the family, the researcher has to understand effective interviewing skills related to family/relationship concepts that show how the relational concepts and theories can be applied to any multicultural family. The concept of energy transfer is an important factor to consider when interviewing family members (Rosenblatt, 2013). According to the family system theory, the environment and the family transfer energy among themselves creating a feedback loop (*Environmental Influences*, 1990). It is important to consider that fueling a family by helping them achieve physical and psychological sources of energy through the help of outsiders can help with bringing potential positive reactions of grief for all members involved. The sources of fuel can involve the environment, which uses support groups that input energy into the family so that the family outputs back into the environment via positive behavioral outcomes (Rosenblatt, 2013).

Another relational concept to consider during the interview process is the reality that the dead may still be "alive" to the bereaved victims. Being "alive" does not necessarily mean that the dead come back to life, but that they are active in the family's emotional and psychological lives. In those families where the dead are active members of the family, the dead influence the choices of the family members in their everyday lives. Family systems grief researchers should acknowledge the dead as part of the family to better understand the relationships between the dead and those who are actively present during the interviews. Acknowledging the dead as a member of the family rather than as an idea that used to exist helps the researcher obtain ground in receiving detailed information about the relationships between the dead and the grieving (Rosenblatt, 2013).

Lastly, the "dangerous witch is the cause of death" relational concept is important to consider when assessing the family for effects of grief. This concept defines situations where the family blames another evil object as the reason their loved one is dead. An example of the witch-is-the-cause-of-death concept is a case in which the family blames physician malpractice as the reason of the death. Incorporating blame and "malevolence" assessing strategies to family systems grief can be beneficial in providing assessments and interventions that can be geared toward helping the family move forward in the grieving process. It is important for the researcher to remember to place importance on the assessment of the family's culture during family grief assessments. Not all families are alike, and the approach of assessments used will depend on the affected family's definition of family. Family can be defined as nuclear, multigenerational, or as anything the family understands it to be. Definitions of grief and family vary according to different cultures. Assessment of both before making any conclusions can prove to be beneficial in defining the effects of grief on the family (Rosenblatt, 2013).

According to Carmon et al. (2010), family communications patterns (FCPs) were also found to be important for researchers in assessing the effects of grief on the family. The FCP are patterns that often observe how families communicate with each other within and outside the family. These communications help to mold and influence family behavior.

Using a qualitative research design, Carmon et al. (2010) collected a convenience sample of 203 participants' surveys to assess the effects of FCP on grief. FCP and grief results were analyzed according to the survey results. The study was looking to observe how FCP are related to the victim's views of grief reactions after bereavement. Conversation orientation was found to significantly increase views of personal growth as the main reaction to grief. Families with high-communication abilities showed tendencies toward high self-esteem, low stress, and improved communication skills all of which are vital in achieving positive grief reactions. Aspects of the FCP can prove to be beneficial when assessing the family for effects of grief for the researcher.

Similarly, Gaudio, Zaider, Brier, and Kissane (2011) found that assessing families who are psychologically at risk because of grief and bereavement was of utmost importance to prevent negative grief outcomes. Using the family-focused grief therapy (FFGT) improves overall family functioning by increasing the family closeness, conflict resolution abilities, and open communication of illness-related outcomes. This model has been found to be easily adaptable by health care professionals in the community. FFGT has been found to increase successful engagement and relations of the family. The implementation of the model has also been found to increase the researcher's ability to assess the family history, identity, and formulate focus of therapy for the family's affected families. Using assessments and implementations that are similar to the FFGT model in assessing bereaved families can prove to be advantageous in the study of assessing effects of grief on the family (Gaudio et al., 2011).

Incorporating the family systems theory as well as the aspects of the FCP and FFGT models into the interview and therapy processes can help the researcher in applying proper family assessment and implementation techniques when assessing effects of grief on family members. Understanding different cultural perspective about death and dying can also prove to be beneficial to family systems grief researchers. Lastly, implementing interviews and/or therapies that encourage high communication among family members can point the way for family systems grief researchers in maximizing the research on obtaining information on the effects of grief on the family.

Expected Limitations

Certain limitations exist in the studies related to family system grief assessments. There is a gap in the research relating to family systems theory related to the loss of adult children and the effects of grief on the family system. Research on the effect of grief on parents of older or adult children is particularly limited. The weakening of concepts and/or therapy implemented can happen over time, and there is no effective method of measuring the causes of the weakness. These newfound weaknesses in the family systems grief therapies can lead to ineffective treatment results as well as lack of cohesion to the therapy. There are also some difficulties in processing the work of family systems grief research because most of the analysis is based on the answers of each individual in the family. It may not be possible or practical to interview all members of the community who were considered as part of the family system by the nuclear family. Creating a measure of disparity among the levels of grief can help with realizing the gaps in assessment that exist so that the whole family's views can be better analyzed. Lack of follow-up interventions and control groups creations can act as limitations on intervention of family systems research when it comes to assessing the results. Lastly, more research that includes different cultures, races, and ethnicity needs to be performed to add to the knowledge of how different types of familial systems function during grief in agreement with (Hayslip & Page, 2013).

METHODOLOGY

Design

A qualitative research case study design with a phenomenological approach will be applied. This design will be most appropriate in investigating the effects of grief on the family system. Grief is something experiential and only the person experiencing it can describe it. Not all the effects of grief can be observed, but the victim can describe them and that way enable other people to study them with the hope of gathering information that can be used to prevent or decrease or treat the negative effects of grief in other people who may be faced with similar circumstances.

Sample

The sample consisted of one family system. The criterion for inclusion into the study was that a family should have experienced the death of one of its members.

Setting

Interviews took place in the family's home.

Instruments

The family was encouraged to tell their story.

- Tell me your definition of family.
- Tell me your definition of grief.
- Tell me about the loss of your loved one.
- Tell me about your family before the loss of your loved one.
- Tell me about your family after the loss of your loved one.
- Tell me how you are coping.

Data analysis

Data were analyzed using content analysis. Recorded data were transcribed immediately by one researcher, and then reviewed by the other researcher to prevent bias and promote accuracy. Data were then analyzed separately by each researcher for emerging concepts. Both researchers compared findings and agreed on the concepts.

Rigor

The researchers made an assumption that the interviewees gave an accurate detail of the events and feelings prior to and following the death of the family member. Replicability and reliability will be assessed by reviewing the interviews to ensure that the subjects are giving an accurate depiction regarding the events surrounding the family's grief.

RESULTS

The couple interviewed is from Kenya and the interviewers are also from Kenya. With this in mind, it is safe to assume that the interpretations of the recorded interview were assessed and analyzed taking into consideration the participant's culture, ethical background, and any unspoken cultural or ethical hidden meanings. The data were transcribed by both interviewers from the original recording and compared before the final draft was adopted. The data were analyzed for accurate transcription, and all conclusions were made based on the transcription. Any interpretation made outside the direct dialogue will be explained in this section. The data were analyzed for emerging themes, and these are also listed in this section.

Themes

Certain themes were quite evident following the interview about how death affected the family. Ten themes were noted during the interview. These were family, grief, community, spirituality, emotional distress, denial, communication, financial implications, acceptance, and support groups.

Family

Janet, the mother of the deceased, states that a family

> may consist of a mother, father, maybe children, there are cases where
> there is just a mother and her children there could be a father and his
> children depending on what has happened to the other spouse; and
> there could also be a case where is just two people who are married and
> they have no children and have no desire to have children; and for them
> to call themselves a family it has to be an environment where they all
> feel safe, a place where you always look forward to go back to because
> its home its family. You feel secure and you feel that there is warmth
> within that environment. It makes a family where people take care of
> each other, and without limits I would say.

Stephen, the father of the deceased, adds that,

> I'd say my spouse, and I agree with everything that Janet said, but I'd
> also like to add it's not only your children when kids are involved you
> can have, you know, you can have in the sense of let's say an extended
> family, if my brother in law, you know their children they are my nieces
> and nephews.

Elsewhere during the interview, Stephen added, "We are a close-knit family…I'd say we were a happy family."

Grief

Janet describes grief as

> An emotion after someone has had a loss, and can be expressed in many
> ways. There is a feeling of sadness, sometimes someone feels depressed
> over a long period of time when you think of your loss that has brought
> in the grief, and it comes, it changes things around in a family situation.
> And grief, when there is loss, sometimes people are never the same
> again, it takes a while to come out of it, maybe with lots of encourage-
> ment from friends and family and it's hard to express grief. It's one of
> those things that sits deep down in your heart, that only the person who
> is experiencing it knows deep down in their hearts, what it's like. But
> the expressions of course could be sadness, depression, lack of interest
> in your normal daily activities, sometimes it can manifest in some, you

could even get sick from grief if it takes too long; and it's one of those things that is hard to explain.

Stephen adds that,

> I think it's very personal, no two people can ever grief the same way because everybody is an individual and when tough times come, we all react differently. You know, there is that emotional aspect and that emotional aspect can go into some physical aspect in your life, and your finances can be altered because you are going through grief. Emotionally you can seem to be the same around people, but behind closed doors, there's things and feelings that happen, you know you have your sadness, you know I've seen people cry, I've seen people who've gone through big changes in their lives such as death and they are always smiling but you can tell something's off.

Community

One of the recurring concepts is the role community plays in times of grief. According to Janet,

> During times of grief, more often than not, they will bring in food, they will bring in resources just to support the family to make sure that they are not thinking about that extra burden of maybe what the visitors will be fed, where the finances will come from, for after a loss as it is expected everything changes, and the greater community comes in to help the family to go through this time of grief, and, but, there comes a time when they leave and when they leave, then you are left alone, then I think that's when now you experience what grief is because everybody is gone, people have to go back to their work, people have to go back to their businesses and it's a moment of truth when now, reality hits that it's really happened, and it's true, that someone has gone and now you are on your own; because friends and family have come to support you for that period of time but they have to go, now it's from there on that you have to deal with it and it's tough.

According to Stephen,

> Coz I think also after that period where you have family and friends come over you know that support, once everything kind of goes back to reality where you know they have to keep on going on with their lives

and in our culture we don't really talk about that anymore, talk about the situation that happened, so it's something that you have to deal internally I'd say with your close family and loved ones; umm, after I guess after the mourning period where you have a lot of support from people, once that phase is done you kind of have to deal with it behind closed doors.

Spirituality

Spirituality is one concept that was evident. According to Janet,

> One great resource is prayer, I believe in prayer and friends and family have been very supportive on that aspect and I believe above all things that, that has been my greatest strength. Prayer, prayer, prayer from friends and family, sometimes you are not able to pray for yourself, and all you can do is just sit; but someone, somewhere praying with you gives you strength, so but for them to pray with you they have to know what's going on in your life; so you kind of have to have a support group; maybe here or in my native country; but prayer has been a great resources.

Emotional Distress

Both parents express frustration, doubt, sadness, desperation, disappointment, and helplessness resulting from high hopes suddenly shattered. Janet stated:

> It was and still remains very hard because though there was some cancer involved and we all felt like we were headed in the right direction with chemotherapy and then we went on to oral chemotherapy and the reports were looking so good; and it looked like she was on the way to recovery. Every report from every corner looked bright and promising until that morning when the call and it was like, it was devastating. That was a young life and I would say at the prime age where someone is trying to now get a, I mean, get your life together and start living, you have children who you have left behind it was, it was hard, it was hard to imagine how to go on after that; and I can only say, it was, it was tough, it's still tough but by the grace of God I guess every day we go through it and we go through the motions and we just have to be strong.

Stephen added:

> What makes it a little, well, we have unanswered questions because when this whole ordeal started, it started out as gallbladder cancer and then she had stents put in she went through chemo and month before she passed away she had a permanent stent put in and then she was getting healthier, more energetic, and then one morning everything just kind of disappeared, and coming to find out on the autopsy her liver had, 95% was gone. and it's tough being told by these doctors that everything is going well and yet are actually seeing an improvement in your loved one and out of nowhere it's a whole different body system that was affected and nobody was able to catch it so you know there is some unanswered questions over there.

Denial

Denial about the diagnosis is a common theme that was clearly demonstrated by the parents. According to Janet,

> Cancer is one of those things, the name itself is a stigma, so when we sat in the doctor's office that morning to get the results of the, what do they call it, where they take out, ooh, the biopsy and the doctor said that the biopsy has come out positive, there is something going on, a tumor and we needed to move fast, it was a shock, and not only to her but to us as a family and having had no incidence of cancer in the family, the immediate family, that was a shocker to us and we almost didn't know what to do.

Stephen added:

> It's something you don't expect and especially to somebody who's that young, you know and in our culture when you hear something about cancer or, you know, any terminal illness; you don't think about the young, you think it's somebody who's older you know, just normal wear and tear of the body, but somebody in your early 30s getting cancer, it's just not unheard of so, there was a little bit of, I guess denial, frustration, and just trying to figure out, now that we had this information, what do, what can we do about it.

Stephen also adds:

> I would say, take it one day at a time; but and sometimes it's hard but you have accept the fact that, you know, she's gone and initially that denial, you know, you go to bed and you wake up expecting to see her, expecting to hear her, or even if it's just a phone call.

Communication

The theme of communication came up a few times. Stephen stated:

> I think we just have to be supportive and communication is really big in times like this because we wanna make sure that we are on the same page, coz even sometimes us as individuals may go through something, what I may thinking, or what I may be feeling may be different from what she is, so we have to make sure that if there is any issues that we are going through, you can, I can still feel be open to talk to her and, you know vice versa.

When asked if they feel like they practice good communication at this time, Janet's response was:

> Yes, we have, we have been able to practice that and it has worked. Yeah and it has helped to deal with this grief process and, yea, being supportive of each other and sharing our thoughts together.

On the other hand, Janet stated:

> It was very difficult for us to break the news to the children, even when the onset of the disease that she was sick, and now here comes the death; how do we face these young children? It was a difficult time.

Stephen also added:

> One thing is in situations like this you need support of others to go through it, and sometimes just human nature you might feel like you are on your own but there is always somebody, someone who is willing to help and all it takes is for you to communicate and seek for that help.

Financial Implications

Financial involvement was also noted during the interview. An example of this is noted when Janet began:

> I think death within a family changes the whole family dynamics, I think we, we have never been the same, there are issues that come and go, there are financial implications, there is the emotional aspect where everybody has been affected and sometimes you really don't know how the children are taking it, they are young, they have lost a mother and she was all they knew, and we have lost a child and, I mean, we can never, no longer see her smile, hear her cheerful voice and, it's just one of those tough things in life that; it changes everything, life is never the same again, in all aspects of life, the emotional aspect, the financial, even as a community, I mean when you come, we cannot see her anymore. So it's one of those things that affects us and it's hard on everybody, and as we talk my greatest concern is for the children, how, how, how are they handling it, how are they coping, it's not easy for them.

Acceptance

The theory of acceptance is another theme that occurred throughout the interview.

> During the interview, Janet stated:

> But, there comes a time when they leave and when they leave, then you are left alone, then I think that's when now you experience what grief is because everybody is gone, people have to go back to their work, people have to go back to their businesses and it's a moment of truth when now, reality hits that it's really happened and it's true, that someone has gone and now you are on your own.

Stephen continued:

> Coz I think also after that period where you have family and friends come over you know that support, once everything kind of goes back to reality where you know they have to keep on going on with their lives and in our culture we don't really talk about that anymore, talk about the situation that happened.

He also adds that:

> As time goes by you realize that's something that can no longer happen, so, I mean when the memories come back you just have to cherish them and, you know, like I said, take it one day at a time and just working through this.

Janet also stated:

> All I'd want to say is that it's tough and it's never easy, but it's one of those things, you know death, that changes your life, but like he said, take it by the day, and we gonna move on.

Support Group

Another theme addressed during the interview was the importance of a support group.

Janet stated:

> One great resource is prayer, I believe in prayer and friends and family have been very supportive on that aspect and I believe above all things that, that has been my greatest strength. Prayer, prayer, prayer from friends and family, sometimes you are not able to pray for yourself and all you can do is just sit; but someone, somewhere praying with you gives you strength, so but for them to pray with you they have to know what's going on in your life; so you kind of have to have a support group; maybe here or in my native country; but prayer has been a great resources.

Stephen continued:

> Yeah, don't try to go through a situation like this by yourself. Sometimes I know it might feel like you are lonely, but there is always somebody out there who is willing to help. It may be close friends, it doesn't have to be immediate family, it could be, you know, just your extended family as well, but one thing is in situations like this you need support of others to go through it, and sometimes just human nature you might feel like you are on your own but there is always somebody, someone who is willing to help and all it takes is for you to communicate and seek for that help.

DISCUSSION

For this particular family, there were many themes that were associated with grief. The two concepts discussed as the focal points that connect family and how they were affected with grief stem from two theories: the family systems theory and the Kübler-Ross's stages of grief.

During the interview, Janet and Stephen stated that there is "no limitation" to what they consider family. Through the help of their extended family as well as the community, they were able to cope and deal with the loss of their daughter. They not only consider their immediate family (husband–wife, daughter) as family, but anyone who is "supportive" and that they get along with well. The cohesiveness of Janet's and Stephen's family to the community is evident in their reliance on, and interaction with the community as a whole. Considering this, and looking at Janet's and Stephen's "family" as the Kenyan community at large, the major finding was that death in their family made a huge impact in their lives. The family systems theory states that actions of one family member affects all family members in the family system. Janet's and Stephen's daughter's death affected all members of the community family as evidenced by the love and emotional, spiritual, and financial support given to Janet and Stephen by the community. The community family cried with them, encouraged them, and gave them financial resources to help cope with the death of their daughter. Although Janet and Stephen were a subsystem within the entire community family, their loss was transferred and shared by each and every member of the community that participated in supporting and loving them. They described their family as having no boundaries, and the concept of interdependence within the community was clearly evident throughout the interview. According to Kiiru (2014), the grief process in Kenyan culture:

> Does not burden an individual alone; it is a shared responsibility geared towards calming and comforting the kin of the departed. In the end, the society becomes a therapeutic support group that helps the bereaved process the loss and resume normal activities. (p. 304)

It is evident that positive feedback and input from the community helped this family cope with the death and loss of their daughter creating an opportunity for positive outcomes, which is in agreement with Rosenblatt (2013).

Any loss affecting an individual is considered as a loss to the entire community. Janet's and Stephen's daughter was part of their community. Because of her death, the entire community system as a family lost an active participating member. According to Janet, wherever they go and whatever they do, they will never get to see her. Seeing her in that context could also be extended to mean participate with, share life with, enjoy with, or just talk with their loved one. It is evident that the family systems theory applies to this family, and the effects of such are noted in the ripple effects that followed her death. The members of the community came together to shield the family from the effect of such great loss. Grief, which is a sense of loss, was not only experienced by Janet and Stephen, but by the whole community family. According to Kiiru (2014), in many communities in Kenya, the community has a greater discretion and power over the bereaved family, to the extent that even the wishes of the bereaved family or the deceased can be overridden by the community if they are in conflict with the beliefs of the indigenous community. This particular community plays a major role in the lives of its members.

Kubler-Ross describes the stages of grief as denial, anger, bargaining, depression, and acceptance. While narrating their story, Janet and Stephen explained how they went through certain types of emotional distress while grieving for their daughter. They described going through periods of denial, sadness, depression, and uncertainty. There was also a notion of anger and frustration that was implied in the uncertainty about their daughter's health related to miscommunication from health care providers.

Although the couple did not necessarily list the stages of grief in any particular order, feelings of denial, anger, depression, and acceptance were evident during the interview. The couple stated that although it has been hard to cope and deal with the loss of their daughter, they had to come with terms of "reality" and accept that their daughter is gone. They also had to come to terms with the "reality" that their lives must go on regardless of the death. According to the couple, once someone dies, and the "mourning" period is over, they do not talk about the death anymore. Stephen explained that any other emotions that they experienced after that period had to be dealt with "behind closed doors." This shows that despite the fact that the family did go through some periods of acceptance of the death of their daughter, residual emotions of denial, anger, bargaining, or depression may have resurfaced afterwards. It is safe to conclude that grief in this family is an ongoing process at this time and that it relates perfectly to the Kubler-Ross grief model and the stages of grief. They are clearly attempting to attain an equilibrium balancing the disruption the death brought on their family regarding financial, psychological, and emotional well-being. Their grieving process does not fit into any linear pattern but appears to enter randomly into different stages at different times.

A sense of passing the blame to cope with the death of a loved one was also seen during the interview. According to Rosenblatt (2013), families sometimes use the "witch is the cause of death" concept when trying to deal with the loss of a loved one. They blame another "evil" or transfer the blame of a death to another object. Janet and Stephen reported miscommunication between them and the health care providers. They reported seeing improvement in their loved one and then "out of nowhere" their daughter died. According to Kiiru (2014), in Kenyan culture, families whose young people died considered their children bewitched. During the interview, a sense of blame was placed not on the cancer itself, but on the doctors who did not communicate efficiently. A gap in communication between the parents and their daughter's doctor was implied. There was possibly no full disclosure of the prognosis of the patient; a communication barrier, misunderstanding between the health provider and the bereaved family or the parents were in denial. For example, the emotional distress that arose out of miscommunication by the health care provider would be eliminated, or minimized, if the family was given a clear understanding of the patient's prognosis.

Application of the FCP and FFGT by the provider would possibly have eliminated or greatly improved the outcome for this family in the period before and after the death of their daughter. Similar therapies to FCP and FFGT would have greatly enhanced communication between the provider and the family, and within the family during and after the course of treatment. Effective communication and group therapy would have also enhanced coping after the death of the patient and mitigated the effects of death and grief on the family. Effective communication would also have addressed the question of the stigma associated with the diagnosis of terminal illness and greatly decreased the effects of emotional distress brought on by death and grief.

The interviewees expressed that there would be some financial restructuring in the family as well. Questions about the way forward with the grandchildren after the death of their mother were raised in the course of the interview. The family's financial structure and the multigenerational structure would possibly be affected in that the grandchildren would need to be assisted and possibly assimilated into the grandparents' family, and this is in agreement with Rosenblatt (2013).

Lastly, the couple did state that they believe in prayer support groups as a means of coping. The couple emphasized the importance of spirituality in their lives as well as the importance of support groups. They consider their friends, family, and the community at large as their support group. It is, therefore, evident that the role of support groups and community therapy like actions played a big role in helping this family cope with the loss of their loved one.

SUMMARY

The cumulative effects of grief on the family system found in this study were evident throughout the interview. There was evidence that the community as a support group proved to be beneficial to the bereaved family in providing financial, moral, and spiritual support. The community enabled the family to quickly regain its equilibrium. Although the family had no negative outcomes from the loss of their daughter, it is still dealing with some residual effects brought on by the death. The death within the family sent ripple effects across the community. This shows that the community was an active part of their family as well.

The Kubler-Ross model can be used as a guide to understanding grief in families as it appears to address universal concepts. However, all the grieving process stages as described in the original work are not evident to all people, cultures, or communities universally. In the present study, the family experienced most of the stages envisaged by the model except for bargaining.

Moreover, although the family systems theory was written based on a culture different from the participant's culture, the theory fit in perfectly when aligned with the effects of grief among immediate family members as well as the community family. According to Carmon et al. (2010), coping effectively with the loss of a loved one can prevent mental health and social problems later on. The couple's coping mechanisms such as spirituality, participating in support groups, accepting community resources, and effective communication among family members assisted the family in coping effectively with the loss of their daughter without any negative outcomes.

IMPLICATIONS

Because of the lack of extensive research in the family grief systems regarding the grieving process in different cultures, this research study will add evidence-based knowledge to the existing literature regarding family grief systems. The FNP can play a major role in reducing risk factors that can lead to loss, stress, grief, anxiety, depression, death, and other negative physical or emotional problems. The FNP can do so by educating the patient and family regarding diagnosis and prognosis of any medical conditions. Education will help the patient and family to anticipate and cope with illnesses and death, if it is inevitable. The FNP can use assessment tools to assess the patient, the patient's family members, and the community.

Adoption of FCPs and FFGT and tailoring them to the needs of individual patients and families is important for every FNP. These tools are useful for research that will enhance nursing practice, as well as the patient's and family's health outcomes. Recognition and utilization of available support groups would greatly help patients and their families cope with illness or death. The FNPs as health care providers are usually trusted and easily assimilated and integrated into the family. This trust would make it easier for them to steer the family and community throughout the process of recovery as well as death, if inevitable. FNPs are best placed to carry out research and share their findings to improve evidence-based practice. The evidence-based research will also provide opportunities for qualitative and quantitative work that could lead to the development of relevant tools, therapies, and education material. The material may be used for nursing practice as well as the entire medical fraternity. Even though the results of this case cannot be generalized, some of the lessons learned can be applied to help other people who might find themselves in similar situations in the future.

LIMITATIONS

The findings of this research cannot be generalized. The interviewers' interactions with the larger Kenyan community could also have introduced some bias, although it also allowed them to have a better understanding and interpretation of the emerging themes and concepts. No tools were used by the researchers to analyze the effects of grief on the family. Standardized tools may be helpful in understanding the extent of grief and its effects. Moreover, the couple has been bereaved for less than a year, and the process of grieving may not be completed. Currently, the effects of the death may not have been fully appreciated.

RECOMMENDATIONS

Lack of longitudinal research data to investigate changing patterns of grief at different stages of grief is needed. Most family systems grief research is often qualitative or quantitative. A mixed method analysis would be beneficial in assessing any gaps the two designs may pose. Because of the attributes of grief research being more narrative than they are quantitative, family systems grief research could benefit from a study that is quantitative in nature and can quantify its results.

REFERENCES

Bolden, L. A. (2007). A review of on grief and grieving: Finding the meaning of grief through the five stages of loss. *Counseling and Values, 51*(3), 235–237.

Bowen, M. (2004). *Family theory in clinical practice.* Lanham, MD: Rowman and Littlefield.

Carmon, A. F., Western, K. J., Miller, A. N., Pearson, J. C., & Fowler, M. R. (2010). Grieving those we've lost: An examination of family communication patterns and grief reactions. *Communication Research Projects, 27*(3), 253–262. Retrieved from http://dx.doi.org/10.1080/08824096.2010.496329

Environmental influences: Family systems theory. (1990). Retrieved from http://www.d.umn.edu/~kbrorson/TSWadapted/resources/PDFS/FamilySystemsTheory.pdf

Gaudio, F. D., Zaider, T. I., Brier, M., & Kissane, D. W. (2011). Challenges in providing family-centered support to families in palliative care. *Palliative Medicine, 26*(8), 1025–1033. Retrieved from http://dx.doi.org/10.1177/0269216311426919

Hayslip, B., & Page, K. S. (2013). Family characteristics and dynamics: A systems approach to grief. *Family Science, 4*(1), 58–58. Retrieved from http://dx.doi.org/10.1080/19424620.2013.819679

Holtslander, L. F., & McMillan, S. C. (2011). Depressive symptoms, grief, and complicated grief among family caregivers of patients with advanced cancer three months into bereavement. *Oncology Nursing Forum, 38*(1), 60–65. Retrieved from http://dx.doi.org/10.1188/11.ONF.60–65

Kiiru, M. (2014). Going gentle into that good night: Indigenous therapy on death in Kenya. *Procedia-Social And Behavioral Sciences, 114.* 4th World Conference on Psychology, Counseling and Guidance (WCPCG-2013), 293–310. Retrieved from http://dx.doi.org/10.1016/j.sbspro.2013.12.702

Kübler-Ross, E. (1969). *On death and dying.* New York, NY: Routledge.

Rosenblatt, P. C. (2013). Family grief in cross-cultural perspective. *Family Science, 4*(1), 12–19. Retrieved from http://dx.doi.org/10.1080/19424620.2013.819226

TRAGEDY TO TRIUMPH: LIFE HISTORY OF AN OLDER WOMAN LIVING WITH AIDS

Tracey Couse and Kelly Heard

*A*pproximately, 33% of people now living with HIV/AIDS in the United States are older than 50 years of age (Psaros et al., 2015). Studies have shown that the life expectancy of a person living with HIV is equivalent to that of an individual without HIV, living with another chronic illness (Nakagawa et al., 2012). The Centers for Disease Control (CDC) estimates that 15% of the new cases of HIV and 24% of persons living with HIV are adults who are 50 years and older (CDC, 2008). The majority of HIV studies have been with men, but there are a growing number of women diagnosed with HIV (Psaros et al., 2015). Research has shown that women tend to cope less effectively with a HIV diagnosis and suffer greater disease-related symptoms and mortality (Bianco, Heckman, Sutton, Watakakosol, & Lovejoy, 2011). There are minimal data published on the coping strategies of older women living with HIV (Grodensky et al., 2015; Slomka, Lim, Gripshover, & Daly, 2013). Discovering and understanding effective coping strategies of older women successfully living with HIV may help guide interventions across the life spans of the growing number of women diagnosed with HIV and improve outcomes.

PROBLEM STATEMENT

The purpose of this study is to interpret the self-described life story of an older woman with a diagnosis of HIV in order to understand the psychosocial factors related to successful management of HIV in the long term. Specifically, the research question is: What psychosocial factors encourage success in overcoming the diagnosis of HIV in a woman as she ages? This topic is significant because there is a growing aging population, an increasing number of HIV-diagnosed women, and decreased HIV-related outcomes for women with this diagnosis (Bianco et al., 2011; Psaros et al., 2015). Themes and issues identified here may guide interventions across life span for women aging with HIV or any chronic illness. The challenges of older women living with HIV have not been well separated from those of men (Grodensky et al., 2015). Finally, psychosocial experiences of older women living with HIV have not been fully described (Grodensky et al., 2015).

ASSUMPTIONS

The main assumption, as in any qualitative study is that the person will tell the truth as she sees it. We have no reason to believe she did not.

DEFINITIONS

For the purposes of this study, *long term* refers to patients who have been diagnosed with HIV for more than 5 years and are now living with the disease past the age of 50 years. *Psychosocial* is defined as "a term referring to the mind's ability to, consciously or unconsciously, adjust and relate the body to its social environment" (Gale Encyclopedia of Medicine, 2008). It is in the psychosocial realm that *coping* exists, which encompasses the spiritual, emotional, and cognitive processes that individuals use to adapt and come to terms with their lives and challenges. Fang et al. (2015) define *resilience* as involving two components including the exposure to significant adversity and the ability to positively adapt despite the adversity. Finally, *successful management of HIV* is defined as accepting the diagnosis and performing necessary self-care and health management tasks contributing to long-term survival.

LITERATURE REVIEW

Numerous studies have investigated successful coping mechanisms in older HIV-positive adults living with the disease. One of those themes was optimism. Carrico and Moskowitz (2014) used a cohort study to demonstrate a link between positive affect and engagement in care through increased treatment adherence. Emlet, Tozay, and Raveis (2011) showed optimism as a major coping theme of adults aging with HIV using semi-structured interviews. A thematic review by Roger, Mignone, & Kirkland (2013) found that older adults deal with living with HIV through well-being promotion. Finally, McIntosh and Rosselli (2012) used a meta-analysis and specifically looked at older women living with HIV. They found that positive reframing promoted psychological adaptation for this population studied.

The concept of resilience also repeatedly surfaced in the literature. Dale et al. (2014) found that women living with HIV scoring high in resilience were more likely to adhere to healthy behaviors such as following a healthy diet, exercising, keeping doctors' appointments, and taking their medications consistently. Even in spite of sexual abuse or multiple abuses, high resilience predicted high Highly Active Antiretroviral Therapy (HAART) medication adherence (Dale et al., 2014). A study by Emlet et al. (2011) found that the majority of subjects older than 50 years had experiences of resilience and strength while living with HIV.

Another recurrent coping theme was social support. Access to social support has been widely studied as part of adherence, increased quality of life, and an important tool for coping with the disease. Webel, Dolansky, Henry, and Salata (2012) studied self-management techniques in women with HIV and found that 21% of their participants believed that attending support groups is an important strategy in self-management. Webel et al. (2013) concluded that improving social capital and incorporating social roles into the daily health activities of women living with HIV may improve their health. Slomka, Lim, Gripshover, and Daley (2013) studied coping in long-term survivors. They found social support to be a basic element of coping and that many participants saw their health care providers as part of their social support network. Cote et al. (2015) found that valuing interpersonal relationships was one of the seven themes to come out of their study on the lived experience of HIV long-term nonprogressors.

The concept of self-efficacy has been studied as a coping strategy. Tyer-Viola et al. (2014) measured self-efficacy using the Adherence Self-Efficacy scale. They were able to determine that adherence, self-efficacy, and depression symptoms predict medication adherence in women. Nokes et al. (2012) also found that self-efficacy was a strong predictor of combined antiretroviral therapy (cART) adherence behavior in their large cross-sectional and descriptive study. Nokes describes how self-efficacy is "an antecedent skill" needed for optimum treatment adherence ultimately assisting this older population with disease coping.

A final recurrent coping theme in the older HIV population was spirituality. Kremer and Ironson (2014) found that spirituality was mainly beneficial for women, heterosexuals, and African Americans. It is a major source of positive coping. Spirituality was described as a source of comfort, empowerment, growth, gratitude, and community support. Kremer and Ironson (2014) found that if clinicians simply asked about spirituality it would help patients cope with trauma. Another study by Molzahn et al. (2012) found three spirituality themes that emerged from their study of people living with serious illnesses. These themes are reflecting on spiritual, religious, and personal beliefs; crafting beliefs for their own lives; and finding meaning and transcending beyond words. Slomka et al. (2013) also noted the prevalence of religion and/or spirituality as a coping mechanism for long-term HIV survivors in their study. Grodensky et al. (2015), who performed semi-structured interviews of women with HIV, who were 50 years and older, found that "spirituality provided great support for all participants."

After performing this review, the authors have found that the literature has extensively documented HIV-coping and many related aspects, especially for those younger than 50 years of age and for men. However, though there have been studies performed on aging with HIV and the unique challenges people living with HIV (PLWH) face as they grow older, very few have been done on the older population, and even fewer on women aging with HIV. Many factors make this population of older women increasingly susceptible to infection with HIV including physiological changes during menopause, decreased perception of risk, decreased use of condoms, and decreased knowledge of risk (Durvasula, 2014). Although the negative implications of an HIV diagnosis on older women have been noted in the literature (Bianco et al., 2011; Durvasula, 2014; Psaros et al., 2015), effective methods used by patients to overcome this diagnosis have not. Chambers et al. (2014) pointed out that qualitative literature could explore the lived experiences of older PLWH, especially in areas of physical health, antiretroviral therapy (ART) adherence, and sexual health. Chambers also points out that most of the studies so far have been on homosexual or bisexual men. The studies on physical health focus on illness not wellness, and there is a lack of intervention research designed for older PLWH, especially women.

METHODOLOGY

The described study is a focused ethnographic study using a life-history format. The life-history technique is a method commonly used in ethnography that provides understanding of a culture through the eyes of a willing representative who communicates their life story to the researcher (de Chesnay, 2005, 2015). Like all life stories, the one under study is told by the researchers, compiled from data obtained from the informant that is interpreted and translated by the researchers (de Chesnay, 2015). The "culture" under study can be described as the older female population living with HIV in the United States. The purpose and goal of this methodology is to provide an in-depth understanding of the psychosocial factors that encourage success in overcoming the diagnosis of HIV in a woman's long-term management of her HIV status. The participant was purposively recruited through a contact at a clinical site. Institutional review board (IRB) approval was obtained followed by informed consent. There are three common data collection methods used in life histories including semi-structured interviews, genograms, and timelines (de Chesnay, 2015). The authors used all three methods to construct the participant's life history. The semi-structured interview guide was developed using guidelines articulated by de Chesnay (2015). Questions were open-ended to minimize the risk of biasing the informant and allow unique themes to emerge. The data were collected over a 90-minute interview to minimize informant burden, and the interview was performed in her home to provide comfort and privacy. The genogram and timeline are not included in this study to protect the identity of the participant. Although the results are not generalizable, the gathered data can be used to obtain a better understanding of this population of women, help to create care interventions for women across the life span living with HIV, and possibly individuals with other chronic illnesses.

RESULTS

The sample for this study is comprised of a single participant. The participant was purposively sampled to participate in the semi-structured interview because of her life story. Inclusion and exclusion criteria do not apply. Means of recruitment was through a contact at a clinical site. The participant is a longtime survivor of HIV infection with progression to AIDS and serves as a clinician in a HIV clinic in the southeast United States. The rationale for choosing the participant included researcher interest and the participant's unique circumstances as a woman successfully thriving long term with a diagnosis of HIV. Pseudonyms are being used for her and the members of her family to protect their privacy.

The participant, Sue, is a Caucasian female in her late 50s who was born and raised in New York City. She graduated from nursing school in 1978 and became a born-again Christian in 1979. Sue married her first husband, Mark, in 1980. Mark was also a new Christian and had homosexual relations before their marriage. Sue and Mark had their first child, David, in 1982. Sue was very late going into labor with David, causing Mark to confess that he had cheated on Sue and had a homosexual affair in her last trimester. David was born healthy and Sue chose to forgive Mark for his infidelity and they moved on. They then relocated to Atlanta in 1985. Shortly after arriving in Atlanta they had their second son, Luke. Luke became ill at age 15 months with enlarged lymph nodes and was misdiagnosed as having Burkitt's lymphoma. After being in and out of the hospital for several months, he died at age 20 months in July of 1987. Posthumously, Luke was diagnosed with HIV creating the need for Sue, Mark, and David to be tested. Sue was already pregnant with their third child when she discovered that she and Mark were both positive. David, the eldest son, tested negative. Sue's daughter and third child, Beth, was born in December of the same year. Beth, who also contracted HIV, became ill with cytomegalovirus (CMV) at around 7 to 8 weeks of age and at this point Sue felt the need for help and support. She and Mark went and confided in their pastor what was happening to them and to Beth. The pastor and the whole church became extremely supportive of Sue and Mark, offering practical help and emotional and spiritual support.

Beth spent most of her life sick and hospitalized, and died by age 17 months in 1989 with AIDS-CMV. When she buried Beth, Sue's grief was not only that she had lost another child, but that she would never have any more, knowing that the HIV she carried had infected and killed her other two children. Mark's health began declining in 1990 and by 1995 he had AIDS-dementia and was admitted to hospice. He died secondary to an AIDS-related illness in 1996. In addition to her grief over losing Mark, she also feared being alone for the rest of her life. She never thought she would marry again due to her diagnosis. After Mark was admitted to hospice and after he died, Sue turned her full attention to her own health, losing 75 pounds. Her days revolved around frequent consumption of antiretroviral medications, which had to be taken 1 hour before or 2 hours after eating. Although it was a grueling medication regimen, it assisted with her weight loss. Sue and David changed churches around this time because the pastor of their church had left and the church culture had changed. As always, Sue was very open about her diagnosis and did not hide it from her new group of friends. She met John, her second husband, in that group who was not deterred by her diagnosis. Sue and John were married in 2000, and she acquired five children from that marriage, which helped to fill the vacuum left by losing two of her own. Sue currently works at a local infectious disease clinic and counsels

HIV-diagnosed patients. She uses her own story, where appropriate, to help encourage those who are struggling.

The 1.5-hour-long tape-recorded interview of Sue's HIV journey was carefully transcribed to 16 single-spaced pages. A detailed content analysis was performed. From the transcript, sections were identified for thought processes that were then translated to themes and concepts. This process continued until the authors reached saturation. Five main concepts surfaced from the interview: faith, social support, knowledge, hope/optimism, and resiliency.

The first identified theme is faith. Sue became a Christian in the late 1970s, and she credits her faith for carrying her through all the difficulties.

> So if I had to say one thing that has really kept me through the whole thing is just my faith. If I had not become a Christian way back when I was twenty-something odd years old....I was raised in the Catholic church but Catholics believe just be good...don't kill anybody. ... Anyhow, every church has got Jesus on the cross but nobody really ever said that that was for *you*....So when that really became a reality, I had a literal turning of my life. I was just a crazy rotten sinner and just became a born again Christian and it was night and day. My family just really didn't even know how to deal with it. They really didn't because they just couldn't believe how I had changed, for the good, but nevertheless it was hard for them to see such a contrast.

She demonstrated regular acts of forgiveness in the name of God the Father as she was able to forgive her husband's acts of homosexuality and his infection of three family members with HIV.

> I never blamed Mark. The whole time with this whole thing I never, we never got into a fight, well I can't say never, during the majority of the time, I never argued with him and never said, "If it wasn't for you doing this, this would have never happened." I never, because I'm like, this man suffered so much over the weight of being the one that could have been responsible for this whole thing!

She did not seek prenatal care for her first born, David, but laid her faith in God for his "health" at birth, saying "Anyway I know it sounds foolish, but I had faith that if we were walking with the Lord he would be with us. He would deliver our baby just like we had seen him deliver so many other babies in the church." She turned to God to speak to her on major life events like moving to another city. She expressed "peace" during the last few dying hours of her son.

> I had peace, you know. I knew when I came home from the hospital and then was going right back again, I knew it was going to be that night. I wasn't like crazy emotional on the way back to the hospital, I just had peace, because I knew it was the inevitable.

Sue found "grace" in a negative HIV diagnosis for her eldest son, after learning that she, her husband, and her second born had contracted the virus. She talked about praying throughout the interview, even praying for her third child to be a girl as the first two were boys. She believed that the kindness of her congregation demonstrated to her family was an outward expression of God's love. Sue found kindness in the Lord for letting her family members die around the same month so she did not have to mourn three times a year. She believed her stepchildren were "gifts from God." In wrapping up the interview, she talked about "apprehending God's grace" for what she went through:

> We have a really, really, really incredibly strong God. We really do, we really do. A lot of people say, "I don't know if I could do it." Excuse me? You don't know what you can handle until you're faced with the situation. I used to take offense at people saying that because I'm just like, "I'm no different than you or anyone else. I'm flesh and blood skin." ... We all have to apprehend grace for whatever we're called to face, you know what I mean? So it's wrong for somebody to say I don't think I could do that, well, you're not being asked to do that. You have to apprehend grace for what you're being asked to do.

The second theme was social support. Social support was found in many facets of her life. Sue was close to her parents who provided emotional support and comfort to her especially during times of illness and death. Her husband, Mark, had a large family, which became a goal of their own. Sue, her husband, and son followed some church friends and moved to another city and even lived with them for a few months after the move. Sue mentions other dependable friends who would do anything for them, like drive them to the hospital in the middle of the night.

Sue also found social support in her church. Sue and her husband confided in multiple pastors who provided counsel, direction, and support. One pastor was willing to lose his congregation to support Sue and Mark knowing the stigmatizing effects of their diagnosis. He said, "I don't care if I lose my whole congregation, we are going to stand by you two. You've been through enough." This pastor also counseled Mark with his "homosexuality struggle" and her son with the loss of his father. Their fellow parishioners provided physical and emotional support to the family addressing their many needs as she describes after Beth got sick:

> I can't even describe to you the outpouring of love once these people got the letter [describing their situation to the church]. People dropping by and just money showing up and just the support we got from people was just incredible. Outpouring of support and love. And this is in 1987. I was amazed. When I think about it, I am still amazed that the people of this congregation pulled it together, they dug deep. They just really found the love of God, put skin on Jesus.

Sue also found social support in her dealings with multiple health care facilities and organizations. She referred to key health care providers who cared for her and her family during the difficult times like the midwife who delivered one of her babies or the pediatrician who helped break the news to Sue's parents that she, her husband, and her daughter had HIV. She made lifelong nursing friends as a result of her tragedies, including the hospital and home health nurses who cared for the two children who eventually died. She praised a local legal aid company that financially and legally assisted her in obtaining disability. She found support in various community organizations like the Ronald McDonald House where she and her family spent many months and in Flight Angels, who saved her child's life on one of many urgent visits to a specialty hospital.

> Forget the name of the organization of that flies people all over the country that have medical conditions—is it Flight Angels? These pilots volunteer their time, that have small engine planes and they fly people all over the country. We had a really good social worker at Scottish Rite and we'd made friends with the nursing staff there too. So there were a lot of really good people that were involved with us at the time.

A third theme that surfaced in her life story was education/knowledge. Sue earned her nursing degree in 1978. She had a passion for midwifery and a desire to obtain this degree. She was able to save her one son Luke, who became unconscious during his short life.

> [We were] at the house we were renting, and he just stopped breathing. It was he just stopped, boom. He was sitting in his high chair. He was

like 16 or 17 months old. And he just stopped breathing at the table. I was like "Mark, call 911!" I started CPR and got him breathing again, rushed him up by ambulance to Scottish Rite.

She credits her medical experience for her ability to actively participate in the critical care needed for her acutely ill children. "So she [Beth] had to go back on Progestimil feedings at home, oh they were awful, with the pump at home. It was a good thing I was a nurse because it was easy to figure it out and stuff." She gives credit to her medical knowledge for being able to question health care providers on diagnoses and treatment plans ensuring the best care for her family members. She gives credit to her medical training for allowing her to be the sole care provider of her husband, who was suffering from HIV dementia, until it became too dangerous to do because of his aggression,

So then Mark's health really started to fail and I can't even begin to tell you the different diseases and infections that he had. I know he did have Kaposi Sarcoma. He had a central line put in for whatever we were doing—I can't even remember the illnesses to be honest with you. It's just a whole big blur. But the one thing that was really, really bad was that he got HIV-dementia...And it got to be so bad that I could no longer take care of him, because he was combative.

The fourth theme extracted from Sue's life story was hope/optimism. Sue demonstrated optimism and hope of a great life after marrying Mark, who put his homosexuality behind them once they became Christians. Sue was optimistic for a home birth of her first born, David, even in the absence of prenatal care. Due to a late delivery, he was born in the hospital with the umbilical cord wrapped around his neck. The baby ended up being healthy. With the presence of a healthy newborn, she was hopeful the family would have a happy life in spite of Mark's confession he had an extramarital affair in the last trimester of the pregnancy. After her second son died from a long illness, she remained optimistic due to the hope of a new baby ahead, as she was pregnant with their third child. "Now we are like the first or second week of August, just trying to get our life back together. Let's put this behind us. We have the hope of a new baby ahead of us. It's not good [Luke's death], but this is good." She found optimism in the fact that her eldest son tested negative for HIV, even when she and her husband were positive for the virus. Sue found hope and optimism in many of the people who surrounded her. After Sue's third child, and only daughter, became acutely ill at 8 weeks of age and possibly carried HIV, Sue was optimistic of a good outcome because the pediatrician was also an infectious disease specialist, saying "Beth was born and she had this respiratory infection. The good thing about it was from, like birth, her pediatrician was an infectious disease doctor." Sue expressed great hope in the new AZT treatment trial that Beth was receiving even though her daughter had been ill and hospitalized for more than half her life. She remained hopeful after confessing her family's diagnosis to their pastor, who offered them his full support even if it meant the loss of his congregation. Additionally, Sue demonstrated optimism after all the tragedy and death because she had a supportive church. She also expressed hope and optimism after getting herself healthy again, "So I got healthy, my T-cells went up, my viral load, you know, got suppressed and I got a new lease on life." In the face of losing two children and her husband, she remained hopeful for a good life for herself and her remaining living son.

All of these concepts illustrate Sue's resiliency, which is the last theme. She picked herself up after each loss and moved forward with hope. She had to deal with insanity with her husband, but even in the midst of it she would not give up on him or her marriage, as illustrated in the following quote:

> I don't know, I had put up with so much (tearfully) 'cause he had really gotten very combative and violent. He had guns in the house and that was why I had to get him away from the house because I was afraid he was going to kill himself or kill me or David or something. It was just ... We had to call the police to get them to come to the house. I mean it was just really bizarre the stuff we had to put up with. But I mean I just made my decision 'til death do us part and that's the way it's gonna be. I don't care and he used to ask me, "We're getting a divorce! That's it I'm divorcing you!" I'm like, "No you're not. No you're not. I have power of attorney over you and you are not divorcing me!" Because I knew if he did he would not have a proper burial and I was just not going to stand for that.

DISCUSSION

Sue was not a stranger to big life changes. This included her faith. She became a born-again Christian well into her twenties. She proudly stated that her new found faith, more than 30 years ago, was a huge turning point for her and her life, which set the stage and foundation for her subsequent years. She beat the odds of transforming her life early. Sue's ability to overcome such a major life change that was rich in support and inspiration gave her the confidence and tools she needed to overcome her diagnosis of HIV. Spirituality is documented as an important factor in aging and those with chronic illness and helps buffer people from related stressors (Cuevas, Vance, Viamonte, Lee, & South, 2010; DeGrezia & Scrandis, 2015). This strong tie to faith usually increases after a diagnosis of HIV. This was not the case for Sue. Her faith and relationship with God was well established before her diagnosis and they continue to be predominant players in her life today. Spirituality and faith in God, remain well documented and a major coping mechanism described in many studies of HIV-infected persons including older women (Cuevas et al., 2010; Degrezia & Scrandis, 2015; Grodensky et al., 2015;). Her faith in God gave her the strength, self-esteem, hope, and optimism she needed to face life with a HIV diagnosis head on.

Sue's faith always remained strong and never wavered. Even after the death of her two youngest children and husband at the hands of AIDS-related illnesses, she never questioned God. Her faith persevered and she trusted in God that it all had meaning and purpose. Studies describe spirituality and cite a faith in God as coping mechanisms for dealing with a HIV status. These same studies report that verbally acknowledging God's participation in one's life creates confidence (DeGrezia & Scrandis, 2015). Her faith gave her the strength and confidence to go on in the face of much negativity. She managed to remain hopeful for her and her son's future life. DeGrezia also describes how faith in God can give purpose in life and often prepares HIV-diagnosed people for their future work (2015). This is not the case for Sue. Although she works as a HIV counselor, she did not credit God for this direction of her life. Regardless, Sue's faith was a major coping mechanism and continues to be today. She possessed a strong sense of spirituality and prayed often, which provided a buffer for her to stressors and promoted confidence in her ability to overcome difficult situations. These related concepts are well described by Grodensky et al. (2015).

Throughout her described life story there is the common thread of constant social support during the evolution of her diagnosis. Sue says she was always forthcoming about her HIV status to her social circle. This was not entirely the case for her parents or extended family. She spared them the truth about how she and her family acquired HIV. She protected them from that information to keep the family strong and united. Her immediate family was the foundation of her drive to cope. It was her devotion and fundamental support of her sick family that gave her purpose during her early diagnosis and the first decade thereafter. Having a purpose after a HIV diagnoses is a described positive coping mechanism in the literature (DeGrezia & Scrandis, 2015).

The other components of Sue's extensive social system provided her with unconditional love, acceptance, and physical support. This came in the form of Sue's second family, her church. Her pastors also provided counsel, advice, and an outlet for her in that she obtained reassurance, encouragement, and the sense of feeling listened to and understood. Those diagnosed with HIV expressing increased satisfaction in these areas are related to more effective coping, leading to increased quality of life, and decreased risk-taking behaviors (Ashton et al., 2005).

Sue also found social support and comfort in many key health care providers that devoted critical medical care as well as emotional support to her and her family. She befriended many of these important players who remain a part of her life and social circle today. There appears to be limited studies in the literature on the value of health care providers and their relation to providing coping skills to HIV-diagnosed populations. The few studies that mention this, state how participants are not satisfied with their providers and the care or support extended (DeGrezia & Scrandis, 2015). Overall, satisfaction with social support is a strong predictor of health outcomes (Ashton et al., 2005). It seems highly plausible that Sue's extensive social system provided the support and coping mechanisms needed to keep her healthy.

Coming full circle, Sue plays an important social support service, herself, to the HIV-infected population. She uses her knowledge, experience, and optimism to educate and counsel the newly diagnosed and those living with HIV/AIDS, on a daily basis. She has devoted the last 10 years of her life to this cause. Educating others regarding the diagnosis and successful living, as well as providing emotional support, is a common coping mechanism described in the literature (DeGrezia & Scrandis, 2015; Psaros et al., 2015). That being said, Sue does not let her diagnosis define her, and she preaches this ideology to her patients. Sue says she thinks about her HIV/AIDS for a minute each day when she takes her pills, otherwise she leads a normal healthy life without the focus being on her HIV.

Sue's medical knowledge through her nursing education and experience helped her to cope with taking care of her family members and to cope with her own diagnosis. There is a great deal in the literature regarding knowledge and education about HIV as a prevention strategy, but knowledge as a coping mechanism in PLWH is rarely discussed. One study by Kumar, Mohanraj, Rao, Murray, and Manhart (2015), done in South India, found that due to the shame and stigma of having HIV there, knowledge of the disease was poor. However, when these PLWH began understanding their disease, they developed a new sense of confidence and realized that they could continue to live fairly healthy lives. Ribeiro, Sarmento e Castro,

Dinis-Ribeiro, and Fernandes (2014) found that knowledge played a significant role in improving HAART adherence in the HIV patients to whom they administered a psycho-educational program. Although Psaros et al. (2015) have shown that older women have a fear of the uncertainty of the disease course, this was not the case for Sue due to her personal knowledge. She believed and still teaches that if one takes her meds regularly, she can stay healthy. Sue also discussed at one point that she became healthier after her diagnosis than she was before. Her knowledge facilitated her HAART adherence.

Buscher, Kallen, Suarez-Almazor, and Giordano (2015) found that PLWH for a longer period of time (15 years or more) felt more pride in surviving HIV and had more feelings of hope. Though she would fit that description now, Sue was diagnosed in 1987 when there was much fear surrounding the disease, little was known about it, and there were no long-term treatment options. Sue's hope seemed to stem from her faith and her dogged determination to move forward, saying after her husband died, "somehow, some way, I found the strength to be better through that whole thing." Puig-Perez et al. (2015) found that "higher optimism was associated with better physiological adjustment to a stressful situation." Sue had the ability to be optimistic even in the worst circumstances. Her optimistic outlook appears to stem from her belief that God is in control and everything happens for a reason. She never gave up hope and never stopped being optimistic about her life getting better.

Sue's hope and optimism were closely related to and a part of her resilience. Fang et al. (2015), in their resilience study of older adults living with HIV, found that hope/optimism was a significant factor in their model of resilience. Sue's entire story is an illustration of resilience. One can hardly imagine more adversity coming into a life than the loss of two children and a husband to HIV, and then having to deal with one's own diagnosis and treatment for HIV. Yet Sue has overcome her adversities, getting remarried and resuming her nursing career as a HIV educator. Psaros' study (2015) mentions contributing to HIV prevention and awareness as an important means of coping with HIV.

The authors observed that Sue only mentioned her own struggle with her diagnosis of HIV in one brief paragraph of the interview when she struggled with her medication regimen. She was so focused on caring for her ailing family members that she hardly focused on her own diagnosis until they had passed away. Webel and Higgins (2012) found that for most of the women who mentioned their role of mother/grandmother, their children/grandchildren were a source of inspiration and purpose for them. Sue never talked about being stressed about her diagnosis or being consumed by it or afraid of it. It appears that the tragedy she faced in losing her family members made her HIV diagnosis seem like a minor life problem in comparison. In the few references to her diagnosis, she put God and her family in the same sentence, keeping everything in perspective.

RECOMMENDATIONS FOR FUTURE RESEARCH

The participant of this study was unique because she was diagnosed early in the evolution of HIV. Additionally, she was one of the first to traverse the path of living with HIV over time. Studying this participant and women like her is necessary to gather information for providers so they can optimally care for a growing, aging women's HIV population as well as the newly diagnosed. Further studies could include a series of life stories of similar groups of women to see if common or new themes arise. Especially interesting would be to compare the stories of newly diagnosed against those with a long history of being diagnosed. Studies looking at quantification assessment of coping strategies would contribute to intervention design. Other research that applies the knowledge learned from the current study to design and test interventions would add to the knowledge base of this population of patients.

As a result of this study, medical providers, including nurse practitioners, can learn from the roles that faith, social support, knowledge, hope, and resilience played in this particular woman's life. Encouraging patients to reconnect with their church, synagogue, or mosque is a good way for them to access spiritual and social support. Providers should also have lists of support groups available to provide to this population of patients (DeGrezia & Scrandis, 2015). Teaching patients about their HIV may assist them with medication adherence and overall coping. Engaging patients to care for their own health is favored by these patients (DeGrezia & Scrandis, 2015). Hope stems from optimism that the future will be better. If patients understand that with proper medication adherence and coping skills, they can live full lives, they may be more hopeful moving into the future. Most importantly, women like Sue need to be treated holistically for all their health needs, ensuring that they are women first and not defined by a diagnosis.

SUMMARY

In answering the question, "What psychosocial factors encourage success in overcoming the diagnosis of HIV in a woman as she ages?" the authors have looked at one woman diagnosed nearly 30 years ago. Although Psaros (2015) found that older women living with HIV experience a process of acceptance over time with their diagnosis, this was not the case for Sue. She had so much tragedy to deal with that she never voiced struggling with accepting her own diagnosis. She alludes to the fact that it was like anything else in life, no bigger or worse, and she did not dwell on it. In her early life, it was experiencing the tragic events of losing two of her children and then her husband, her training as a nurse, her extensive social network, her strong faith in God, and her strong desire and hope for a better future, that helped her successfully survive and cope with her HIV diagnosis for so long. Later in life, and currently, it is celebrating her newfound family that compensates for all her losses and helps her successfully age in the presence of her HIV status.

REFERENCES

Ashton, E., Vosvick, M., Chesney, M., Gore-Felton, C., Koopman, C., O'Shea, K., ... Spiegel, D. (2005). Social support and maladaptive coping as predictors of the change in physical health symptoms among persons living with HIV/AIDS. *AIDS Patient Care and STDs, 19*(9), 587–598.

Bianco, J. A., Heckman, T. G., Sutton, M., Watakakosol, R., & Lovejoy, T. (2011). Predicting adherence to antiretroviral therapy in HIV-infected older adults: The moderating role of gender. *AIDS and Behavior, 15*(7), 1437–1446.

Buscher, A. L., Kallen, M. A., Suarez-Almazor, M. E., & Giordano, T. P. (2015). Development of an "Impact of HIV" instrument for HIV survivors. *Journal of the Association of Nurses in AIDS Care, 26*(6), 720–731.

Carrico, A. W., & Moskowitz, J. T. (2014). Positive affect promotes engagement in care after HIV diagnosis. *Health Psychology: Official Journal of the Division of Health Psychology, American Psychological Association, 33*(7), 686–689.

Centers for Disease Control & Prevention (2008). *Persons 50 years and over.* Retrieved from http://www.cdc.gov/hiv/pdf/library_factsheet_HIV_among_person-saged50andolder.pdf

Chambers, L. A., Wilson, M. G., Rueda, S., Gogolishvili, D., Shi, M. Q., & Rourke, S. B.; Positive Aging Review Team. (2014). Evidence informing the intersection of HIV, aging and health: A scoping review. *AIDS and behavior, 18*(4), 661–675.

Cote, J., Bourbonnais, A., Rouleau, G., Couture, M., Masse, B., & Tremblay, C. (2015). Psychosocial profile and lived experience of HIV-infected long-term progressors: A mixed methods study. *Journal of the Association of Nurses in AIDS Care, 26*(2), 164–175.

Cuevas, J., Vance, D., Viamonte, S., Lee, S., & South, J. (2010). A comparison of spirituality and religiousness in older and younger adults with and without HIV. *Journal of Spirituality in Mental Health, 12*(4), 273–287.

Dale, S., Cohen, M., Weber, K., Cruise, R., Kelso, G., & Brody, L. (2014). Abuse and resilience in relation to HAART medication adherence and HIV viral load among women with HIV in the United States. *AIDS Patient Care and STDs, 28*(3), 136–143.

De Chesnay, M. (2005). "Can't keep me down": Life histories of successful African American adults. In M. de Chesnay (Ed.), *Caring for the vulnerable* (pp. 221–232). Sudbury, MA: Jones and Bartlett, Inc.

De Chesnay, M. (2015). *Nursing research using life history: Qualitative designs & methods in nursing.* New York, NY: Springer Publishing Company.

DeGrezia, M. G., & Scrandis, D. (2015). Successful coping in urban, community-dwelling older adults with HIV. *The Journal of the Association of Nurses in AIDS Care: JANAC, 26*(2), 151–163.

Durvasula, R. (2014). HIV/AIDS in older women: Unique challenges, unmet needs. *Behavioral Medicine (Washington, D.C.), 40*(3), 85–98.

Emlet, C. A., Tozay, S., & Raveis, V. H. (2011). "I'm not going to die from the AIDS": Resilience in aging with HIV disease. *The Gerontologist, 51*(1), 101–111.

Fang, X., Vincent, W., Calabrese, S. K., Heckman, T. G., Sikkema, K. J., Humphries, D. L., & Hansen, N. B. (2015). Resilience, stress, and life quality in older adults living with HIV/AIDS. *Aging & Mental Health, 19*(11), 1015–1021.

Gale encyclopedia of medicine. (2008). Retrieved from http://medical-dictionary.thefreedictionary.com/psychosocial

Grodensky, C. A., Golin, C. E., Jones, C., Mamo, M., Dennis, A. C., Abernethy, M. G., & Patterson, K. B. (2015). "I should know better": The roles of relationships, spirituality, disclosure, stigma, and shame for older women living with HIV seeking support in the South. *The Journal of the Association of Nurses in AIDS Care, 26*(1), 12–23.

Kremer, H., & Ironson, G. (2014). Longitudinal spiritual coping with trauma in people with HIV: Implications for health care. *AIDS Patient Care and STDs, 28*(3), 144–154.

Kumar, S., Mohanraj, R., Rao, D., Murray, K. R., & Manhart, L. E. (2015). Positive coping strategies and HIV-related stigma in south India. *AIDS Patient Care and STDs, 29*(3), 157–163.

McIntosh, R. C., & Rosselli, M. (2012). Stress and coping in women living with HIV: A meta-analytic review. *AIDS and Behavior, 16*(8), 2144–2159.

Molzahn, A., Sheilds, L., Bruce, A., Stajduhar, K., Makaroff, K. S., Beuthin, R., & Shermak, S. (2012). People living with serious illness: Stories of spirituality. *Journal of Clinical Nursing, 21*(15–16), 2347–2356.

Nakagawa, F., Lodwick, R. K., Smith, C. J., Smith, R., Cambiano, V., Lundgren, J. D.,...Phillips, A. N. (2012). Projected life expectancy of people with HIV according to timing of diagnosis. *AIDS (London, England), 26*(3), 335–343.

Nokes, K., Johnson, M. O., Webel, A., Rose, C. D., Phillips, J. C., Sullivan, K.,...Holzemer, W. L. (2012). Focus on increasing treatment self-efficacy to improve human immunodeficiency virus treatment adherence. *Journal of Nursing Scholarship: An Official Publication of Sigma Theta Tau International Honor Society of Nursing/Sigma Theta Tau, 44*(4), 403–410.

Psaros, C., Barinas, J., Robbins, G. K., Bedoya, C. A., Park, E. R., & Safren, S. A. (2015). Reflections on living with HIV over time: Exploring the perspective of HIV-infected women over 50. *Aging & Mental Health, 19*(2), 121–128.

Puig-Perez, S., Villada, C., Pulopulos, M. M., Almela, M., Hidalgo, V., & Salvador, A. (2015). Optimism and pessimism are related to different components of the stress response in healthy older people. *International Journal of Psychophysiology, 98*(2 Pt. 1), 213–221. Retrieved from http://dx.doi.org/10.1016/j.ijpsycho.2015.09.002

Ribeiro, C., Sarmento, E., Castro, R., Dinis-Ribeiro, M., & Fernandes, L. (2014). Effectiveness of psycho-educational intervention in HIV patients' treatment. *Frontiers in Psychiatry, 5,* 198.

Roger, K. S., Mignone, J., & Kirkland, S. (2013). Social aspects of HIV/AIDS and aging: A thematic review. *Canadian Journal on Aging = La revue Canadienne du vieillissement, 32*(3), 298–306.

Slomka, J., Lim, J. W., Gripshover, B., & Daly, B. (2013). How have long-term survivors coped with living with HIV? *The Journal of the Association of Nurses in AIDS Care, 24*(5), 449–459.

Tyer-Viola, L. A., Corless, I. B., Webel, A., Reid, P., Sullivan, K. M., & Nichols, P.; International Nursing Network for HIV/AIDS Research. (2014). Predictors of medication adherence among HIV-positive women in North America. *Journal of Obstetric, Gynecologic, and Neonatal Nursing: JOGNN/NAACOG, 43*(2), 168–178.

Webel, A. R., Cuca, Y., Okonsky, J. G., Asher, A. K., Kaihura, A., & Salata, R. A. (2013). The impact of social context on self-management in women living with HIV. *Social Science & Medicine (1982), 87,* 147–154.

Webel, A. R., Dolansky, M. A., Henry, A. G., & Salata, R. A. (2012). A qualitative description of women's HIV self-management techniques: Context, strategies, and considerations. *The Journal of the Association of Nurses in AIDS Care: JANAC, 23*(4), 281–293.

Webel, A., & Higgins, P. (2012). The relationship between social roles and self-management behavior in women living with HIV/AIDS. *Women's Health Issues, 22*(1), 27–33.

CHAPTER SIXTEEN

THE UNDER-12 RULE: A REVIEW ON THE PEDIATRIC LUNG ALLOCATION POLICY

Amy P. Pope

*T*he case of Sarah Murnaghan sparked a major controversy in 2013. Sarah, a 10-year-old girl with cystic fibrosis (CF), was given weeks to live by her transplant surgeons if a lifesaving bilateral lung transplantation operation was not implemented. Her family initiated a media firestorm accusing the Organ Procurement and Transplantation Network's (OPTN) policies on pediatric lung allocation to be discriminatory toward age (Lupkin, 2014). The policy at the time of the controversy stated that those children requiring lung transplantation receive lungs from a donor of a similar age (0–11 years) and were given either a priority 1 or 2 rating instead of a lung allocation score (LAS), which is what candidates older than 12 years of age are given (Snyder et al., 2014).

The case of Sarah led to a temporary restraining order invoked by the Philadelphia district court Judge Baylson, which resulted in a year's suspension in the under-12 rule created by OPTN in 2005 (Halpern, 2013). This overruling allowed Sarah and 12 other children to be placed on two waiting lists: the pediatric and the adult lung transplant lists (Aleccia, 2014). However, the only child to receive adult-sized organs after the overruling was Sarah (Aleccia, 2014).

PURPOSE

The purpose of this chapter is to identify how the under-12 rule in place for pediatric patients requiring a lung transplantation came to fruition and how the aftermath of the media exposure on Sarah Murnaghan's case affected the policy. Fieldwork on the subject is outlined, as well as a thorough literature review on the topic related to pediatric lung transplantation and allocation and an evaluation of the ethical implications of the policy is conducted.

Fieldwork Plan

This project was initiated by an interest in transplantation and the policies associated with this surgical intervention. The author was familiar with adult heart transplant patients and the associated policies due to her work as a bed-side critical care RN; however, the desire to understand the pediatric aspect of transplantation was present. When the discovery was made on Sarah Mur-naghan's story, the project developed into an interest of understanding the process of changing an established policy, particularly, in the case of one that is ethically driven.

Fieldwork activities included the completion of thorough research on Sarah and her case through media outlets, YouTube videos, and scholarly papers. A review of past and present OPTN policies was also completed with the emphasis on lung transplantation. The minutes of an emergency meeting held by the OPTN and the associated documents were reviewed, and this provided the author with OPTN's stance on the issue as well as valuable correspondence between OPTN and the Department of Health and Human Services secretary, Katherine Sebelius. Lastly, two prominent members of the transplant community were contacted, resulting in an e-mail conversation regarding the medical field's opinion on the contro-versy and policy change.

Relevance to Nursing

Health care policy is central to a nurse's approach to care. As Milstead (2013) notes, a nurse holds multifunctional roles as, "provider of care, educator, administrator, consultant, researcher, political activist, and policymaker," and with these multiple roles, any change in health care policy affects nurs-ing care (p. 2). The under-12 rule was accused of being discriminatory by the Murnaghan family in 2013, which violates the American Nurses Association (ANA, 2001) *Code of Ethics* principle that states that nurses are to act without discrimination toward each individual patient despite their "social or eco-nomic status, personal attributes, or the nature of health problems" (p. 7). With this allegation, nurses should take part in the evaluation of this policy and others similar to determine the truth and work in a team approach to propose revisions.

Additionally, the scarcity of organs creates ethically charged debates on how to appropriately allocate the resource. Despite advances in medical technology in recent years, there is still a need for transplantation for certain illnesses, which require stringent guidelines and long waiting lists for those needing the intervention. Therefore, the need to have a team of transplant experts to create allocation policies is imperative to ensure ethical and objective guidelines are in place. OPTN was designated as this source in 1984 (Mueller, 1989); yet in the case of Sarah, the lack of frequent policy review on OPTN's part resulted in charges of discrimination.

Moreover, due to this resource shortage, nursing needs to be cognizant of the issues surrounding organ transplantation, whether it be for a child or an adult. The lack of available organs and the ethical principles of utility and justice surrounding organ allocation make it difficult to provide the desired treatment to every patient. Though nurses are ethically bound to each individual patient, they are also responsible for ensuring care is distributed fairly and appropriately to those who need it the most.

Nurses are a prevalent persona in the health care arena, helping to develop and implement laws and legislation related to health care. Therefore, when a politically charged controversy arises, such as Sarah's, nursing needs to become an active player in not only the delivery of care, but ensuring the policies involved are ethically and legally appropriate.

THE HISTORY OF LUNG ALLOCATION POLICIES

The National Organ Transplantation Act (NOTA) of 1984 was written and made into law during a time when organ transplantation was fairly new and mainly used for the wealthy, as Medicare only provided reimbursement for kidney transplants (Mueller, 1989). There were also, similar to today's transplant climate, scarce resources, which resulted in those who had money or political power to purchase organs through illegal avenues, like the black market. In the hopes to illegalize black market organ trades, NOTA was signed into law by President Ronald Reagan in 1984.

Additionally, NOTA established a contract between the U.S. government and the private agency, OPTN (Colvin-Adams et al., 2012). During the early years of transplantation, there were transplant programs and centers scattered across the United States with no overseeing body (Mueller, 1989). This created a lack of cohesiveness among programs as well as the inability to appropriately allocate organs and to collect data on transplant recipients. Therefore, the contract between the United States and OPTN established the

OPTN as the overseeing body of the nation's transplant programs and centers. These entities use the OPTN and its union with the United Network for Organ Sharing (UNOS) for national policies, wait-list placement, and national statistics and data analysis on organ transplantation (Devito, 2014).

Jumping ahead 20 years to 2005, a review of the lung allocation policies at that time was completed by the OPTN. Before 2005, lung donations were allocated based on a person's length of time on the waiting list as well as proximity to the donor hospital, not by severity of their disease (Colvin-Adams et al., 2012; Sweet, 2009; Tomlinson, 2013). Therefore, the need was realized to change this policy, and the LAS was initiated into practice (Colvin-Adams et al., 2012; Sweet, 2009; Tomlinson, 2013). This score provided information regarding the severity of the candidate's disease as well as their survivability after transplantation (Sweet, 2009). However, this was only for adult candidates, as those younger than 12 years were "felt to be significantly different than older patients" because of the differences in disease states as well as in size and stature (Sweet, 2009, p. 809). However, children were given a wider geographical boundary than their adult counterparts: 1000-mile radius from pediatric donor hospital compared with a 500-mile radius from an adult donor (Sokohl, 2010; Sweet, 2009).

After the institution of the LAS in adult patients, it soon became noticeable that children needed to have a change in policy as well, as they were still being transplanted based on waiting time. Therefore, the pediatric policy was reviewed in 2010 and rewritten to incorporate medical urgency by using a priority rating 1 or 2 (Sokohl, 2010). A child with a medical urgency need for transplantation was given a priority 1 rating, and this was based on clinical information or an exception made by the regional lung review board (LRB; Sokohl, 2010). The under-12 rule was the policy until 2013 when the Murnaghan family demanded a change.

As has been pointed out, a judge invoked a temporary restraining order on this pediatric allocation policy and allowed Sarah and 12 other children to become exceptions to this rule (Aleccia, 2014; Halpern, 2013). With this restraining order in place, OPTN held an emergency meeting on June 10, 2013, to review the policy and brainstorm ideas for proposing a revised pediatric lung allocation policy (Organ Procurement & Transplantation Network & United Network for Organ Sharing Executive Committee, 2013). The OPTN was given 1 year to revise the policy or allow the restraining order to expire, which would result in the reestablishment of the under-12 rule (Snyder et al., 2014).

On June 23, 2014, it was made into a permanent OPTN policy to allow children who were deemed an exception to the rule to be placed on the adult transplant list in addition to the pediatric list (Organ Procurement & Transplantation Network, 2015a). The new policy allows the transplant surgeon the ability to make the decision whether or not the child would be successful with an adult donor transplant with the provision of objective data to the LRB to prove his or her case. Once the LRB receives the information, they have 7 days to determine if the child is an exception. If it is denied, the surgeon may then request an exception from the Thoracic Organ Transplantation Committee. Once the child is considered an exception, they are given a LAS and placed on the adult waiting list as well as the pediatric list.

Forthcoming will be a literature review on the Murnaghan case; however, during the author's fieldwork, an investigation on medical opinion regarding this policy change was conducted. Two prominent members of the transplant community were questioned on the current policy state of pediatric lung allocation. One member, a director of a southeast lung transplant program, who was also a member of the thoracic organ transplantation committee at the time of the controversy, supplied this answer via e-mail communication:

> It is a very complex discussion that balances the subjectivity of wanting to do everything possible to transplant patients with the objective issues of organ allocation and [the] fact that most transplant centers are not going to put adult lungs into pediatric recipients. There are very few pediatric lung transplants performed in the United States annually. This coupled with the fact that many of the patients under 12 years of age cannot perform some of the tests needed for the adult Lung Allocation Score and the fact that most adult lungs would not fit in a pediatric chest make the argument somewhat mute. Essentially, you would not be benefitting many patients by changing the rule. That being said, my thoughts were that if a lung transplant program wanted to use adult lungs for a pediatric recipient they should be allowed to and the decision should be up to the transplant program as well as the regional lung review board who could approve any deviation from the standard protocol. (personal communication, 2015)

Another expert in the field of transplantation who is a nurse and president and chief executive officer (CEO) of an organ donation and allocation program in Maryland provided a similar description on his opinion on the policy change:

> It's just [an] opinion, but I don't think medical policy should be written by the courts, which is essentially what happened in this case. I do

agree that size and other clinical factors appear to be more relevant in matching lung donors to recipients then age is, so there is probably a better system in place now. (personal communication, 2015)

As it can be deduced from the aforementioned opinions, though the involvement of the legal system was felt to be a disregard for the transplant community's expertise, the change in policy was warranted and allows for greater access to a scarce resource for pediatric patients who may have been disadvantaged in the previous policy.

Curiosity was ignited beyond the medical field's opinion on this case as the research is limited in objective data on outcomes and usefulness of the LAS for pediatric patients. Due to the small amount of pediatric lung transplantations done per year, there has not been the ability to objectively declare that this allocation method is appropriate for this age group (Organ Procurement & Transplantation Network & United Network for Organ Sharing Executive Committee, 2013). At the time of this writing, there are 1,638 individuals on the lung transplant waiting list, 16 of whom are pediatric patients (Organ Procurement & Transplantation Network, 2015b). As of April 23, 2015, an inquiry from UNOS found, from the dates June 10, 2013 to April 3, 2015, that there were 14 patients listed as an exception to the rule, and two of these patients younger than 12 years received a lung transplant from a donor aged 18 years or older between June 10, 2013 and January 31, 2015 (Beeson, personal communication, 2015). Due to the timing of Sarah's transplant in June 2013, it can be concluded that one of these two patients is Sarah. Therefore, only one other child has benefitted from the change in policy. However, this policy change is still very new, and time will provide the ability for more objective data collection and analysis on the implications of pediatric patients being made exceptions to the under-12 rule.

LITERATURE REVIEW ON THE MURNAGHAN CASE

There has not been much written in regard to scholarly work on the Murnaghan case, despite an amplitude of media coverage and political involvement during 2013. The back and forth between political leaders is captured on news outlets across the nation, yet little has been objectively investigated in this case. The ethical issues and the objective data available associated with the Murnaghan case is discussed further in the following sections.

Ethics

Sarah and her plight created an emotional and visceral response that many condoned the overturning of the under-12 rule. However, Secretary Sebelius is quoted as saying, "I don't want to live in a world where we choose who lives and dies" (Toomey, 2013). Though this is a valid point in other aspects of health care, it is not fully applicable in this particular situation, as organ transplantation and allocation policies are written to determine who is sicker or who has waited the longest to receive an organ. With this statement in mind, it is important to discuss the ethical principles associated with organ allocation.

These principles mentioned include utility and justice. Veatch, Haddad, and English (2010) define utility as "the state of being useful or producing good" (p. 434), which means that the resource is being allocated in a way that is the most useful as well as it provides the most benefit and the least amount of harm to the individual or community. Veatch et al. (2010) also define justice as the "fairness in distributing goods and harms" (p. 12). They discuss these principles in regard to organ transplantation and identify that there can be the creation of a conflict when it seems fair to allocate an organ to one person, yet it would offer the most benefit when allocated to a different person (Veatch et al., 2010).

The OPTN's standing policy, or final rule, requires that a balance between utility and justice be in place for all organ allocation and that all established policies demonstrate the best use for donor organs (Organ Procurement & Transplantation Network, n. d.). The emergency meeting held by the OPTN/UNOS Executive Committee (2013) supplied a document outlining the two ethical principles and provided examples of different interpretations for the principles.

In regard to utility, the OPTN/UNOS Executive Committee (2013) stated that this is a key element to organ allocation as the amount of recipients far outweighs the amount of available organs, requiring the initiation of the goal to provide the organ to a person who will maximize the use of the donation. This best use comes from the predicted outcomes of the transplant and is typically based on objective data; however, the committee prefaces that the lack of pediatric data results in the inability to fully objectify the outcomes (Organ Procurement & Transplantation Network & United Network for Organ Sharing Executive Committee, 2013).

Furthermore, the committee identifies a term known as "fair innings" in regard to justice in organ allocation (Organ Procurement & Transplantation Network & United Network for Organ Sharing Executive Committee,

2013, p. 71). The OPTN/UNOS Ethics Committee notes that this form of justice is one that advocates for pediatric allocation as it is defined as providing each individual with a full life in terms of number of healthy years lived (Organ Procurement & Transplantation Network, n. d.). However, the Executive Committee (2013) provides the point that this is a relevant issue for all ages; for example, a person who is a mother and a wife deserves a long, healthy life just as a pediatric candidate does. They note that this form of justice creates conflict with "other justice considerations such as equality of opportunity" (Organ Procurement & Transplantation Network & United Network for Organ Sharing Executive Committee, 2013, p. 71).

The Executive Committee (2013) concludes that the "special review, appeal, or exception to allocation policies based on a particular candidate's circumstance" is in direct conflict with OPTN/UNOS policies and the overall aim to remain fair in regard to organ allocation (p. 72). Despite this statement, they did revise the under-12 rule to allow exceptions for pediatric children in dire situations and provided a greater ability for a child younger than 12 years to receive an organ donation. Although, these exceptions are only provided if the clinical data are present to illicit the need for an adult donated organ transplant.

Similarly, Raju (2013) and Halpern (2013) discuss the ethical implications created by providing Sarah with special treatment. Raju (2013) discusses the issues with transplantation of adult organs into children as it has been statistically found that there is less than one in three chance of survival 10 years posttransplantation. He also provides a point that not all children have the financial and political power that the Murnaghan family had, which creates an unfair advantage for those with these types of power. However, his argument does not contain the fact that 12 other children were made an exception to the under-12 rule during 2013, which is more than half of the 20 pediatric candidates listed on the waiting list (Lupkin, 2014).

In addition to Raju, Halpern (2013) discusses the unfair advantage the Murnaghan family possessed creating a new precedent within the transplant community: allowing exceptions for those who request it without a thorough review of the data, literature, and ethics associated with the policy. He suggests ensuring policies are based on empirical and evidence-based data as well as the use of a simulation model used by the Scientific Registry for Transplant Recipients (SRTR), which identifies how access and outcomes affect a transplant (Halpern, 2013).

Overall, ethics play a large part in not only Sarah's case, but in all policies associated with organ allocation. It is imperative to maintain the balance between the principles of utility and justice to ensure that the greater good and most benefit is being achieved. It can be a difficult burden for those responsible for organ allocation, particularly when children are involved. Yet, it is a responsibility that is essential to providing the fair and just care necessary to organ transplant patients.

Objective Medical Data

In response to the controversy Sarah's story ignited, Snyder et al. (2014) published an article outlining how to equitably allocate organs in regard to this case as well as their opinion on the validity of the Murnaghan's case. Snyder et al. (2014) investigated and compared the pediatric and adult waiting list mortality and time spent on the list. The findings resulted in an insignificant difference between these two concerns that were used in the suit against OPTN from the Murnaghan family (Snyder et al., 2014). The inconsistency among the data the politicians used to argue Sarah's case included data from candidates ages 0 to 5 years, which has higher mortality and waiting time compared to ages 6 to 11 years. In fact, Snyder et al. (2014) found that ages 6 to 11 years had very similar wait-list mortality rates as well as time spent waiting for a transplant to those 18 years and older. They concluded that the argument made on behalf of the Murnaghan family was moot, as the objective data was used incorrectly (Snyder et al., 2014).

In response to Snyder et al.'s (2014) argument, Sweet and Barr (2014) wrote an editorial stating the mortality rates and time frame spent on the waiting list might not be significant, but that does not mean that the Murnaghan's case is invalid. They provided information outlining how children are not given access to adolescent lungs, as the policy states they should (Sweet & Barr, 2014). Priority is supposed to be given to adolescents, then children, then adults; however, Sweet and Barr (2014) stated that 90% of adolescent lungs are matched to adult candidates. Therefore, they provide recommendations for improving pediatric outcomes by opening the donated supply of adolescent lungs to children before adults as well as relaxing the 1,000-mile geographical boundary for pediatric organ allocation (Sweet & Barr, 2014).

Recently, Snyder et al. (2014) presented a poster on the implications of this policy change for children aged 9 to 11 years. It found that allowing access to adolescent and adult donors increased the pediatric donor pool by a factor of 10 resulting in a 750-person donor pool (Snyder et al., 2014). This is a significant finding as this increases a pediatric candidate's access to lungs dramatically. However, Snyder et al. (2014) present the caveat that not all children are suitable for adult lung donation, particularly due to size and blood type matching and potential other variables.

Lastly, a law note was written by Devito (2014) that provided an in-depth look at the history of the OPTN, an analysis of Sarah's case, as well as three potential suggestions for solving an issue similar to the Murnaghan case. Devito's (2014) first solution emphasized allowing courts and judiciary reviews to be conducted on government-contracted private agencies, such as OPTN, in regard to policy review, revision, and permanent changes. Second, she recommended allowing the private agency to conduct the review without government encroachment; and finally, she suggested creating a joint effort by the courts and the agency to review and revise policies in question. She discusses how the second solution is not ideal, as those involved may not be able to visualize flaws in policies that they created. She also discusses how primarily using the justice system to evaluate private policies infringes on the autonomy and expertise of that agency. Therefore, Devito (2014) concludes that a team approach between the justice system and private agency is the best solution and notes that this is the solution that was used in the Murnaghan case.

However, due to the limited life span given to Sarah, the courts made a rash decision, and the OPTN was unable to thoroughly review and evaluate the policy before the restraining order was invoked. Unfortunately, in cases involving a scarce resource, time is usually of the essence, and a joint effort is not feasible. Therefore, a proactive measure on behalf of OPTN would be to frequently review allocation policies to ensure the instillation of ethical principles inherent to organ allocation and confirm that the resource is being used to its maximum potential.

SUMMARY

In conclusion, Sarah Murnaghan may have created a controversy in the fight to save her life, but it was an issue that needed to be addressed to ensure that the policy was fair and nondiscriminatory. Because of her family's suit against OPTN and the reversal of the under-12 rule, today Sarah is thriving with her double lung transplant provided by an adult donor. At times, it takes a controversial move to create change for the better, and the ability for pediatric candidates to apply for an exception allows greater access to a life they did not have before Sarah. Now, children waiting for lung transplants have greater hope to growing up and developing socially and physically that once may have been only a wish.

REFERENCES

Aleccia, J. (2014). Lung transplant rule that saved Sarah is final. *NBC News*. Retrieved from http://www.nbcnews.com/health/health-news/lung-transplant-rule-saved-sarah-final-n138086

American Nurses Association. (2001). *Code of ethics for nurses with interpretive statements*. Silver Spring, MD: American Nurses Association.

Colvin-Adams, M., Valapour, M., Hertz, M., Heubner, B., Paulson, K., Dhungel, V.,...& Israni, A. K. (2012). Lung and heart allocation in the United States. *American Journal of Transplantation, 12*(12), 3213–3234.

DeVito, M. (2014). The judge put me on the list: Judicial review and organ allocation decisions. *Case Western Reserve Law Review, 65*(1), 181–207. Retrieved from http://eds.a.ebscohost.com.proxy.kennesaw.edu/eds/pdfviewer/pdfviewer?sid=23f-c0e6f-e40a-42e6-bd1f-c92691f41372%40sessionmgr4005&vid=7&hid=4102

Halpern, S. D. (2013). Turning wrong into right: The 2013 lung allocation controversy. *Annals of Internal Medicine, 159*(5), 358–359. Retrieved from http://eds.a.ebscohost.com.proxy.kennesaw.edu/eds/pdfviewer/pdfviewer?sid=f7d-b2ee2-a48c-4884-a1eb-dd0b9702e651%40sessionmgr4005&vid=13&hid=4108

Lupkin, S. (2014, June 16). Sarah Murnaghan breathing completely on her own. *ABC News*. Retrieved from http://abcnews.go.com/Health/sarah-murnaghan-breathing-completely/story?id=24161157

Lupkin, S. (2014). How many children benefited from lung transplant rule tweak? *ABC news*. Retrieved from http://abcnews.go.com/Health/children-benefited-lung-transplant-rule-tweak/story?id=23065716

Milstead, J. A. (2013). *Heath policy and politics: A nurse's guide* (4th ed.). Burlington, MA: Jones & Bartlett Learning.

Mueller, K. J. (1989). The national organ transplant act of 1984: Congressional response to changing biotechnology. *Policy Studies Review, 8*(2), 346–356. Retrieved from http://eds.a.ebscohost.com.proxy.kennesaw.edu/eds/pdfviewer/pdfviewer?sid=01755f09–3df2–4475-b88a-ae31523af1ff%40sessionmgr4002&vid=3&hid=4102

Organ Procurement & Transplantation Network. (2015a). *Data: Organ by age*. Retrieved from http://optn.transplant.hrsa.gov/converge/latestData/rptData.asp

Organ Procurement & Transplantation Network. (2015b). Policy 10: Allocation of lungs. *Policies, 122*–150. Retrieved from http://optn.transplant.hrsa.gov/contentdocuments/optn_policies.pdf

Organ Procurement & Transplantation Network. (n. d.). *Ethical principles of pediatric organ allocation*. Retrieved from http://optn.transplant.hrsa.gov/resources/ethics/ethical-principles-of-pediatric-organ-allocation/

Organ Procurement & Transplantation Network & United Network for Organ Sharing Executive Committee. (2013). *OPTN UNOS executive committee meeting materials*. Retrieved from http://optn.transplant.hrsa.gov/contentdocuments/optn_exec_comm_mtng_materials_06–10–13.pdf

Raju, S. (2013). Adolescent organ donation at the children's hospital of Philadelphia. *Penn Bioethics Journal, 8*(2), 10. Retrieved from http://eds.a.ebscohost.com .proxy.kennesaw.edu/eds/pdfviewer/pdfviewer?sid=23fc0e6f-e40a-42e6-bd1f-c92691f41372%40sessionmgr4005&vid=28&hid=4102

Snyder, J., Skeans, M., Heubner, B., Leighton, T., Hertz, M., & Valapour, M. (2014, July 29). *Lung donor availability and implications for pediatric candidates aged 9–11 years.* Retrieved from http://www.srtr.org/publications/content/posters/2014/Lung_Donor_Availability_and_Implications_for_Pediatric_Candidates_Aged_9-11_Years.pdf

Snyder, J. J., Salkwoski, N., Skeans, M., Leighton, T., Valapour, M., Israni, A. K., . . . & Kasiske, B. L. (2014). The equitable allocation of deceased donor lungs for transplant in children in the United States. *Am J Transplant, 14*(1), 178–183.

Sokohl, K. (2010). A review of the recent thoracic organ allocation changes. *UNOS Update.* Retrieved from http://www.unos.org/docs/Update_NovDec10_Thoracic.pdf

Sweet, S. C. (2009). Update on pediatric lung allocation in the United States. *Pediatr Transplant, 13*(7), 808–813.

Sweet, S. C., & Barr, M. L. (2014). Pediatric lung allocation: The rest of the story. *American Journal of Transplantation, 14*(1), 11–12.

Tomlinson, T. (2013). *Lungs for Sarah Murnaghan raise ethical questions* [Web log post]. Retrieved from http://msubioethics.com/2013/06/27/lungs-for-sarah-murnaghan-raise-ethical-questions

Toomey, P. (2013). *The Today Show highlights Sarah Murnaghan.* Retrieved from https://www.youtube.com/watch?v=_zwnOESuTjo

Veatch, R. M., Haddad, A. M., & English, D. C. (2010). *Case studies in biomedical ethics.* New York, NY: Oxford University Press.

CHAPTER SEVENTEEN

THE HEALTH CONSEQUENCES OF MOTHERS USING DRUGS AND THE LEGAL SYSTEM'S CALL TO ACTION

Kathy Barnett

The National Institute on Drug Abuse (2014) reports that an estimated 23.9 million Americans aged 12 years and older have abused drugs in the past month. It is estimated that only about 2.5 million or 1% of all those addicted to drugs received treatment at a specialty facility (National Institute on Drug Abuse, 2014). To combat this ever-evolving drug problem, health policies are being developed on the national, state, and local levels. These drug policies are focused in three areas. The first type of health policy is designed to prevent drug use. The second type of health policy concentrates on providing services to treat those with chronic substance abuse. Finally, the third type of drug policy is related to controlling the supply of drugs such as incarceration for someone caught selling drugs (Barbor et al., 2010). Barbor et al. (2010) list drug use as the eighth leading cause of disease, death, and disability in developed countries of the world. Because of the significant health impact drug use has not only on the health and well-being of the substance abuser, but also on the "public good" of the nation, successful health policies play a vital role in the drug epidemic (Barbor et al., 2010, p. 1137). This chapter discusses the health implications of chronic substance abuse and one local judicial system's call to action in creating a family drug court to ameliorate substance abuse.

SUBSTANCE ABUSE AND ITS IMPACT ON SOCIETY

Drug use has both significant negative health consequences as well as financial implications to the nation including drug-related automotive accidents, spread of infectious disease, and suicide and unintentional death (Barbor et al., 2010). Substance use also plays a major role in most acts of violent crime and property crime (Barbor et al., 2010). The National Criminal Justice Reference Service (NCJRS, 2015) estimates that the social and health consequences of illicit drug use, including drug-related illness, death, and crime, cost the nation approximately $66.9 billion annually.

Drug use during pregnancy contributes to serious problems and birth defects for the unborn child (Sachdeva, Patel, & Patel, 2009). Infants born to mothers using opioids go through a long process of withdrawal from the opioids after birth. Drug-exposed infants are considered to be at high risk from exposure in utero, and this exposure may be further exacerbated by their living conditions after discharge from the hospital because of the parent's drug lifestyle (NCJRS, 2015). One study referenced by the NCJRS (2015) showed an increase in infant mortality from 10.7 per one thousand for non-drug users compared with the infant mortality of 14.9 per thousand for those who admitted to using drugs during the pregnancy.

Conners et al. (2003) estimate that 6% of all children in America have a parent who is in need of treatment for illicit drug use. Children whose parents are addicted to drugs experience negative health and behavior consequences. A study conducted by Conners et al. (2003) suggests that children of those addicted to drugs are placed at "increased vulnerability for physical, academic, and socioemotional problems" (p. 752). Children living with a parent who uses drugs are more likely to be victims of domestic violence, have sleep disturbances, anxiety, and depression (Conners et al., 2003). Moreover, the children of substance abusers are more likely to have eating disorders and commit suicide (Conners et al., 2003). Many children grow up to continue the cycle of drug abuse that they saw during their childhood growing up with a parent abusing drugs.

The U.S. government recognizes the nation's drug problem as one of the leading health problems in the country. In 2011, the Obama administration requested $20 million or a 40% increase in funding for drug treatment programs as an alternative to funding for prisons (Humphreys & McLellan, 2010). This increase in funding was designated to be used to train probation officers and judges on how to operate drug court programs.

DEVELOPMENT OF DRUG COURTS

In response to the nation's increasing drug problem, several judicial systems across America are using a nontraditional court system called drug courts to treat those with substance abuse instead of the traditional judicial system using incarceration as a punishment. The first drug court was established in Miami, Florida, in 1989 (McKean, 2014). By 2005, more than one thousand drug court programs were in operation across the country (McKean, 2014). The purpose of a drug court is to place drug addicts who have committed a nonviolent crime into a treatment program instead of incarceration. Drug courts focus on combining accountability to the criminal justice system with a substance-abuse treatment plan. Typically, the drug user is arrested for a nonviolent crime related to drug use such as committing thefts or buying drugs (McKean, 2014). If the addict is eligible for drug court, the requirements for the program are explained to the accused, and the drug user can choose to enter the treatment program instead of incarceration. Treatment includes long-term substance abuse treatment, random drug tests, and accountability to the judge and court. If the addict agrees to enter the program and completes the program successfully, many times the criminal charges will be dropped, or the criminal case dismissed.

Because of the success of the drug court model, judicial systems across the country began to adapt the model for use with parents of minor children addicted to drugs. These parents did not necessarily have to be involved in a crime, but instead were brought into court because of delinquency of their minor children related to their drug use. This new model of drug court is known as a family drug court. The first family drug court was created in 1995 in Reno, Nevada (Marlowe & Carey, 2012). Today, nearly 300 family drug courts are in operation across the United States. These programs use the judicial court system in combination with a substance-abuse treatment plan to collectively ameliorate substance abuse issues and reunite children in foster homes with a drug-free parent. Unlike the traditional drug court model where the incentive for participation might be to have their criminal record cleared of charges and the participant avoid incarceration, the family drug court model is designed to provide incentives for participation and reduce the time the participant's children spend in foster care (Marlowe & Carey, 2012). Several pathways to entering into the family drug court program exist. One path to entering the program is when child protective services have removed the child from the home because of delinquency of the minor children related to the parent's drug use. In order for the parents to regain custody of their minor children, they are required to attend the family drug court program. Another pathway to entering the court system is when a mother tests positive for drugs at the birth of her baby or her infant has had a positive drug screen right after delivery. Others have entered the system because their children have been involved in criminal activity and are seen in juvenile drug court. If the judge determines the juvenile is not being well cared for because of the mother's or father's drug addiction, or the mother or father admits to drug use, the judge may order the parent to attend the family drug court program. Finally, some mothers and fathers enter the program through the traditional adult drug court. The mother or father has committed a nonviolent crime related to drug use and because they have minor children, the judge orders the parent to the family drug court program.

The Success of Family Drug Court

One large county in the southeast United States started a successful family drug court program in 2006. In 2015, an interview was conducted with the judge who initiated the local family drug court program, as well as a parent attorney, a child protective services attorney, the coordinator of the family drug court as well as the juvenile drug court coordinator. Because of confidentiality, the name of the county court, and all of those interviewed have been changed to protect their identification. The Central County family drug court was started by Judge Cheryl Thomas in 2006. Over the years, several hundred mothers and fathers have participated in the 2-year family drug court treatment program. When Judge Thomas was first elected to the county judge position, she saw a need to keep nonviolent drug offenders with minor children out of the jail system and instead offer treatment for their addiction so that the families could be reunited. Soon after taking office, Judge Thomas began researching drug court models to determine which system would work best for her county. After many hours of meeting with legislators, community members, and judges from across the country, Judge Thomas created the county's first family drug court program. This program is designed to keep mothers and fathers with drug addiction out of the prison system and instead provide them the substance-abuse treatment necessary to get healthy and reunite the children that have been placed in a foster home. Judge Thomas explains:

> Many of the parents that enter my court room are reluctant to enter treatment but because they don't want to lose their children permanently, they agree to my treatment plan. The mission is to keep these parents out of jail and get them the treatment they need for their addiction and to eventually reunite them with their children.

The judge reports that one third of all the participants in the county's family drug court system enter the system through a criminal court case. The other two thirds enter the system through the civil route where child protective services has become involved because of delinquency from the parent's drug use. Child protective services will remove the children from the parents and place them in foster care. In order for the parent to regain custody of their children, the parent must enter the family drug court program and agree to the treatment guidelines recommended by the judge. If the parent chooses to not participate in the recommended treatment plan, the parent may permanently loose custody of their children.

Once a parent agrees to the judge's treatment program, it is a 2-year commitment. First, the parent enters a residential treatment program. The parent's attorney, Renee Werner, explains that for several months the parent receives counseling on drug addiction, parenting, marriage counseling, group therapy, high school equivalency training (GED), and employment training. Random drug screens are performed to verify compliance. The participant is required to appear in family court on a weekly schedule. The judge assesses the progress of the participant and when the participant has been successful with their treatment plan, the judge provides positive encouragement and praise. After successfully completing the residential treatment portion of the program, the participant moves into outpatient housing and continues to meet for group therapy and substance-abuse counseling several hours a day. During this time, participants are assisted with finding a job and performing community service. Child protective services begin to reinstate visitation with the parent and the child. The children receive play therapy and counseling to help them transition through this period. Once the participant completes the outpatient treatment program, the participant begins to look for permanent housing. The participant is held accountable by attending required family drug court sessions so that the judge can evaluate the participant's success. After a participant moves into his or her own home, a parole officer is assigned to monitor the participant's activities and administer random drug screens for up to a full year. This officer provides surveillance of the participant's behavior and activities to report compliance of the participant back to the judge. The officer will visit the participant's home without notice to make sure the participant is remaining drug free. Mary Smith, the family drug court coordinator, says this holds the participant accountable long after they stop their residential treatment when temptations to reuse drugs are at its highest. At the end of the 2 years, the participants graduate from the program. The members of the drug court help these parents celebrate their sobriety and the new healthy life they have created for their family. Each year graduates of the program from the first drug class in 2006 to the present graduating class gather for a family reunion to celebrate the years of sobriety and living a healthy lifestyle as a family with other graduates and staff of the family drug court.

Mary Smith, family drug court coordinator, contributes the team approach to the success of the program.

> The family drug court team consists of the judge, the parent attorney, the attorney for child protective services representing the child, family therapist, a case manager, the family drug court coordinator, treatment providers, a parole officer and a peer specialist. The peer specialist is a former drug addict and graduate of the family drug court program. She is a valuable member of the team because the participants can really relate to her. She can speak personally of the experience, and the participants can see her success. The family drug court team really wants to see these moms and dads do well and complete the program. We cheer them on every step of the way.

Another factor that adds to the success of the program is a local nonprofit organization in the community that has teamed up with the family drug court to provide services from the community. Mary Smith explains how valuable the collaboration between the family drug court and the nonprofit organization is in the success of the participants. The nonprofit organization helps supply goods such as clothing, furniture, and other household materials needed by the graduates to start their new sober life. Each year the nonprofit group collects Christmas presents for the children of the family drug court participants that are in foster care. A local church buses the family drug court children and their parents in for an annual Easter Egg Hunt. The nonprofit organization raises money to help the parents obtain necessary items as they transition through the program. If a participant in the program has secured a new apartment to move into but cannot afford the high costs of the initial start-up fees for utilities, the nonprofit organization may help pay those start-up fees. Moreover, the nonprofit organization collects furniture and clothing to help the parent and child begin their new life in their new home.

Judge Thomas remarks on a new garden the nonprofit has just created to benefit the participants of the program.

> A local church has donated two empty lots for a garden. One will be a vegetable garden, and the other will be a flower garden with benches. Participants in the family drug court will be encouraged to work in the garden with volunteers from the church to learn how to grow vegetables that they can then take home for consumption.

The family drug court received its initial start-up funding from a federal grant. This 2-year grant was then renewed for a third year. After the third year, all funding for this program has come from the state legislators (Judge Thomas, personal statement, 2015). Judge Thomas reports that recently, the state legislator contributed over $900,000 to help fund transportation needs of the program. The parent attorney, Renee Werner, rates the county's lack of public transportation as the biggest obstacle faced by the participants in the program. Because the county lacks a public train system or bus system, participants find it difficult to attend counseling sessions, group therapy, and their court appearances. The parent attorney tells of one girl's difficulties:

> For one participant in the program, her dad drops her off at a bus stop at 6 a.m. She rides the bus for nearly 3 hours before arriving for her substance-abuse group therapy class at 9 a.m. Then after it is over, she spends 3 more hours on the bus headed home.

The money the state legislators assigned for transportation will help with bus vouchers, taxi vouchers, and enable the treatment facility to arrange for vans to provide transportation for participants who lack a means to otherwise attend court appointments and treatment sessions.

Another reason this county's family drug court is so successful is because of the regional service boards created from House Bill 100 in 1993 (Mary Smith, personal statement, 2015). Funding for these resources has provided space in treatment facilities that the judge can utilize for participants in the family drug court. Several treatment facilities exist in the community for various populations including pregnant women, mothers with minor children, teenagers, and men. Although these programs all operate at a filled capacity, placement options are available for those in need. These facilities provide not only substance-abuse treatment but also services for some minor mental health issues, behavioral health care services, and introduce skills to help the participants gain employment.

The Central County family drug court program has seen much success over the years. Mary Smith, the family court coordinator, reports that out of several hundred participants that have graduated from the program, only five have reappeared in the family drug court needing further substance-abuse treatment. Hundreds of children have been returned to their parents because of this program and the successful rehabilitation of the parents. However, even with the success of this program, there are some cases where the parents struggle. Some are just unable or unwilling to finish the program. Other participants violate the provisions required with the program. Renee Werner explains implication for violations of the treatment program. During the initial visit to family drug court, the participant agrees to a set of rules and signs an agreement with the judge in order to enter into the program. If during the 2 years of participation in the treatment program, any of the conditions are violated, the participant may now be found in contempt of court. Violations may include staying out after curfew, a positive drug screen, drugs found in the apartment, having members of the opposite sex in the apartment, and so forth. If the participant violates the program rules and is found in contempt of court, the participant may be subject to jail time. After serving jail time, the judge will work with the substance abuser to restart the treatment program.

Research Supports the Family Drug Court

Literature suggests that family drug courts have significantly better outcomes compared with other family reunification services (Marlowe & Carey, 2012). Oliveros and Kaufman (2011) argue that the family drug court model is one of the most effective programs for treating substance abuse in regards to the child welfare population. Marlowe and Carey (2012) found that family drug court's participants were 20% to 40% more likely to reach family reunification that those substance abusers not involved in the family drug court. Children of participants spent significantly less time, averaging several fewer months, in foster care than those not involved in the family court program (Marlowe & Carey, 2012).

Marlowe and Carey (2012) argue that the success of the family drug court program is because of the participants interactions with the judge. The participants feel empowered by the judge, and this empowerment leads the participant to work harder in their treatment program and their own recovery, which produces greater long-term success (Marlowe & Carey, 2012).

The family drug court model has also contributed to significant financial savings for many states. In the state of Georgia, it costs $20 per day for a bed in a treatment facility compared with $51 a day for a bed in state prison (Rankin & Teegardin, 2012). Rankin and Teegardin (2012) also report that drug courts saved the state of Georgia an average of $14 million in 2009. In 2010, a Georgia State audit found that 29% of all state prison inmates with substance-abuse problems committed another crime within 2 years of release compared with only 7% of all those who graduated from a drug court treatment program (Rankin & Teegardin, 2012).

Even with the reported success of the family drug court model in the health of the substance abuser, in the health of the substance abuser's minor children, and in the financial implications to the nation, more research needs to be conducted to evaluate the effectiveness of the family drug court model (McKean, 2014). With long-term monitoring of the participants in family drug court, it can be determined if the graduates relapse and commit further crimes or maintain their drug-free lifestyle.

Judge Thomas also suggests long-term research could be important to evaluate the children of the graduates:

> I would like to see if the cycle of addiction has been broken for the children of those whom have graduated from this program.

Additional long-term research tracking of not only the graduates but also their children would help to validate the effectiveness of the program and may provide additional, much-needed resources for funding of the family drug court program.

SUMMARY

Over the past 20 years, the family drug court has emerged as one of the most promising models for improving treatment retention and reuniting families in the child welfare system (Oliveros & Kaufman, 2011). One local county, Central County, has seen the success of the family drug court program and the impact it has had on not only the participants and their children, but on the community as well. Further research is needed to examine the long-term implications to not only the participants but also their children. This research could help determine if the family drug court has the ability to break the cycle of substance abuse passed from generation to generation. The success of the family drug court of Central County should be used as a prescription for other communities across the country. The expansion of this successful program may increase the effective treatment of substance abusers, protect vulnerable children, and reunite families across the nation.

REFERENCES

Barbor, T., Caulkins, J., Edwards, G., Fischer, B., Foxcroft, D., & Humphreys, K. (2010). Drug policy and the public good: A summary of the book. *Addiction, 105*, 1137–1145.

Conners, N. A., Bradley, R. H., Mansell, L. W., Liu, J. Y., Roberts, T. J., Burgdorf, K., & Herrell, J. M. (2003). Children of mothers with serious substance abuse problems: An accumulation of risks. *The American Journal of Drug and Alcohol Abuse, 29*(4), 743–758.

Humphreys, K., & McLellan, A. (2010). Brief intervention, treatment, and recovery support services for Americans who have substance use disorders: An overview of policy in the Obama administration. *Psychological Services, 7*(4), 275–284.

Marlowe, D., & Carey, S. (2012). *Research update on family drug courts.* Alexandria: National Association of Drug Court Professionals.

McKean, J. (2014). Drug courts. In *Salem Press encyclopedia.* Retrieved from http:// www.encyclopedia.com/topic/Drug_Courts.aspx

National Criminal Justice Reference Service (NCJRS). (2015). *America's drug abuse profile.* Retrieved from http://www.ncjrs.gov/htm/chapter2.htm

National Institute on Drug Abuse, National Institute of Health. (2014). *Drugfacts: Nationwide trends.* Retrieved from http://www.drugabuse.gov/publications/ drugfacts/nationwide-trends

Oliveros, A., & Kaufman, J. (2011). Addressing substance abuse treatment needs of parents involved with the child welfare system. *Child Welfare, 90*(1), 25–41.

Rankin, B., & Teegardin, C. (2012). *Drug court: Saving money, saving lives.* Retrieved from http://www.ajc.com/news/news/local/drug-court-saving-money-saving-lives/nQRrb

Sachdeva, P., Patel, B. G., & Patel, B. K. (2009). Drug use in pregnancy; a point to ponder! *Indian Journal of Pharmaceutical Sciences, 71*(1), 1–7.

LIST OF JOURNALS THAT PUBLISH QUALITATIVE RESEARCH

Mary de Chesnay

Conducting excellent research and not publishing the results negates the study and prohibits anyone from learning from the work. Therefore, it is critical that qualitative researchers disseminate their work widely, and the best way to do so is through publication in refereed journals. The peer-review process, although seemingly brutal at times, is designed to improve knowledge by enhancing the quality of literature in a discipline. Fortunately, the publishing climate has evolved to the point where qualitative research is valued by editors and readers alike, and many journals now seek out, or even specialize in publishing, qualitative research.

The following table was compiled partially from the synopsis of the previous work identifying qualitative journals by the St. Louis University Qualitative Research Committee (n.d.), with a multidisciplinary faculty, who are proponents of qualitative research. Many of these journals would be considered multidisciplinary, although marketed to nurses. All are peer reviewed. Other journals were identified by the author of this series and by McKibbon and Gadd (2004) in their quantitative analysis of qualitative research. It is not meant to be exhaustive, and we would welcome any suggestions for inclusion.

An additional resource is the nursing literature mapping project conducted by Sherwill-Navarro and Allen (Allen, Jacobs, & Levy, 2006). The 217 journals were listed as a resource for libraries to accrue relevant journals, and many of them publish qualitative research. Readers are encouraged to view the websites for specific journals that might be interested in publishing their studies. Readers are also encouraged to look outside the traditional nursing journals, especially if their topics more closely match the journal mission of related disciplines.

NURSING JOURNALS

Journal	Website
Advances in Nursing Science	www.journals.lww.com/advancesinnursingscience/pages/default.aspx
Africa Journal of Nursing and Midwifery	www.journals.co.za/ej/ejour_ajnm.html
Annual Review of Nursing Research	http://www.springerpub.com/annual-review-of-nursing-research.html
British Journal of Nursing	www.britishjournalofnursing.com
Canadian Journal of Nursing Research	www.cjnr.mcgill.ca
Hispanic Health Care International	http://www.springerpub.com/hispanic-health-care-international.html
Holistic Nursing Practice	www.journals.lww.com/hnpjournal/pages/default.aspx
International Journal of Mental Health Nursing	www.onlinelibrary.wiley.com/journal/10.1111/(ISSN)1447-0349
International Journal of Nursing Practice	www.onlinelibrary.wiley.com/journal/10.1111/(ISSN)1440-172X
International Journal of Nursing Studies	www.journals.elsevier.com/international-journal-of-nursing-studies
Journal of Advanced Nursing	www.onlinelibrary.wiley.com/journal/10.1111/(ISSN)1365-2648
Journal of Clinical Nursing	www.onlinelibrary.wiley.com/journal/10.1111/(ISSN)1365-2702
Journal of Family Nursing	http://jfn.sagepub.com/
Journal of Nursing Education	www.healio.com/journals/JNE
Journal of Nursing Scholarship	www.onlinelibrary.wiley.com/journal/10.1111/(ISSN)1547-5069
Nurse Researcher	http://journals.rcni.com/journal/nr
Nursing History Review	www.aahn.org/nhr.html
Nursing Inquiry	www.onlinelibrary.wiley.com/journal/10.1111/(ISSN)1440-1800
Nursing Research	www.ninr.nih.gov
Nursing Science Quarterly	http://nsq.sagepub.com/
Online Brazilian Journal of Nursing	www.objnursing.uff.br/index.php/nursing

Journal	Website
The Online Journal of Cultural Competence in Nursing and Healthcare	www.ojccnh.org
Public Health Nursing	www.onlinelibrary.wiley.com/journal/10.1111 /(ISSN)1525-1446
Qualitative Health Research	www.qhr.sagepub.com
Qualitative Research in Nursing and Healthcare	www.wiley.com/WileyCDA/WileyTitle/product Cd-1405161221.html
Research and Theory for Nursing Practice	www.springerpub.com/product/15416577#.Ueab lTvvv6U
Scandinavian Journal of Caring Sciences	www.onlinelibrary.wiley.com/journal/10.1111 /(ISSN)1471-6712
Western Journal of Nursing Research	http://wjn.sagepub.com

REFERENCES

Allen, M., Jacobs, S. K., & Levy, J. R. (2006). Mapping the literature of nursing: 1996–2000. *Journal of the Medical Library Association, 94*(2), 206–220. Retrieved from http://nahrs.mlanet.org/home/images/activity/nahrs2012selectedlist nursing.pdf

McKibbon, K., & Gadd, C. (2004). A quantitative analysis of qualitative studies in clinical journals for the publishing year 2000. *BMC Medical Informatics and Decision Making, 4*, 11.Retrieved from http://www.ncbi.nlm.nih.gov/pmc/articles/ PMC503397

St. Louis University Qualitative Research Committee. (n.d.). Retrieved from http:// www.slu.edu/organizations/qrc/QRjournals.html

ESSENTIAL ELEMENTS FOR A QUALITATIVE PROPOSAL

Tommie Nelms

1. Introduction: Aim of the study
   a. Phenomenon of interest and focus of inquiry
   b. Justification for studying the phenomenon (how big an issue/problem?)
   c. Phenomenon discussed within a specific context (lived experience, culture, human response)
   d. Theoretical framework(s)
   e. Assumptions, biases, experiences, intuitions, and perceptions related to the belief that inquiry into a phenomenon is important (researcher's relationship to the topic)
   f. Qualitative methodology chosen, with rationale
   g. Significance to nursing (How will the new knowledge gained benefit patients, nursing practice, nurses, society, etc.?)
   Note: The focus of interest/inquiry and statement of purpose of the study should appear at the top of page 3 of the proposal
2. Literature review: What is known about the topic? How has it been studied in the past?
   Include background of the theoretical framework and how it has been used in the past.
3. Methodology
   a. Introduction of methodology (philosophical underpinnings of the method)
   b. Rationale for choosing the methodology
   c. Background of methodology
   d. Outcome of methodology
   e. Methods: general sources and steps and procedures
   f. Translation of concepts and terms

4. Methods
    a. Aim
    b. Participants
    c. Setting
    d. Gaining access and recruitment of participants
    e. General steps in conduct of study (data gathering tool(s), procedures, etc.)
    f. Human subjects' considerations
    g. Expected timetable
    h. Framework for rigor and specific strategies to ensure rigor
    i. Plans and procedures for data analysis

WRITING QUALITATIVE RESEARCH PROPOSALS

Joan L. Bottorff

PURPOSE OF A RESEARCH PROPOSAL

- Communicates research plan to others (e.g., funding agencies)
- Serves as a detailed plan of action
- Serves as a contract between investigator and funding bodies when proposal is approved

QUALITATIVE RESEARCH: BASIC ASSUMPTIONS

- Reality is complex, constructed, and, ultimately, subjective.
- Research is an interpretative process.
- Knowledge is best achieved by conducting research in the natural setting.

QUALITATIVE RESEARCH

- Qualitative research is unstructured.
- Qualitative designs are "emergent" rather than fixed.
- The results of qualitative research are unpredictable (Morse, 1994).

KINDS OF QUALITATIVE RESEARCH

- Grounded theory
- Ethnography (critical ethnography, institutional ethnography, ethnomethodology, ethnoscience, etc.)
- Phenomenology
- Narrative inquiry
- Others

CHALLENGES FOR QUALITATIVE RESEARCHERS

- Developing a solid, convincing argument that the study contributes to theory, research, practice, and/or policy (the "so what?" question)
- Planning a study that is systematic, manageable, and flexible (to reassure skeptics):
  - Justification of the selected qualitative method
  - Explicit details about design and methods, without limiting the project's evolution
  - Attention to criteria for the overall soundness or rigor of the project

QUESTIONS A PROPOSAL MUST ANSWER

- Why should anyone be interested in my research?
- Is the research design credible, achievable, and carefully explained?
- Is the researcher capable of conducting the research? (Marshall & Rossman, 1999)

TIPS TO ANSWER THESE QUESTIONS

- Be practical (practical problems cannot be easily brushed off)
- Be persuasive ("sell" your proposal)
- Make broad links (hint at the wider context)
- Aim for crystal clarity (avoid jargon, assume nothing, explain everything; Silverman, 2000)

SECTIONS OF A TYPICAL QUALITATIVE PROPOSAL

- Introduction
  - Introduction of topic and its significance
  - Statement of purpose, research questions/objectives
- Review of literature
  - Related literature and theoretical traditions
- Design and methods
  - Overall approach and rationale
  - Sampling, data gathering methods, data analysis
  - Trustworthiness (soundness of the research)
  - Ethical considerations
- Dissemination and knowledge translation
  - Timeline
  - Budget
  - Appendices

INTRODUCING THE STUDY—FIRST PARA

- Goal: Capture interest in the study
  - Focus on the importance of the study (Why bother with the question?)
  - Be clear and concise (details will follow)
  - Provide a synopsis of the primary target of the study
  - Present persuasive logic backed up with factual evidence

THE PROBLEM/RESEARCH QUESTION

- The problem can be broad, but it must be specific enough to convince others that it is worth focusing on.
- Research questions must be clearly delineated.
- The research questions must sometimes be delineated with sub-questions.
- The scope of the research question(s) needs to be manageable within the time frame and context of the study.

PURPOSE OF THE QUALITATIVE STUDY

- Discovery?
- Description?
- Conceptualization (theory building)?
- Sensitization?
- Emancipation?
- Other?

LITERATURE REVIEW

- The literature review should be selective and persuasive, building a case for what is known or believed, what is missing, and how the study fits in.
- The literature is used to demonstrate openness to the complexity of the phenomenon, rather than funneling toward an a priori conceptualization.

METHODS—CHALLENGES HERE

- Quantitative designs are often more familiar to reviewers.
- Qualitative researchers have a different language.

METHODS SECTION

- Orientation to the method:
  - Description of the particular method that will be used and its creators/ interpreters
  - Rationale for qualitative research generally and for the specific method to be used

QUALITATIVE STUDIES ARE VALUABLE FOR RESEARCH

- It delves deeply into complexities and processes.
- It focuses on little-known phenomena or innovative systems.

- It explores informal and unstructured processes in organizations.
- It seeks to explore where and why policy and local knowledge and practice are at odds.
- It is based on real, as opposed to stated, organizational goals.
- It cannot be done experimentally for practical or ethical reasons.
- It requires identification of relevant variables (Marshall & Rossman, 1999).

SAMPLE

- Purposive or theoretical sampling
  - The purpose of the sampling
  - Characteristics of potential types of persons, events, or processes to be sampled
  - Methods of making decisions about sampling
- Sample size
  - Estimates provided based on previous experience, pilot work, and so on.
- Access and recruitment

DATA COLLECTION AND ANALYSIS

- Types: Individual interviews, participant observation, focus groups, personal and public documents, Internet-based data, videos, and so on, all of which vary with different traditions.
- Analysis methods vary depending on the qualitative approach.
- Add *details* and *more details* about how data will be gathered and processed (procedures should be made public).

QUESTIONS FOR DATA MANAGEMENT AND ANALYSIS

- How will data be kept organized and retrievable?
- How will data be "broken up" to see something new?
- How will the researchers engage in reflexivity (e.g., be self-analytical)?
- How will the reader be convinced that the researcher is sufficiently knowledgeable about qualitative analysis and has the necessary skills?

TRUSTWORTHINESS (SOUNDNESS OF THE RESEARCH)

- Should be reflected throughout the proposal
- Should be addressed specifically, with the relevant criteria for the qualitative approach used
- Should provide examples of the strategies used:
  - Triangulation
  - Prolonged contact with informants, including continuous validation of data
  - Continuous checking for representativeness of data and fit between coding categories and data
  - Use of expert consultants

EXAMPLES OF STRATEGIES FOR LIMITING BIAS IN INTERPRETATIONS

- Planning to search for negative cases
- Describing how analysis will include a purposeful examination of alternative explanations
- Using members of the research team to critically question the analysis
- Planning to conduct an audit of data collection and analytic strategies

OTHER COMPONENTS

- Ethical considerations
  - Consent forms
  - Dealing with sensitive issues
- Dissemination and knowledge translation
- Timeline
- Budget justification

LAST BITS OF ADVICE

- Seek assistance and pre review from others with experience in grant writing (plan time for rewriting)
- Highlight match between your proposal and purpose of competition
- Follow the rules of the competition
- Write for a multidisciplinary audience

REFERENCES

Marshall, C., & Rossman, G. B. (1999). *Designing qualitative research*. Thousand Oaks, CA: Sage.

Morse, J. M. (1994). Designing funded qualitative research. In N. Denzin & Y. Lincoln (Eds.), *Handbook of qualitative research* (pp. 220–235). Thousand Oaks, CA: Sage.

Silverman, D. (2000). *Doing qualitative research*. Thousand Oaks, CA: Sage.

OUTLINE FOR A RESEARCH PROPOSAL

Mary de Chesnay

The following guidelines are meant to be a general set of suggestions that supplements the instructions for the student's program. In all cases in which there is conflicting advice, the student should be guided by the dissertation chair's instructions. The outlined plan includes five chapters: the first three constitute the proposal and the remaining two the results and conclusions, but the number may vary depending on the nature of the topic or the style of the committee chair (e.g., I do not favor repeating the research questions at the beginning of every chapter, but some faculty do. I like to use this outline but some faculty prefer a different order. Some studies lend themselves to four instead of five chapters.)

CHAPTER I: OVERVIEW OF THE STUDY
(or Preview of Coming Attractions)

This refers to a few pages that tell the reader:

- What he or she is going to investigate (purpose or statement of the problem and research questions or hypotheses).
- What theoretical support the idea has (conceptual framework or theoretical support). In qualitative research, this section may include only a rationale for conducting the study, with the conceptual framework or typology emerging from the data.
- What assumptions underlie the problem.
- What definitions of terms are important to state (typically, these definitions in quantitative research are called *operational definitions* because they describe how one will know the item when one sees it. An operational definition usually starts with the phrase: "a score of … or above on the [name of instrument]"). One may also want to include a conceptual definition, which is the usual meaning of the concept of interest or a definition according to a specific author. In contrast, qualitative research

usually does not include measurements, so operational definitions are not appropriate, but conceptual definitions may be important to state.

- What limitations to the design are expected (not delimitations, which are intentional decisions about how to narrow the scope of one's population or focus).
- What the importance of the study (significance) is to the discipline.

CHAPTER II: THE REVIEW OF RESEARCH LITERATURE
(or Why You Are Not Reinventing the Wheel)

For Quantitative Research

Organize this chapter according to the concepts in the conceptual framework in Chapter I and describe the literature review thoroughly first, followed by the state of the art of the literature and how the study fills the gaps in the existing literature. Do not include nonresearch literature in this section—place it in Chapter I as introductory material if the citation is necessary to the description.

- Concept 1: a brief description of each study reviewed that supports concept 1 with appropriate transitional statements between paragraphs
- Concept 2: a brief description of each study reviewed that supports concept 2 with appropriate transitional statements between paragraphs
- Concept 3: a brief description of each study reviewed that supports concept 3 with appropriate transitional statements between paragraphs
- And so on, for as many concepts as there are in the conceptual framework (I advise limiting the number of concepts for a master's degree thesis owing to time and cost constraints.)
- Areas of agreement in the literature—a paragraph, or two, that summarizes the main points on which the authors agree
- Areas of disagreement—where the main issues on which the authors disagree are summarized
- State of the art on the topic—a few paragraphs in which the areas where the literature is strong and where the gaps are, are clearly articulated
- A brief statement of how the study fills the gaps or why the study needs to be conducted to replicate what someone else has done.

For Qualitative Research

The literature review is usually conducted after the results are analyzed and the emergent concepts are known. The literature may then be placed in Chapter II of the proposal as shown earlier or incorporated into the results and discussion.

CHAPTER III: METHODOLOGY (or Exactly What You Are Going to Do Anyway)

- Design (name the design—e.g., ethnographic, experimental, survey, cross-sectional, phenomenological, grounded theory, etc.).
- Sample—describe the number of people who will serve as the sample and the sampling method: Where and how will the sample be recruited? Provide the rationale for sample selection and methods. Include the institutional review board (IRB) statement and say how the rights of subjects (Ss) will be protected, including how informed consent will be obtained and the data coded and stored.
- Setting—where will data collection take place? In quantitative research, this might be a laboratory or, if a questionnaire, a home. If qualitative, there are special considerations of privacy and comfortable surroundings for the interviews.
- Instruments and data analysis—how will the variables of interest be measured and how will sense be made of the data, if quantitative, and if qualitative, how will the data be coded and interpreted—that is, for both, this involves how the data will be analyzed.
- Validity and reliability—how will it be known if the data are good (in qualitative research, these terms are "accuracy" and "replicability").
- Procedures for data collection and analysis: a 1-2-3 step-by-step plan for what will be done.
- Timeline—a chart that lists the plan month by month—use Month 1, 2, 3 instead of January, February, March.

The aforementioned three-chapter plan constitutes an acceptable proposal for a research project. The following is an outline for the final two chapters.

CHAPTER IV: RESULTS (What I Discovered)

- Some researchers like to describe the sample in this section as a way to lead off talking about the findings.

- In the order of each hypothesis or research question, describe the data that addressed that question. Use raw data only; do not conclude anything about the data and make no interpretations.

CHAPTER V: DISCUSSION (or How I Can Make Sense of All This)

- Conclusions—a concise statement of the answer to each research question or hypothesis. Some people like to interpret here—that is, to say how confident they can be about each conclusion.
- Implications—how each conclusion can be used to help address the needs of vulnerable populations or nursing practice, education, or administration.
- Recommendations for further research—that is, what will be done for an encore?

QUALITATIVE SOFTWARE COMPARISON

Paul Mihas

	ATLAS.ti 6.0	MAXQDA 10	NVivo 9.0	Dedoose
Website	www.atlas.com	www.maxqda.com	www.qsr.com.au	www.dedoose.com
Price	Educational: $585; Student: $120	Educational: $570; Student: $99	Educational: $595; Student: $199 (12-month limit)	6-month contract ($15.95; 12.95) 9-month contract ($12.95; $10.95)
MAC or PC	PC	PC	PC	PC or Mac (platform independent)
File management	• Data stored locally or on network • Compressed backup file (copy bundle file)	• Data stored locally or on network ☺ Can create copy of project file	• Data stored locally or on network • Can create copy of project file	• Data stored on Web • Backup stored on Web
Multimedia	☺ Audio, video, graphic	• Can link to audio, video, and graphic files	☺ Audio, video, graphic	• Under development. Will link audio, video, and graphics (tentatively in 2011)
Document types	☺ Rich text files, txt, doc, pdf	☺ Rich text files, doc, docx, pdf	☺ Rich text files, txt, doc, pdf	• docx, doc, txt
Table import	• Table import possible but results are awkward	• Table import not possible	☺ Ability to import spreadsheets and database tables	• Table import not possible
Geo-coding functionality	☺ Geo-coding facility creates screenshots from any Google Earth view and assigns them as graphical primary documents	• Allows links to Google Earth maps	• Allows links to Google Earth maps	• Allows links to Google Earth maps

Extended audio capability	• Allows importing of transcribed audio files from F4 software • Text to media synchronization	• Can import and code audio	• Can import and code audio	• Under development
Text segment is an object	• Can visually present text segments (separate from codes)	NA	NA	• Can visually present text segments (separate from codes)
Making diagrams	• Diagrams can include documents, codes, segments, and memos • Can link major project objects including segments • Limited range of color and shape	• Diagrams can include documents, codes, and memos • Can link major project objects, except segments • Links in diagram are not recognized elsewhere in the project • Limited range of color and shape	• Diagram can include documents, codes, and memos • Can link major project objects, except segments • Wide range of color, shape options	• No diagramming feature (but bubble plots are available)
Demographics	• Demographics stored as document "families"	• Table of variables	• Enter variables, link values • Apply to cases	• Table of variables
Code book evolution	• Sortable alphabetical or hierarchical code list	• Primary display is hierarchical	• Primarily hierarchical node structure	• Primary display is hierarchical
Code application	• Drag-and-drop from code list • Other options available (menu, tool bar, right click)	• Drag-and-drop codes from code list • Can add weight to codes	• Drag-and-drop code from code list • Other options available (menu, right click)	• Drag-and-drop codes from code list • Can add weight to codes

(continued)

	ATLAS.ti 6.0	MAXQDA 10	NVivo 9.0	Dedoose
Code display	☺ Codes are visible in margin ☺ Code display in margin is active • Can change color of text • Can assign color to codes	☺ Can assign color to codes ☺ Codes are visible in margin • Code display in margin provides basic information	☺ Can control color of codes • Start and stop of code application visible via "coding stripes" • Vertical layout is difficult to read	• Cannot control color of codes • Codes are visible, but only by hovering on excerpt bracket
Memo writing	☺ Can write project-wide memos or memos attached to segments (called "comments") ☺ Can retrieve memos and comments with coded segments	☺ Can write project-wide memos or memos attached to segments • Can retrieve memos on sections of data without coded segments	☺ Can write project-wide memos or annotations attached to segments • Can write comments to specific project items (docs, text segments, codes) • Can view annotations with coded segments	• Can write comments to specific project items (docs, text segments, codes, variables)
Code review	☺ Can review and adjust code application • Can print report of codes ☺ Can simulate "index card on kitchen table" view • Can print report of codes for a demographic	☺ Can review and adjust code application • Can print report of codes ☺ Output feature allows visual review of codes and comment writing • Can print report of codes for a demographic	☺ Can review and adjust code application • Can print report of codes • Can use model feature for visual review of codes • Can print report of codes for a demographic	• Can review and adjust code application • Can print report of codes • Can print report of codes for a demographic

Matrices	• Can output frequency table of documents and codes ⊚ Can output table of codes co-occurring with other codes	⊚ Can output frequency table of documents and codes ⊚ Can output table of codes co-occurring with other codes ⊚ Can jump from cell of table to textual content	⊚ Can output frequency table of documents and codes ⊚ Can output table of codes co-occurring with other codes ⊚ Can jump from cell of table to textual content	⊚ Can output frequency table of documents and codes ⊚ Can output table of code and code weights ⊚ Can output table of codes co-occurring with other codes ⊚ Can jump from cell of table to textual content
Filtering	⊚ Can filter to set of documents, demographics, and/or codes	⊚ Can filter to set of documents, demographics, and/or codes	⊚ Can filter to set of documents, demographics, and/or codes	⊚ Can filter to set of documents, demographics, and/or codes
Code connections	⊚ Boolean (and, or, not, xor) ⊚ Proximity searches (near) ⊚ Combination searches of codes and demographics	⊚ Boolean (and, or, not, xor) ⊚ Proximity searches (near) ⊚ Combination searches of codes and demographics	⊚ Boolean (and, or, not, xor) ⊚ Proximity searches (near) ⊚ Combination searches of codes and text ⊚ Combination searches of codes and demographics	• Boolean (and, or) ⊚ Code weight bubble plot ⊚ Code frequency bubble plot ⊚ Code weight statistics

(continued)

	ATLAS.ti 6.0	MAXQDA 10	NVivo 9.0	Dedoose
Working with quantitative data	☺ Can import quantitative data from spreadsheet or use manual entry ☺ Can export quantitative data to spreadsheet ☺ Can output code frequencies	☺ Can import quantitative program from spreadsheet program or use manual entry ☺ Can export quantitative data to spreadsheet program ☺ Can output code frequencies	☺ Can import quantitative program from spreadsheet program or use manual entry ☺ Can export quantitative data to spreadsheet program ☺ Can output code frequencies	☺ Can import quantitative program from spreadsheet program or use manual entry ☺ Can export quantitative data to spreadsheet program ☺ Can output code frequencies
Merge	• Can merge different projects where division of labor is guided by division of documents, codes, or both	• Can merge different projects where division of labor is guided by division of documents, codes, or both.	• Can merge different projects where division of labor is guided by division of documents, codes, or both.	• Under development. No merge function at this time.
Team work: Simultaneous access	• Projects cannot be accessed at the same time by different users	• Projects cannot be accessed at the same time by different users	☺ Simultaneous access in real time (with the purchase of NVivo Server)	☺ Simultaneous access in real time
Intercoder reliability	• Can import an Atlas.ti file into a separate program, CAT, to calculate intercoder statistics and kappas	• Can generate report that gives agreement percentages per code	• Can generate report that gives agreement percentages and kappas per code	• Still under development. Will be able to generate report that gives agreement percentages (must first create a "training session" with specific excerpts)

Color filtering	• No color filtering available	☺ Can filter codes in the margin based on colors	• No color filtering available	• No color filtering available
Document color report	• No color report available	☺ Can create a report of codes based on their color attributes	• No color report available	• No color report available
Text comparison chart (by color)	• No color comparison chart available	☺ Can create a table showing different documents and different codes, based on their color attributes	• No color comparison chart available	• No color comparison chart available
Weighting text segments	• No weighting feature available	☺ Can assign a weight to a code application • Can create various reports based on code weights	• No weighting feature available	☺ Can assign a weight to a code application ☺ Can create various reports / charts based on code weights
Lexical searching	• Can auto-code based on words and phrases	☺ Can auto-code based on words and phrases ☺ Can create customized dictionary using MaxDictio	☺ Can auto-code based on words and phrases ☺ Can easily create a code based on a word in a frequency list	• No auto-coding feature

• Adequate / ☺ Excellent

Source: Paul Mihas, Odum Institute: Paul_Mihas@unc.edu

INDEX

Abbott, A. A., 23
Abma, T., 25
Abrahamson, K., 21, 36
accommodation, 58
acute/inpatient care, studies
    Adams et al., 14
    Dionne-Odom et al., 13
    Droskinis, 16
    Fleiszer et al., 16–17
    Hoyle and Grant, 15
    Ireland et al., 17–18
    Lines et al., 19
    Maxwell et al., 18
    Nesbitt, 14
    Popejoy et al., 19
    Powell, 16
    Rudolfsson, 14–15
    Stetler et al., 17
    Tobiano et al., 18–19
    Velloso et al., 18
    White et al., 15
Adams, J. A., 14
Adaptive Leadership, 14
advantages, of case study research, 63
Agis, F. I., 162
Al Awaisi, H., 28
Al Rubaie, T., 61
Alves, M., 18
Amella, E., 21
Anderson, R. A., 14
Angell, R. C., 7

anonymity, 4–5
Anthony, S., 11–12, 13, 35
archival records, 5, 6
Arling, G., 21
Arnaert, A., 34
assimilation, 58
ATLAS.ti 6.0, 280–285
Ayala, R. A., 24
Ayers, T., 192

Bachi, K., 164, 165–166
Bailey, C., 23
Bailey, D. E., 14
Bailey, S., 187
Baillie, L., 18
Bakitas, M., 13
Bandura, A., 58
Bani-issa, W., 33
Barbor, T., 251
Barr, M. L., 247
Batchelor-Aselage, M., 21
Baxter, P., 11, 35
Becker, H. S., 7
Beddingham, E., 29
Belanger, L., 193
Bender, J. L., 193
Bertoti, B. D., 162
Blanchard, C., 193
Boblin, S., 17
Bolden, L. A., 200
Bracke, P., 24

breast cancer awareness among Muslim
Omani women, case study
addressing trustworthiness issues,
133–134
author's reflection and summary,
134–135
case choice, 121
design, 120–121
gathering and triangulating data,
122–123
government breast health policy, 116–117
impact of study, 134–135
literature review, 118–120
need for, 115–116
nongovernmental breast health
efforts, 117–118
process, 118–134
reporting findings, 124–133
summarizing and synthesizing
data, 123–124
Brier, M., 203–204
Brooks, F., 24
Bruner, J., 58
Burton, D., 62
Buscher, A. L., 234

Calaminus, G., 187
canine partners in health care, case study
design, 147
discussion, 153
instruments and data analysis, 148
literature review, 145–146
methodology, 147–148
purpose, 145
results, 148–153
sample, 147
settings, 147
structure
physician's office, 148–150
rehabilitation unit, 150–152
themes, 152–153
Carey, S., 258
Carmon, A. F., 203, 217
Carrico, A. W., 222
case histories, 2
case work, 2

Casey, D., 35
Castro, R., 233
Ceci, C., 18
Chaboyer, W., 18–19
Chambers, L. A., 224
Chambers-Evans, J., 34
Chan, Z. C., 12
Chang, S. M., 27
Change Theory, 23
Charns, M. P., 17
Coatsworth, J. D., 192
Colley, H., 61
coming home, veterans with PTSD
adapting to life at home, case
study, 99–100
attachment bonds, shift in, 108–109
case exemplars, 109–113
case study method, 102–104
comparison approach, 103–104
compensatory survival behaviors,
106–107
data collection, 103
discussion, 113–114
ethical issues, 104–105
focus of the study, 103
heightened fear response theme,
105–106
inclusion/exclusion criteria, 103
literature review, 100–102
research method, 104–105
research themes, 105–109
social disengagement and attachment
difficulties, 107–108
community/outpatient care, studies
Abbott et al., 23–24
Lewin, 23
Mizutani et al., 22
Procter et al., 24
Rose and Yates, 23
Sandy et al., 22
Whiffin et al., 23
concept, of case study research, 2
conducting case study research,
89–90, 96–97
case
bounding, 91–92

defining, 90–91
    selection, 92–93
    challenges, 96
    CSR contribution, 95–96
    data
        analysis, 94–95
        collection, 94
        recruitment strategy, 93
        sample inclusion/exclusion
            criteria, 93–94
    discussion, 95–96
    literature review, 92
    rigor, 95
Connally, F., 25
Conners, N. A., 252
consent form format, 52–53
constructivism, 58–59
Cooke, H., 28
Cote, J., 223
Courneya, K. S., 186, 193
Court-Appointed Special Advocates for
    Children (CASA), 81
Crandall, B., 13
Crawford, P., 28
Creswell, J., 121
cross-case analysis, 67–68
Cruickshank, M., 29, 33

Dale, S., 223
Daly, B., 223
Danielsen, S., 193
data analysis, 4, 67
data collection, 4, 35, 67
    issues, 35
Davila, H. W., 21
de Chesnay, M., 175, 188, 225
de Jong, G., 25
De Rouck, S., 26
DeCrane, S., 21
Dedoose, 280–285
definitions, case study research, 62–63
DeGrezia, M. G., 232
Denis, J., 16–17
DeVito, M., 248
Dhital, D., 25
Dillon, J., 170–172

Dinis-Ribeiro, M., 234
Dionne-Odom, J. N., 13
direct observation, 5, 6
do Prado, M. L., 33
documents, 5, 6
Dolansky, M. A., 223
Dorman Marek, K., 19
Droskinis, A., 16
drug policies, 251, 259
    drug courts
        development of, 252–254
        research support, 258–259
        success of, 254–259
    substance abuse and its impact on
        society, 251–252
Durvasula, R., 224

Eeltink, C. M., 187
Eisenhardt, K. M., 66–68
Ellis-Hill, C., 23
Emlet, C. A., 222–223
English, D. C., 245
ethical issues, 4–5
ethnographic case study, 4, 5
evaluation, 73

Family Group Conferencing (FGC)
    approach, 25–26
Fang, X., 222, 234
Fernandes, L., 234
field notes, 65–66
Fisher, J., 107
Fleiszer, A. R., 16–17
Foa, E., 105
Fobair, P., 193
Fosså, S. D., 186
Foucault, M., 18
Fuji, K. T., 23
Furness, T., 25

Galt, K. A., 23
Garrow, D., 21
Gaudio, F. D., 203–204
Georgia Department of Human Services
    (DHS), 73
Gerring, J., 62

Giles, T. M., 19
Giordano, T. P., 234
Gjerset, G. M., 186
Glasersfeld, E., 59
Glesne, C., 63
Goffman, E., 7
Gomm, R., 63
Goopy, S., 27
Gordon, K., 193
Gorman, J. R., 187
Grace, P. J., 13
graduate students, case study methods
    for, 139
  clinical case studies versus research
    case studies, 139–140
  curriculum, 140–143
  doctoral course in health policy, 142–143
  master's degree sequence, 140–141
Granados, C. A., 162
Grant, A., 15
Gredler, M. E.
Greer, B., 7
Gripshover, B., 223
Grodensky, C. A., 224, 232

Haddad, A. M., 245
Hakanson, M., 164
Hakim, C., 63
Hallberg, L., 164–165
Halpern, S. D., 246
handler's perspective of equine-
    facilitated therapy study, 155,
    167–168
  challenges, 162–163
  data analysis, 159
  design, 158
  discussion, 163–166
  implications, 167
  instruments, 158–159
  literature review, 156–157
  methodology, 158–159
  observations, 161–162
  problem statement, 155–156
  results, 160–163
  rigor, 159
  sample, 158

  settings, 158
Hawthorne, L., 30
Hegenbarth, M., 34
Hembree, E. A., 105
Henry, A. G., 223
Henshaw, L., 29
Hentz, P., 1, 3
Herman, J., 113
Higgins, P. A., 234
Hodgkin's lymphoma survivor
    study, 185, 195–196
  conceptual definitions, 186
  data analysis, 188–189
  discussion, 192–193
  fertility, 187
  implications, 194–195
  instrumentation, 188
  literature review, 186–187
  methodology, 187–189
  physical activity study, 186
  procedures, 188
  QOL indicators, 187
  recommendations for future research,
    195
  research question, 185
  results, 189–192
  rigor, 188
  sample, 187–188
  significance, 186
  social support, 187
Hodkinson, P., 61
Holtslander, L. F., 200
Hope Box, 73–74, 87–88
  case study methodology
    design, 74–75
    sample, 75
    setting, 76
  case study results, 76–87
  mission and structure, 74
Horowitz, S., 146
Houghton, C., 35, 61
Hoyle, L., 15, 30
Huberman, M. A., 121
Hughes, W. C., 7
Hutchinson, P. J., 23
Hutton, A., 32–33

in-depth and inside view of the
      phenomenon, 1
institutional review board (IRB), 4
instructional models,
      of learning, 60
interviews, 5, 6
Ireland, S., 17, 36
Ironson, G., 224
Ivie, B., 79

Jack, S., 11–12, 13, 35
Jadad, A. R., 193
James, D., 61
Jarrett, N., 23
Johnston, D. A., 27
Jones, B., 193
Jones, M. L., 8

Kallen, M. A., 234
Kaufman, J., 258
Keats, M. R., 193
Kelton, M., 32–33
Kendall, S., 24
Kgole, J. C., 22
Kiiru, M., 214, 215, 216
Kirkland, S., 223
Kirkpatrick, H., 17
Kissane, D. W., 203–204
Klepping, L., 140
Koeppen, S., 84–87
Koplow, S. M., 20
Kozak, M. J., 105
Kremer, H., 224
Krumwiede, K. A., 31, 36
Krumwiede, N. K., 31
Kumar, S., 233

Lave, J., 60
Lea, J., 29, 33
Lee, M. R., 170
Lewin, K., 23–24
Leys, M., 26
life history of a combat veteran
      suffering from PTSD and TBI,
      study of, 169, 182–183
   assumptions, 171

definitions, 171–172
discussion, 179–182
literature review, 172–175
methodology, 175
problem statement, 169–170
results, 175–179
life history of an older woman
      living with AIDS,
      221, 235–236
   assumptions, 222
   conceptual definitions, 222
   discussion, 231–235
   literature review, 222–224
   methodology, 224–225
   problem statement, 221–222
   recommendations for future
      research, 235
   results, 225–231
Lim, J. W., 223
Lines, L. E., 19
literature review, 57
long-term/elder care, studies
   Abrahamson et al., 21
   Koplow, 20
   Mamier and Winslow, 20
   Tayab and Narushima, 20–21
   Zapka et al., 21–22
loss of a child study, 199, 217
   acceptance, 212–213
   communication, 211
   community, 208–209
   data analysis, 206
   denial, 210–211
   design, 205
   discussion, 214–217
   emotional distress, 209–210
   expected limitations, 204–205
   family, 207
   financial implications, 212
   grief, 207–208
   grief related to the family
      systems theory, 201–204
   implications, 217–218
   instruments, 205
   limitations, 218
   literature review, 199–201

loss of a child study (*cont.*)
  methodology, 205–206
  recommendations, 218–219
  relevance to nursing, 201
  results, 206
  rigor, 206
  sample, 205
  setting, 205
  spirituality, 209
  support group, 213
  themes, 206–213
lung allocation policies,
    history of, 241–244

Madisetti, M., 21
Magwood, G., 21
Mamier, I., 20
Manhart, L. E., 233
Mannix, T., 19
Marlowe, D., 258
Martiniano, S. C., 32
Masten, A. S., 192
Mavundla, T. R., 22
MAXQDA 10, 280–285
Maxwell, E., 18, 36
McCarl, L. I., 169
McDonnell, A., 8
McGillis Hall, L., 30
McIntosh, R. C., 223
McKenna, B., 25
McKeown, M., 25
McLaren, S. M., 18
McLaughlin, M., 193
McMillan, S. C., 200
McMurray, A., 18–19
McQuestion, M., 29
Medina, J. L., 33
memos, and reflexivity in research, 65
mental health nursing care, studies
  de Jong et al., 25–26
  McKenna et al., 25
  McKeown et al., 25
  Morris, 26
  Sercu et al., 24–25
Merriam, S. B., 120
Mignone, J., 223

Miles, M. B., 121
Milstead, J. A., 240
Mizutani, M., 22
Mohanraj, R., 233
Molzahn, A., 224
Monster (movie), 3
Moore, J., 29, 36
Morris, M., 26
Moskowitz, J. T., 222
Mueller, C., 21
multiple case studies, 8
Munt, R., 32–33
Muntaner, C., 30
Murnaghan case. *See* pediatric lung
    allocation policy, case study
Murphy, K., 35
Murray, K. R., 233
Murray, L., 34

Narushima, M., 20
Nelson, S., 30
Nesbitt, J., 14
Newton, J. M., 61
Nokes, K., 223
nursing education issues, studies
  Bani-issa and Rempusheski, 33
  Hegenbarth et al., 34
  Martiniano et al., 32
  Pront et al., 32–33
  Waterkemper et al., 33–34
nursing journals, 261–263
nursing studies, using qualitative case
    study methodology, 11–12
NVivo 9.0, 280–285

object of study, 6
  examples, 6–7
obstetric fistula case study, proposal for
  consent form format, 52–53
  data analysis, 48–49
  design, 45
  instruments, 47–48
  literature review, 44–45
  procedures, 48
  purpose of the study, 43–44
  sample, 45–46

semi-structured interview guides, 47–48
setting, 46–47
timeline, 49
Ogden, P., 107
O'Grady, L., 193
Oliveros, A., 258
Olmert, M. D., 170
ontology and epistemology, 60
Owen, P., 29

Pandit, N. R., 68
Park, M., 25
participant observation, 5, 6
pediatric lung allocation policy, case
    study, 239
conclusion, 248
ethics, 245–247
field work, 240
history of lung allocation
    policies, 241–244
literature review, 244–248
objective medical data, 247–248
purpose, 239–240
relevance to nursing, 240–241
peripartum/perinatal care, studies
Chang et al., 27
De Rouck and Leys, 26–27
Johnston, 27
personal perspective, on case study
    research (CSR), 55–56
advantages of CSR, 63
case study building, 66–69
definitions of CSR, 62–63
historical perspective, 61–62
learning, study on, 59–60
methodology, 64–65
philosophy of practice, 56
reasons for using CSR, 56–58
reflexivity in research, 65–66
unit of analysis, 64
Peshkin, A., 63
Pesut, B., 15
philosophical derivation, case study
    research, 2–4
physical artifacts, 5, 6
Piaget, J., 58, 59

Pierce, J. P., 187
Pollock, K., 28
Popejoy, L. L., 19
Powell, I., 16, 36
Prentice, D., 29
Primary Nursing/Collaborative Practice
    framework, 23
Procter, S., 24
professional development/workplace
    issues, studies
Al Awaisi et al., 28
Hoyle, 30
Krumwiede et al., 31
Lea and Cruickshank, 29
Moore et al., 29–30
Ramos et al., 31–32
Salami et al., 30–31
Stacey et al., 28–29
Whitehead et al., 29
Pront, L., 32–33
Pryjmachuk, S., 28
Psaros, C., 234, 235–236
Puig-Perez, S., 234

qualitative case study methodology
    (QCSM), 11–12, 89
acute/inpatient care, 13–19
challenges and opportunities, 12
common and emerging themes, 36–37
community/outpatient care, 22–24, 36
current state, 13–34
long-term/elder care, 20–22, 36
mental health nursing care, 24–26, 36
methodological considerations, 34–35
nursing education issues, 31–34, 36
nursing studies (*see* nursing studies,
    using qualitative case study
    methodology)
peripartum/perinatal care, 26–27, 36
professional development/workplace
    issues, 27–31, 36
rationale for using, 34–35
qualitative perspective, case study
    research, 2
qualitative software, 280–285
quantitative research, 89

Raju, S., 246
Ramos, F. S., 31, 32
Rankin, B., 258
Rao, D., 233
Raveis, V. H., 222–223
Rawe, S., 34
Read, S., 8
reasons for choosing case study
    research, 1, 8
Reibnitz, K. S., 33
Rempusheski, V. F., 33
replication, in multiple case studies, 8
research evidence types, 5–6
research proposals
  advice on, 272
  assumptions, 267
  challenges for qualitative
    researchers, 268
  components, 272
  data collection and analysis, 271
  essential elements for, 265–266
  examples of strategies for limiting
    bias in interpretations, 272
  introducing the study, 269
  kinds of qualitative research, 268
  literature review, 270
  methods, challenges, 270
  methods section, 270
  outline
    discussion, 278
    methodology, 277
    overview of the study, 275–276
    results, 277–278
    review of research literature, 276–277
  problem/research question, 269
  purpose, 267
  purpose of the qualitative study, 270
  qualitative research, 267
  qualitative studies are valuable for
    research, 270–271
  questions for data management and
    analysis, 271
  questions to answer, 268
  sample, 271
  sections of, 269
  trustworthiness, 272

review, of case study research, 5–7
Ribeiro, C., 233
Richer, M., 16–17
Rickard, W., 18
Ritchie, J. A., 16–17
Robertson, K., 17
Roger, K. S., 223
Roper, K., 193
Rose, P., 23
Rosenberg, A. R., 193
Rosenberg, J. P., 2
Rosenblatt, P. C., 214, 216
Rosselli, M., 223
Rotherbaum, B. O., 105
Rowe, J., 27
Rudolfsson, G., 14–15
Rush, K. L., 15
Russell, C., 137
Rycroft-Malone, J., 17

Safe Haven Law (Georgia), 82–83
Salami, B., 30
Salata, R. A., 223
Sandy, P. T., 22
Sarmento, E., 233
Schout, G., 25
Scott-Cawiezell, J., 19
Semenic, S. E., 16–17
Sercu, C., 24
Shaw, C., 6–7
Shaw, D., 35
Short, J., 192
Shubert, J., 181
Simmons, M., 29
single case studies, 8
situated learning, 60
Skovlund, E., 186
Slomka, J., 223, 224
Snyder, 247–248
social constructivism, 58–59
social reality, 60
Stacey, G., 28
Stake, R. E., 11, 17, 25, 35,
    90, 91, 120
Stetler, C. B., 17
Strauss, A. L., 7

strength, of case study research, 3
Su, H. I., 187
Suarez-Almazor, M. E., 234
sustainability, 73
Sweet, S. C., 247

Tayab, A., 20
teaching case, 2
Teegardin, C., 258
Thorsen, L., 186
Thygeson, M., 14
Tobiano, G., 18–19
Tozay, S., 222–223
Turolla, T., 76–84
Tyer-Viola, L. A., 223

unit of analysis, 3–4, 36, 64

Van der Kolk, B., 103
Van Gelderen, S. A., 31
Van Maanen, J., 65
Veatch, R. M., 245
Velloso, I., 18
Vygotsky, L. S., 58, 59

Walsh, M., 62
Waterkemper, R., 33
Webel, A. R., 223, 234
Wenger, E., 60
Wharton, C., 193
Whiffin, C. J., 23
White, C., 15
Whitehead, B., 29
Whitsett, S. F., 193
Whyte, W. F., 3, 7
Willis, D. G., 13
Wilson, P. M., 24
Winslow, B. W., 20
within-case analysis, 67
Worms, K., 165

Yates, P. M., 2, 23
Yi-Frazier, J. P., 193
Yin, R. K., 5, 6, 11, 12, 15, 22, 35, 62–63, 67, 90–91, 94, 95, 96, 120
Yount, R. A., 170, 172–173

Zaider, T. I., 203–204
Zapka, J., 22

Printed in the United States
By Bookmasters